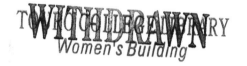

Aphasia and Related Neurogenic Language Disorders

Third Edition

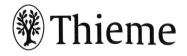

Aphasia and Related Neurogenic Language Disorders

Third Edition

Leonard L. LaPointe, Ph.D.

Francis Eppes Professor of Communication Disorders
Department of Communication Disorders
Florida State University
Tallahassee, Florida

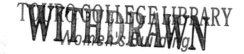
Thieme
New York · Stuttgart

WB

Thieme New York
333 Seventh Avenue
New York, NY 10001

Editor: Melissa Von Rohr
Assistant Editor: Jennifer Berger
Editorial Assistant: Judith Tomat
Director, Production and Manufacturing: Anne Vinnicombe
Senior Production Editor: David R. Stewart
Marketing Director: Phyllis Gold
Director of Sales: Ross Lumpkin
Chief Financial Officer: Peter van Woerden
President: Brian D. Scanlan
Compositor: Compset, Inc.
Printer: Sheridan Books, Inc.

Library of Congress Cataloging in Publication Data is available from the publisher

Important note: Medical knowledge is ever-changing. As new research and clinical experience broaden our knowledge, changes in treatment and drug therapy may be required. The authors and editors of the material herein have consulted sources believed to be reliable in their efforts to provide information that is complete and in accord with the standards accepted at the time of publication. However, in view of the possibility of human error by the authors, editors, or publisher of the work herein, or changes in medical knowledge, neither the authors, editors, or publisher, nor any other party who has been involved in the preparation of this work, warrants that the information contained herein is in every respect accurate or complete, and they are not responsible for any errors or omissions or for the results obtained from use of such information. Readers are encouraged to confirm the information contained herein with other sources. For example, readers are advised to check the product information sheet included in the package of each drug they plan to administer to be certain that the information contained in this publication is accurate and that changes have not been made in the recommended dose or in the contraindications for administration. This recommendation is of particular importance in connection with new or infrequently used drugs.

Some of the product names, patents, and registered designs referred to in this book are in fact registered trademarks or proprietary names even though specific reference to this fact is not always made in the text. Therefore, the appearance of a name without designation as proprietary is not to be construed as a representation by the publisher that it is in the public domain.

Printed in the United States of America

5 4 3 2 1

TNY ISBN 1–58890–226–9
GTV ISBN 3–13–747703–4

2/26/07

To all of the courageous souls with aphasia who have faced the stormy seas.
And to Corinne, who has supported my efforts to navigate.

In Memoriam

Carol Frattali, our cherished colleague and friend, died on July 13, 2004 during the production of this edition. She was a valued contributor to this book, and the care and insight she brought to all of her work is evident in the chapter she wrote with her colleague Jordan Grafman. Her contributions to our book and to our profession will be archived and remembered.

Contents

Foreword ix

Preface to the Third Edition xi

Preface to the Second Edition xiv

Contributors xviii

1. Foundations: Adaptation, Accommodation, *Aristos* 1
    Leonard L. LaPointe

2. Functional Neuroimaging: Applications for Studying Aphasia 19
    Cynthia K. Thompson

3. Social and Life Participation Approaches to Aphasia Intervention . . . 39
    Roberta J. Elman

4. Language and Discourse Deficits Following Prefrontal
    Cortex Damage 51
    Carol Frattali and Jordan Grafman

5. Naming and Word-Retrieval Problems 68
    Anastasia M. Raymer

6. Acquired Dyslexias: Reading Disorders Associated with Aphasia . . . 83
    Wanda G. Webb

7. Acquired Neurogenic Agraphias: Writing Problems 97
    Malcolm R. McNeil and Chin-Hsing Tseng

8. Broca's Aphasia 117
    Kevin P. Kearns

9. Wernicke's Aphasia 142
    Isabelle Caspari

10. Conduction Aphasia 155
    Nina Simmons-Mackie

11. The Transcortical Aphasias 169
    *Ann Marie Cimino-Knight, Amber L. Hollingsworth,
    and Leslie J. Gonzalez Rothi*

12. **Global Aphasia** 186
    Michael Collins

13. **Dementia** 199
    Michelle S. Bourgeois

14. **Right Hemisphere Syndrome** 213
    Margaret Lehman Blake

15. **Traumatic Brain Injury** 225
    Brenda L.B. Adamovich

16. **Pragmatics** 237
    Heather Harris Wright and Marilyn Newhoff

17. **Family, Caregiver, and Clinician Resources** 249
    Adrienne Blanchard

    Index 259

Foreword

Of offering more than I can deliver,
I have a bad habit, it is true. But
I have to offer more than I can
deliver to be able to deliver what
I do.

—Ken Kesey

Not so with the Third Edition of *Aphasia and Related Neurogenic Language Disorders*. The editor, Leonard L. LaPointe, and his cadre of contributors deliver exactly what the title offers. Herein is an abundance of fact on the nature and management of aphasia and related language disorders to put the student's train on the right track, make the academician's course content current, and give clinicians ample thought and activity to manage their patients effectively.

Like its predecessors, the Third Edition provides the pathophysiology, nature, appraisal, and treatment for a variety of aphasias—Broca's (Kearns); Wernicke's (Caspari); conduction (Simmons-Mackie); transcortical (Cimino-Knight, Hollingsworth, and Gonzalez Rothi); and global (Collins). Similarly, associated neurogenic communication disorders—dementia (Bourgeois), right hemisphere syndrome (Blake), traumatic brain injury (Adamovich)—found in previous editions receive a description, methods for evaluation, and suggested treatments. And, as before, specific deficits—naming and word-retrieval problems (Raymer), acquired dyslexias (Webb), acquired agraphias (McNeil and Tseng), and pragmatic impairment (Wright and Newhoff)—are elaborated through description, evaluation, and treatment.

Dr. LaPointe's opening chapter, Foundations: Adaptation, Accommodation, *Aristos*, points the direction for what follows by reminding us that neurogenic communication disorders transcend being a hole in the nervous system with disrupted phonology, semantics, and syntax. They are problems that reside in people who require not only care, but also being cared about. This social side of fractured communication and its influences on a person's and his or her family's quality of life is elaborated in two new chapters in the Third Edition—Social and Life Participation Approaches to Aphasia Intervention (Elman) and Family, Caregiver, and Clinician Resources (Blanchard). Also new in the Third Edition are chapters on Functional Neuroimaging: Applications for Studying Aphasia (Thompson) and Language and Discourse Deficits Following Prefrontal Cortex Damage (Frattali and Grafman).

Contributors to the Third Edition share their first-hand knowledge and experience. All are clinical investigators, and all are clinicians. Each has spent time in both the laboratory and knee-to-knee with people who display the problems each addresses. Thus, the reader is given a scientific foundation, the best available evidence, and clinical expertise. Essentially, the chapters take us to the edge of what is known about neurogenic communication disorders and supply us with means to function and contribute in a time of expanding boundaries.

Dr. LaPointe ends his chapter by citing John Fowles's book *The Aristos* and stating Fowles' belief that "for every wreck there is a raft." A rough translation of *Aristos*, LaPointe tells us, is "making the best of a given situation." Our attention to the contents of the Third Edition of *Aphasia and Related Neurogenic Language Disorders* will assist us in making the situations we face with our patients better, and will provide a raft to keep us afloat in the depths of today.

Robert T. Wertz, Ph.D., BC-NCD
Senior Rehabilitation Research Career Scientist
VA-Vanderbilt Professor of Hearing and Speech Sciences
Nashville, Tennessee

Preface to the Third Edition

Human footprints on the frosted bridge planking.

Under morning frosts the maple leaves turn scarlet,
In the evening dusk mists grow shadowy.
As the season passes one's grief is not slight;
Sorrows come and memories weigh down.

I follow the moon into the mountains,
I search for clouds to accompany me home.

Things of the past are already long gone
And things to be, distant from imagining
Plum blossoms fallen; gardenia just opening.

The sky where dragons were, moistens hidden
orchids.

A selection of images from classic Chinese poets
(Hsieh Ling-yün; Wan An-shih; Han Shan Te-ching; Po-tzu Ting)
(Owen, 1996).

Since the publication of the first edition of this book we have seen more than a decade pass and have entered a new millennium. Retrospection breeds reflection. The images and metaphors of adversity, trouble, and recovery are just as remarkably transparent in the poets of ancient China as they were in the Navajo chants of the first edition. Although the only thing constant continues to be change, some aspects of human existence remain hauntingly familiar. The dark clouds and mist curtains of hardship and tribulation still exist. Some would say the events of the recent past have changed everything, but indeed they have not. Though we live in a frightening context of apparent increased threat and stress, our ancestors faced challenges equal in magnitude in their minds from solar eclipse, the invention of gunpowder, the crossbow, evil spirits, and unholy diseases. The evolution of humankind has tamed or lessened the significance of many of these early sources of fear, but new anxieties have emerged. The threat of ailment, loss of wellness, and life quality persists in the human body and psyche. Though the carriers have changed—leprosy, typhoid, and tuberculosis do not generate the fear they once did in developed societies—some of the more significant conditions continue to exist. Risk to the brain remains high.

Prevalence estimates of adult-onset brain impairment in the U.S. population at the beginning of the 21st Century are daunting. Over 15 million people in the United States have diagnosed adult-onset brain diagnoses, including 4 million with stroke, 3.7 million with traumatic brain injury, and nearly 4 million with progressive, degenerative neurological diseases, such as Parkinson Disease, multiple sclerosis, Huntington's Disease, and HIV (AIDS). (Data derived from Brain Statistics Table at: http://www.braininjurylawtexas.com/brain_statistics.htm.) An additional 5 million suffer from Alzheimer's and other dementing illnesses.

The United States is not atypical. In established market economies as well as across countries in other parts of the globe, stroke and neurological disease is widespread.

- Data from 22 European countries indicate almost 1 million strokes occurring per year in a population of over 500 million.
- In the United Kingdom, more than 100,000 people a year suffer stroke, 10,000 of whom are still of working age.
- Australia records more than 12,000 people with strokes per year, and stroke is the leading cause of disability there.
- African Americans, indigenous Australians, citizens of developing countries, and members of some ethnic minorities record nearly double the number of strokes per year as Caucasian citizens of industrialized societies.
- Global statistics reveal prevalence of stroke at 4.4 million in the countries of the former Soviet Union; 7.4 million in China; 2.7 million in India; nearly 3 million in Sub-Sahara Africa and the Middle East Crescent; and 1.6 million in Latin America and the Caribbean (Kennedy et al., 2002; Launer et al., 2000).

Few families are untouched by the alarming scope of these conditions. Each of us carries a story of a grandparent, mother, father, or close relative who endured stroke or brain disease and lost the ability to remember, think, or express his or her needs and wants.

This Third Edition of the book continues to address these needs and wants. Experts in the areas of clinical research and in the delivery of clinical services are drawn together to share the very latest on aphasia and related neurogenic language disorders. In this edition we have condensed some chapters and added breadth to the areas of coverage. Additions include chapters on neurobiological aspects of recovery secondary to treatment. The concept that changes actually take place in brain and brain connections as a result of treatment is as exciting as any clinical research initiative of the last decade. Social and group models of intervention and rehabilitation are also awarded coverage in this edition, as is research on the remarkable capabilities and processes associated with the ever so human frontal cerebral lobes. We also have added a chapter on family, caregiver, and clinician resources with considerable emphasis on the technological advances and information resources available on the Internet and World Wide Web.

These chapters are in addition to the previously covered (though in some cases by different authors) material on naming and word-retrieval problems; acquired dyslexia; acquired agraphias; Broca's, Wernicke's, conduction, transcortical, and global aphasia; dementia; right hemisphere syndrome; traumatic brain injury; and pragmatics of communication. This increase in coverage of issues on aphasia and neurogenic disorders of communication approaches the breadth of a handbook for clinicians and researchers and should serve as a valuable learning resource for speech-language pathologists, other rehabilitation specialists, physicians and associated health care personnel, health care reimbursers, and both undergraduate and graduate students interested in the fascinating, if sometimes challenging, world of human communication and cognition caused by brain damage.

Also retained throughout our chapters is the ideal that for every wreck there is a raft. With tragedy rides the promise of recovery, restitution, and adjusted and acceptable quality of life. Perhaps this Third Edition of our book will help. The footsteps of morning perhaps may reveal the hidden orchids, moistened from the sky where dragons were.

I would like to acknowledge with gratitude the expert contributors to all three editions of this book. The perspectives offered by these scholars allow a degree of order to be gleaned from the seeming chaos of these complex neurological disorders.

Leonard L. LaPointe, Ph.D.

References

Brain Statistics Table. Available at: http://www.braininjurylawtexas.com/brain_statistics.htm. Accessed February 26, 2003.

Kennedy, B.S., Stanislav, V., Kasl, L.M., & Vaccarino, V. (2002). Trends in Hospitalized Stroke for Blacks and Whites in the United States, 1980–1999. *Neuroepidemiology, 21,* 131–141.

Launer, L.J., Oudkerk, M., Nilsson, L.G., Alperovitch, A, Berger, K., Breteler, M.M.B. Fuhrer, R., Giampaoli, S., Nissinen, A. Pajak, A., Sans, S., Schmidt, R., & Hofman, A. (2000). CASCADE: A European Collaborative Study on Vascular Determinants of Brain Lesions. *Neuroepidemiology, 19,* 113–120.

Owen, S. (Ed. and Trans.) (1996). *An Anthology of Chinese Literature: Beginnings to 1911.* New York: Norton.

Preface to the Second Edition

Roots, Routes, Chants, and Reasons

In the house made of evening twilight.
In the house made of dark cloud.
In the house made of rain and mist.
Where the dark mist curtains the doorway.
The path is on the rainbow . . . .

Happily I recover.
My eyes regain their power.
My head cools.
My limbs regain their strength.
I hear again.
My voice restore for me.

In the white of the wings are the footsteps of morning.
Wandering on a trail of beauty.
Living again.
May I walk
May I talk.

A selection of Navajo chants from Cronyn (1918).

The Navajo people, in the American Southwest, live in a land that some have said is barren and sparse; cruel and chilled in the winter and dry-parched in the summer. Yet they have found beauty in this land. They have found a way not only to survive but to reveal their optimism about life and their appreciation of the butter-orange sunsets and the subtle earth tones of a hundred shades of brown and coral. This optimism and appreciation is apparent not only in the delicately crafted patterns of their unique weavings, but also in the chants and songs and prayers that shape their relationship to the world and their reactions to the adversities that are inevitable in the course of living. From the chants and songs above we discern not so thinly veiled themes. Dark clouds. Mist curtains. Adversity. Trouble. But also hope. Paths. Recovery. Restoration.

In my view, the metaphor is not stretched too far to reveal some of these same themes and lessons in the harsh reality and eventual restoration of function and attitude that accompanies those struck down with disorders of speech and understanding and writing and reading and memory and perception due to a shattered nervous system. And that is an underlying theme of this book. While one may be dealt a harsh existence by nature or events, there exists always the possibility of hope and effort and restoration. The contributors of the chapters of this book have retained these themes. In fact, the very heart of rehabilitation relies on retention of optimism, appropriate objectives, and the application of studied and enlightened strategies for overcoming significant barriers.

Surfacing in this book are several interwoven and interrelated matters of language, brain, loss, and restoration or adjustment. Foremost among these is the process of human communication, that life's-blood process that allows living and learning and loving. As Colin Cherry has stated, "human language is vastly more than a complicated system of cluckings" (Cherry, 1968). It allows us the means of transacting daily business and getting on with the exchanges necessary to get through a day. Cursing the alarm, calming the parrot, scanning the Enquirer, planning the day, calling in late for work, greeting, reviewing, phoning, writing, thanking, arguing, requesting, arranging, studying, listening, waving, ordering, buying, correcting, revealing, begging, soothing, praising, cooing—all require the subtle manipulations necessary for social interaction. These are taken for granted by most of us because we have lost the memory of the struggle of acquisition. But once this medium of human contact is compromised, by stroke or disease or accident, it is taken for granted no longer and instead is sorely missed. In most cases a monumental struggle ensues to regain the gift. The science and art of that struggle has been the focus of investigation and clinical effort for generations, and recently it has seemed as though thin rays of light have become apparent in the efforts to understand and do something about these complex and variegated disorders.

Primary among the neurogenic disorders that affect language are the aphasias, that group of disruptions that result in convoluted syntax and meaning. More than a million people suffer from aphasia in the United States alone, and each day almost 300 new cases are added to the list. As with so many communication disorders, this condition is ill-recognized and ill-understood by the general public as well as by some professional groups. It is ironic that the public has a greater recognition of Froot Loops, panty hose, and the horrors of pet-induced carpet odor than it does of aphasia. To counter this, an excellent new organization, the National Aphasia Association (http://www.aphasia.org/) has been formed to stimulate and encourage the development and utilization of resources to better serve the needs of individuals and families who have to cope with aphasia.

A rich array of related disorders that may or may not coexist with aphasia also can result from damage to the delicate neurological network that subserves communication function. Increasingly, the communication deficits that result from traumatically induced brain injury, the strange mix of perceptual-linguistic problems that accompany nondominant hemisphere damage, and the clouding of cognition and words created by abnormal aging and dementia have become recognized as equally or sometimes even more devastating than the traditionally recognized forms of aphasia. Traumatic brain injury has been called the "silent epidemic," particularly in the 15 to 24 year age category, and it has been estimated that between 30,000 and 50,000 people per year in the United States sustain a head injury severe enough to impede a return to a normal lifestyle (Schwartz, 1989). Nearly 20% of the elderly population is estimated to suffer from some form of dementia, which almost always affects communication in some way. Against the backdrop of the well-recognized population explosion in this age group, this problem will do nothing but increase in terms of societal cost and human suffering (Albert & Albert, 1984).

In the second edition of this book we continue to update our coverage of neurogenic disorders of communication and cognition. All chapters have been redone to incorporate the very latest in clinical thought and research on each topic. In addition, a new chapter has been added that considers the psychosocial issues that have an impact on individuals and families who must deal with neurogenic disorders. This revision can serve a wide audience. Because each chapter has information on clinical management of the cognitive and communicative disorders pertinent to the disorder type, practicing clinicians will find many suggestions on evaluation, principles of treatment, and specific intervention strategies. The contributors of this work have a rich clinical experience, so their ideas and directions are born of exposure and involvement and not theory alone. This revised edition will continue to serve well as a textbook for undergraduate or graduate courses in aphasia and related disorders. The coverage of related topics such as right hemisphere syndrome, traumatic brain injury, and dementia mean that the puzzles of differential diagnosis of these disorders will be less daunting. Related professionals in medicine and other health care or rehabilitative specialties may benefit also from learning more about the disorders delineated in this book.

Since the publication of the original work, we have seen important changes in the dynamics of health care delivery and reimbursement systems in the United States, with significant impact on rehabilitation professionals, consumers, and structure. Escalating health care costs have dictated the streamlining or in some cases curtailing of services to some groups. Reimbursement-driven changes in the scope of practice of speech-language pathology have altered the nature and very fiber of caseloads in most health care environments. In many clinics and caseloads preoccupation with disorders of swallowing and feeding has assumed dominance; some have said at the expense of other disorders, resulting in a very dissimilar visage to that of even 10 years ago. Further dynamics in health care delivery are predicted to range from significant mutation to catastrophic prophecies of nonphysicians being locked out of managed care organizations. Time will tell. No doubt the 21st century will welcome some golden mean of adjustment rather than radical alteration of health and human services.

Yet the exigencies in the areas of neurogenic communication and cognitive disorders continue to escalate. Over one million people in the United States endure daily struggles with aphasia and its impact on living, loving, and learning. In a National Aphasia Association (NAA) Needs Survey, 90% of all respondents said the public does not understand their needs, and 90% remarked that they feel isolated (Klein, 1996). While the NAA and like groups throughout the globe chip away at public awareness of aphasia and related disorders, the task appears formidable. Approaching the turn of the century, the calamitous epidemic of traumatic brain injury ravages mostly the young population. Automobile and other vehicular crashes, falls, recreation injuries, assaults, and violence account for the leading cause of death and disability in the United States. Dementia, against the backdrop of a graying population, looms as one of the intensifying challenges to society and health care professionals. Right hemisphere neuropathology is becoming recognized for the blow it can impart on normal lifestyle. No longer is it regarded as an unfortunate episode that affects a hemispheric spare tire with little or no residual consequence. All of these disorders are significant issues, and their management is vital to fostering a return to an acceptable quality of life. To anyone interested in working with people with these disorders or curious about the nature and management of language deficits following nervous system damage, this book presents current thinking and practice.

Although these contributors bring diversity and a variety of approaches to these topics, as editor I have attempted to exert some degree of format standardization in the hope that the book would be smooth and perhaps less disjointed across chapters than some contributed works appear. We have asked most to discuss their topic from the perspective of Introduction, Pathophysiology, Nature and Differentiating Features, Evaluation, Treatment, Specific Treatment Tasks, and, finally, Suggested Readings and References. I think this format worked well in the first edition and continues its utility in subsequent editions.

The concepts found in the chants and songs of the Navajo formed a warp of theme for this book. If we can capture and retain some of the dust of optimism about restoration and recovery inherent is these chants and songs and transfer these attitudes and applications to the mist curtains and clouds of people afflicted with neurogenic disorders of communication, we will have retained good reason to look forward to the footsteps of morning.

Leonard L. LaPointe, Ph.D.

References

Albert, P.C. & Albert, M.L. (1984). History and Scope of Geriatric Neurology. In: M.L. Albert (Ed.), *Clinical Neurology of Aging* (pp. 3–8). New York: Oxford University Press.

Cherry, C. (1968). *On Human Communication* (2nd ed). Cambridge, MA: MIT Press.

Cronyn, G.W. (1918). *The Path on the Rainbow.* New York: Boni and Leverright.

Klein, K. (1996). *Aphasia Community Group Manual.* National Aphasia Association.

Schwartz, R. (1989). Early Rehabilitation in Trauma Centers: Have Speech-Language Pathology Services Progressed? *ASHA, August,* 91–94.

Contributors

Brenda L.B. Adamovich, Ph.D.
West Virginia School of Osteopathic
    Medicine
Lewisburg, West Virginia

Margaret Lehman Blake, Ph.D.
Assistant Professor
Department of Communication Disorders
University of Houston
Houston, Texas

Adrienne Blanchard, M.S.
Department of Communication Disorders
Florida State University
Tallahassee, Florida

Michelle S. Bourgeois, Ph.D.
Professor
Department of Communication Disorders
Florida State University
Tallahassee, Florida

Isabelle Caspari, Ph.D.
Speech and Hearing Department
Arizona State University
Tempe, Arizona

Ann Marie Cimino-Knight, M.A.
Doctoral Candidate
Department of Communication Sciences
    and Disorders
University of Florida
Brain Rehabilitation Research Center
Malcolm Randall VA Medical Center
Gainesville, Florida

Michael Collins, Ph.D.
Director, Speech and Language Pathology
Dean Medical Center
Madison, Wisconsin

**Roberta J. Elman, Ph.D., CCC-SLP,
    BC-NCD**
President and Founder
Aphasia Center of California
Oakland, California

Carol M. Frattali, Ph.D., BC-NCD[†]
Research Coordinator
Speech-Language Pathology Section
Rehabilitation Medicine Department
National Institutes of Health
W.G. Madison Clinical Center
Bethesda, Maryland

Leslie J. Gonzalez Rothi, Ph.D.
Center Director and Professor of Neurology
Department of Neurology
University of Florida
Brain Rehabilitation Research Center
Malcolm Randall VA Medical Center
Gainesville, Florida

Jordan Grafman, Ph.D.
Cognitive Neuroscience Section
National Institute of Neurological Disorders
    and Stroke
National Institutes of Health
Bethesda, Maryland

[†]*Deceased.*

Amber L. Hollingsworth, M.A., CCC-SLP
Research Speech Pathologist
Department of Communication Sciences
    and Disorders
University of Florida
Brain Rehabilitation Research Center
Malcolm Randall VA Medical Center
Gainesville, Florida

Kevin P. Kearns, Ph.D.
Professor and Director
Department of Communication Sciences
    and Disorders
MGH Institute of Health Professions
Boston, Massachusetts

Leonard L. LaPointe, Ph.D.
Francis Eppes Professor of Communication
    Disorders
Department of Communication Disorders
Florida State University
Tallahassee, Florida

Malcolm R. McNeil, Ph.D.
Professor and Chair
Department of Communication Science and
    Disorders
University of Pittsburgh
Pittsburgh, Pennsylvania

Marilyn Newhoff, Ph.D.
Dean (Interim), College of Health and
    Human Services
Professor, School of Speech, Language, and
    Hearing Sciences and SDSU/UCSD Joint
    Doctoral Program
San Diego State University
San Diego, California

Anastasia M. Raymer, Ph.D.
Associate Professor
Department of Early Childhood, Speech
    Pathology, and Special Education
Old Dominion University
Norfolk, Virginia

Nina Simmons-Mackie, Ph.D.
Scholar in Residence
Department of Communication Sciences
    and Disorders
Southeastern Louisiana University
Hammond, Louisiana

Cynthia K. Thompson, Ph.D.
Professor
Department of Communication Sciences
    and Disorders, and Neurology
Northwestern University
Evanston, Illinois

Chin-Hsing Tseng, Ph.D.
Professor
Department of Communication Disorders
    and Special Education
National Kaohsiung Normal University
Kaohsiung
Taiwan

Wanda G. Webb, Ph.D.
Assistant Professor
Department of Hearing and Speech Sciences
Vanderbilt University
Nashville, Tennessee

Heather Harris Wright, Ph.D.
Assistant Professor
Department of Rehabilitation Sciences
University of Kentucky
Lexington, Kentucky

1

Foundations: Adaptation, Accommodation, Aristos

LEONARD L. LAPOINTE

I thought they had cut my tongue out. I had gone in for surgery on my wisdom teeth; they had put me under general anesthesia; and I developed a stroke during the surgical procedure. When I awoke and struggled to find words, I thought for sure I had lost my tongue. But it was far worse than that, as I was to find out. My tongue was fine but I couldn't come up with the right words or put them in the right order. And then when I tried to write or read, I had the same trouble. And it sounded like everyone was speaking a language I didn't know. Talk about terrifying! Betty *(LaPointe, 1994)*

And I'm lost . . . I am lost, completely lost; have to get to . . . somewhere, Omaha I think. The radio is out, or rather for some reason picks up only Bucharest. Emily Stilson *(Kopit, 1978)*

A lot of the accident victims I've met will need help the rest of their lives. And most of them ran out of insurance long ago . . . It's been rough. Sometimes I feel like Cha'kwaina, the kachina called One Who Cries. I'll keep trying though. I can still create beauty from silver. I won't lose my spirit. We have a rich tradition of persistence. Maybe by the Hawk Moon I'll be doing better. Bennett *(LaPointe, 1994)*

I cannot read a road map . . . I was good at maps and things . . . now I couldn't even find my way home . . . Also, I can't play chess worth a tinker's damn anymore. I can't seem to figure out the moves or the strategies . . . I guess chess is out. I used to play like a Russian. Now I play like a cushion . . . Can you help me with any of this? Russell *(LaPointe, 1994)*

I'm more happy and content than I ever thought I could be. Life with Carl is different, but just as fulfilling. He now makes the same bed that I used to have to help him into not so long ago . . . I never tried to be strong before . . . I didn't have to. Eileen Wilson *(Ewing & Pfalzgraf, 1990)*

These are the voices of survivors and those close to them. In the ensuing chapters we will learn about a daunting array of communication and cognitive disorders that arise from a shattered or compromised nervous system. Aphasia, in all its variants. Frontal cerebral lobe dysfunction. Right hemisphere syndrome. Traumatic brain injury. The language of dementia. These are described by the experts in our text to render understanding of the nature and characteristics of these disorders, learn about their pathophysiology, and discover some of the clinical hurdles of their assessment and treatment. Although it is a comforting thought to learn that some neuropathologies seem to be declining in incidence (Kennedy et al., 2002), it is equally sobering to learn that survival has increased comparably, with a net result of the existence of more disabled stroke survivors and their family members who require support and assistance (Biegel et al, 1991). Not all who suffer these pathologies of the nervous system retain chronic residuals of the damage. Some recover completely (perhaps as many as 30% of stroke survivors, for example), with no trace of impairment and resume their lives in much the same fashion as before. For the majority, however, recovery is less than complete (Sacco, 1995).

Foundations: Brain Damage and Human Communication

This book provides information that will facilitate a basic understanding of aphasia and related disturbances of communication caused by brain damage. We define aphasia and its characteristics, outline the causes or etiologies of the condition, illustrate the types of impairment that can affect everyday activities and life participation, distinguish it from other communication disorders caused by brain damage, and consider some of the more frequent related or intertwined disturbances such as those that appear in frontal lobe dysfunction, right hemisphere syndrome, traumatic brain injury, and dementia. We also consider in some depth issues that are bound to neurogenic communication disorders, such as the pervasive naming, reading, writing, and pragmatic disruptions that accompany these impairments and degrade a full appreciation of communication activities and life participation.

What Is Aphasia?

Aphasia is an acquired communication disorder caused by brain damage that impairs a person's ability to understand, produce, and use language. In a more general sense, it may disrupt the ability to generate and use symbol systems, for aphasia affects not only written, spoken, and gestural language, but also musical notation, telling time, mathematical operations, and even discerning meaning from rudimentary sources of symbolic information such as traffic signals, emergency vehicle warning sirens, or dealing with money, currency, or playing cards and board games. It is first and foremost a linguistic disorder that throws into disarray the primary linguistic systems of lexical-semantic processing (words and their meanings); syntax (the grammar and rules of a particular language); phonology-graphology (the rules and use of spoken speech sounds or written symbols and letters); and pragmatics (the use of communication in contextual or social situations).

Aphasia is created by damage to areas of the human brain that are intimately involved in dealing not only with linguistic operations, but also with nervous system areas that are intertwined with thinking, memory, control of information processing, and other cognitive functions. The cerebral cortex, along with its important subcortical regions and connections, is for the most part the area of the nervous system that makes us human. We think, we plan, we attend, we organize, we create, we remember, we interact, we listen, we write, we read, and we talk. These are precisely some of the human cognitive and communication activities that can be addressed and changed in aphasia and related neurogenic communication disorders. Figure 1–1 is an illustration of the major cerebral lobes of the brain along with the all important major speech areas, labeled Broca's area and Wernicke's area (A.D.A.M., U.S. National Library of Medicine, 2002).

Communication disorders arise from many sources. Structural abnormalities, genetic and developmental disorders, environmental factors, hearing loss, and psychological dynamics all can create either developmental or acquired problems in the use of speech and language. Aphasia, however, must be tied to demonstrable damage to the nervous system and present certain qualitative characteristics. It is an acquired phenomenon that appears after the miracle of language has been learned and the joys of language have been experienced.

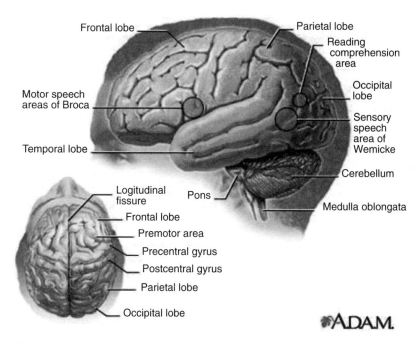

Figure 1–1. Major lobes of the brain with location of important language areas.

Etiologies

Cerebrovascular accident (CVA) or stroke is by far the leading cause of aphasia. A stroke or brain attack is the disruption of the blood supply to the brain. The brain must be continually perfused with the life-giving oxygen and glucose carried by the bloodstream.

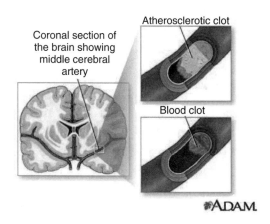

Figure 1–2. Cerebral thromboses or clots.

If nourishment of brain cells or neurons is interrupted for as few as 4 minutes, permanent neuronal death or damage can occur. Blood clots, hemorrhages, and constriction of the blood vessels that supply the brain are common types of CVA. Another important cause of brain damage that can result in aphasia is traumatic brain injury (TBI). Although TBI can cause a constellation of signs and symptoms, it very frequently impairs specific cognitive and communication functions as well. Figures 1–2 and 1–3 illustrate cerebral pathology caused by stroke. Figure 1–2 is a coronal section of the cerebral hemispheres and illustrates two types of thromboses or clots that can create cerebral damage with resulting aphasia. (A.D.A.M., U.S. National Library of Medicine, 2002). Figure 1–3 is a photograph of a brain illustrating the resultant damage from a cerebrovascular accident.

Tumors or abnormal cell growth in the brain can create aphasia. Dementing diseases such as Alzheimer's disease, occasionally Parkinson's

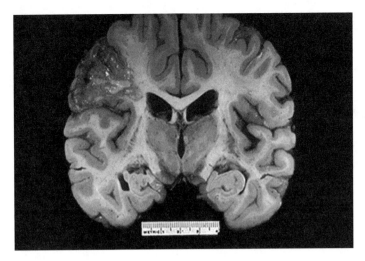

Figure 1–3. Dissected brain (coronal section) with cerebrovascular accident (CVA) damage.

disease, and a vast array of other neurodegenerative diseases can cause diffuse brain damage, or localized damage that subverts connections to other important brain areas, and that impinges upon memory, reasoning, judgment, organizational and planning skills, and specific language functions. The presence of aphasia within the crosshatch of signs and symptoms in diffuse brain damage is a source of controversy among the experts and creates intricate and complicated issues of differential diagnosis.

Modern connectionist theories and models of brain function subscribe to parallel distributed processing and neural networks and suggest that a lot more of the brain is involved in language and symbolic processing than was recognized earlier. On the other hand, selected areas of the brain, especially certain cortical and subcortical areas, consistently surface as being prominent and in some cases dominant. The traditional areas of the dominant cerebral cortex (the left in over 90% of right-handed people) in the anterior frontal lobe (Broca's area), in the posterior temporal lobe (Wernicke's area), and in areas surrounding the supramarginal and angular gyrus region [parietal/temporal/occipital (PTO) cortex] emerge as the most crucial language areas. Damage to these areas does not inevitably result in aphasia, but is most certainly associated with aphasia more frequently than damage to some other neural regions. Nondominant cerebral and subcortical regions are increasingly being implicated in complex and select language and cognitive/perceptual functions as well, attesting to distributed neural regions supporting, augmenting, and sometimes subserving specific symbolic functions. So what emerges is a picture of the dominant (usually left) cerebral hemisphere housing critical brain regions related to aphasia, supported by several other cortical and subcortical areas that can play a role in aphasia as well. The rapidly advancing field of neural imaging will continue to clarify this picture of brain architecture, function, and aphasia.

After the foundations of aphasia and related neurogenic communication disorders are understood, what remains to be emphasized are the people who endure these conditions. One of the central premises of this book is that the conditions described herein are not divorced from the humanity of the individuals who experience them. An adequate philosophy of rehabilitative science must embrace values, attitudes, and teachings that respect and appreciate the unique nature of the individuals with whom we interact. We do not work with diseases, conditions, disorders, or impairments. We deal with these issues within the context of their existence in people and how these individuals are affected in the quality of their activities and life participation. These ideas are a resonant theme throughout the chapters of this book. Communication is importantly related to these psychosocial and humanistic notions, and it is to these issues that we now turn.

The Wreck

Most of the people who experience one of the disorders described in this volume have their lives forever refashioned. The challenge becomes not only how to lessen the effects of the disability, but also how to achieve accommodation and a degree of adjustment to a transformed existence. How does one accept a radically tilted life? How does a family adjust to a burden that may be 10-fold on Friday to what it was last Monday? Is it possible to accept and deal with chronicity and a prodigiously changed existence? These questions border on the darkly philosophical. Can relative happiness be attained/regained? Is life worth living? Is there precedent for dealing with the illness experience and coping with chronicity? Those of us who believe in the tenets of the rehabilitative process must embrace the affirmative. Though the immensity of the struggle is irrefutable, it is possible to make gains and to achieve balance. Internal factors as well as resources in the family, community, and society influence the struggle to cope and the eventual outcome. These elements shape the theme of this chapter. Coping with chronicity is a topic largely missing from many sources. We will explore some of the psychosocial factors that accompany these disorders as well as the attitudes and strategies that allow people who have been dealt a bad break to accommodate, to adjust, and perhaps to accept drastically altered circumstances while retaining a worthwhile quality of life. These are notions that are germane to the subsequent chapters in this book.

Impairment, Disability, Handicap, and Beyond

The social context of neurogenic communication disorders should not be divorced from the clinical aspects, but frequently it is. Others are adamant that the social context, especially the family, must be an integral part of the condition. Some experts go so far as to define the disorders within the context of how they affect families. Wahrborg (1991) defines aphasia as a disruption of family life. Earlier, McKenzie Buck (1968), a speech-language pathologist who suffered a stroke, recovered sufficiently to write an insightful treatise on aphasia, and he viewed the aphasia as a "family disease."

The World Health Organization (WHO, 1980) generated a classification schema that has drawn important distinctions among such terms as *impairment* (the pathology itself); *disability* (the consequences or impact on everyday personal, social, and vocational life); and *handicap* (the value that the individual, family, or community place on the disability, and the degree to which the individual is disadvantaged). Disability and handicap can vary greatly across relatively similar levels of impairment. Further, the levels of disability and handicap can vary a great deal across people, depending on differences in the resources, values, and attitudes of the individual and family. These variants necessitate prudent identification and assessment if suitable plans of intervention are to be formulated. After reconsideration, the WHO has modified its original approach to classification of functioning and disability. Threats (2000) has discussed the changes in the International Classification of Impairments, Disabilities, and Handicaps revision (ICIDH-2). This conceptualization of human functioning and disability and its relationship to health and life quality has permeated rehabilitation science and infused the treatment of aphasia and related neurogenic communication disorders with new principle. Models and theories of aphasia are evolving (Small, 2000). Therapeutic targets and strategies are emerging. Life participation and the social context of the person with aphasia are being acknowledged as important rehabilitation factors (Code, 1996; Holland, 1998; LaPointe, 2002; LPAA Project Group, 2000; Worrall & Frattali, 2000).

The fabric of the perceived disability and handicap suffered by individuals and families with neurogenic disorders is intertwined with a web of psychosocial elements. This is being researched and written about around the globe, including some important work that has come out of Finland (Kauhanen et al, 1999).

With the exception of some slowly progressive dementias, most of the other disorders covered in this book make their appearance suddenly. Life is explosively transformed. It will never be the same. Thrust upon a person and family are mutations in life role and employment, financial stability, living environment, sexuality, leisure lifestyle, social integration, independence, and control (Code, 1999; Sarno, 1993).

All of this may be wrapped in modified mood or personality, perception of stigma, emotional turmoil, and alteration of the very core of identity and self-esteem (Barrett & Gonzalez Rothi, 1998). Ewing and Pfalzgraf (1990) have personalized some of these psychosocial barriers, as well as the struggle and courage involved in the rehabilitative process, by tracing the journey of six men and women who survived stroke. Ed, Betty, Ted, Paula, Tom, and Carl weave important lessons of their emotional reactions, changed relationships, resumption of activities, new responsibilities, and coping strategies. Their stories can be fit alongside those of Tan, Betty Penner, Jimmy Parker, Ken Kimber, Mr. Babcock, Jimmy LaPointe, Dr. Anderson, Martha, Arthur Kopit's father (see below), Emily the Wingwalker, Tom Reyhons, Dr. Ray, Dr. Kelly Hocker, and the thousands of others who trod the path. All had to endure ponderous life adjustments and psychosocial hurdles. We learn from each of them.

The Illness Experience

What is it like to be ill? What is it like to suffer life-altering changes in activities and participation in our world? Our ability to imagine or empathize with those who are chronically disabled is limited. A traditional approach to understanding the illness experience has emanated from the education and focus of health-care professionals on the *disease*. Little emphasis has been placed on the perspective of the *individual* with the disease. Fortunately, trends in some of the health-care literature appear to be developing along paths that try to understand the illness experience and try to develop research directions that incorporate qualitative as well as quantitative research strategies.

Morse and Johnson (1991) have written insightfully about the illness experience. They have proposed models for understanding and studying it and have reported important qualitative research across several different types of chronic illnesses and conditions. They use strategies of ethnographic research with careful attention to in-depth interview methods, participant observation, and what they refer to as "symbolic interactionism," or the experiential aspects of human behaviors. Morse and Johnson explain "grounded theory" as the essence of conducting qualitative research on the illness experience and show how health-care researchers can transcribe, analyze, and interpret informant interviews to reveal themes of coping strategies, social support, and participation in treatment decisions. They catalogue a rich array of descriptions of the illness experience and make no apologies for their intensity or poignancy. The strain of trying to endure, the shock of institutionalization, and the suffering and uncertainty of the illness experience was clearly evident in the reflections of those who were interviewed.

> When you're thrown into a pool, and you can't swim, and you don't have a life preserver, that's the way I felt for a long time. In other words, struggling. It was hard to get up in the morning knowing that you were

going to have another one of those days that was unpredictable.

The pain of watching somebody that you love going through pain, going through agony, that is the hardest part. That is the hardest part of the whole thing to deal with that. That was my hardest part—it wasn't the caring or the cleaning up or the helping her to the washroom or getting the pills. (Morse & Johnson, 1991, p. 338)

Stages

Arising from these experiences is a broader understanding of the illness experience. Morse and Johnson (1991) propose a more comprehensive view of illness, which they call the *illness constellation model*, in contrast with traditional illness views. In this model the experience is viewed from the perspective not only of the physical signs and symptoms, but also of the adaptation and coping behaviors exhibited by the ill person within the social context of the effects of the events on family and friends. Table 1–1 presents an adaptation of Morse and Johnson's conceptualization of the stages that the individual and significant others presumably traverse through the evolution of an illness.

These stages arose from the common themes expressed by patients and their families and friends, who were interviewed in depth throughout the course of the illnesses or conditions. Surely the insights gained from this type of qualitative research can aid us in our task of knowing what to expect and how emotions and behaviors evolve during the course of having to deal with neurogenic conditions. Although each stage may not be represented with the same duration or in precisely the same way across the different neurogenic conditions we encounter (e.g., in stroke the onset is sudden and the stage of uncertainty may be compressed into a matter of seconds or minutes), the fundamental aspects of these stages may have considerable relevance to the conditions with which we deal. No doubt considerable individual variation occurs across individuals and families as well, but an understanding of the major themes that may be represented during the course of illness can be useful to us in predicting and dealing with the reactions of our patients and their families (Table 1–1).

Table 1–1. Stages in the Illness Experience

Stage	Self	Family, Friends
Stage 1 Uncertainty	Suspecting Reading the body Being overwhelmed	Suspecting Monitoring Being overwhelmed
Stage 2 Disruption	Relinquishing control Distracting oneself	Accepting responsibility Vigilance
Stage 3 Regaining self	Making sense Preserving self Renegotiating roles Setting goals Seeking reassurance	Committing to the struggle Buffering Renegotiating roles Monitoring activities Supporting
Stage 4 Regaining wellness	Taking charge Attaining mastery Seeking closure	Relinquishing control Making it through Seeking closure

Adapted from Morse and Johnson (1991).

Stage 1 of the illness experience for many conditions begins with the individual beginning to suspect that something is wrong. Family and friends may be drawn into this process of suspicion, and doubts begin to creep into the thinking of everyone that perhaps something is amiss. If the signs or symptoms are insidious, questions begin to crop up about each subtle change that may be perceived in the body. Family and friends begin to monitor behaviors and tune in with more attention focused on any type of action or sign that may signify deviance from the norm. The ill person listens to his or her body with concern and tries to identify triggers that mark any change in signs or symptoms. Finally, the course of the condition may proceed to a point where the ill person and others become overwhelmed. This is the point where in many conditions "cure shopping" and multiple opinions are sought to add support or validation to the realization that something truly is seriously wrong.

In stage 2, sick people realize that they have no choice. Control must be relinquished, and choices become a medical prerogative. This is the stage where an individual is transformed into a "case" or a "patient." The individual and the family feel the loss of control and a resolution to turn all decision making over to professionals. The sick person feels that he or she is merely an object who is undergoing a process of "having things done to me."

> I can't do anything about it now. I just have to wait for these tests. They're doing some tests. I just get wheeled here and wheeled there. I just have to trust them, I guess. I've had all these doctors and people talking to me. Some are nice. Some could use a few lessons in talking to people who don't know a lot about medical things. It's in their hands now, I guess.

The patient's family and friends in stage 2 feel compelled to accept responsibility. They get on with the tasks of notifying other relatives and friends and in fetching basic items for the patient even though they may be consumed with anxiety and fear. Helping turns into a coping strategy at this point. Responsibilities are clarified and assumed.

> I've got to be strong. I don't want the kids to think we're all falling apart. Now is my chance to do something. He did so much for me for 30 years. I wouldn't want to be anywhere else right now. He needs me. There's an old song that goes "He holds the lantern while his mother chops the wood." Wait a minute. I don't know if that relates to this. What the hell is wrong with me? Well, anyway I'm here, and I've got to be strong and I'll help with this.

Stage 3 is the struggle to regain self. The process may not become actualized or complete during this phase, but now people begin to try to make sense of everything. They mull over and ponder and ask questions about the details of how they behaved during the acute phase. They review the events in their minds and examine in excruciating detail the events leading up to the illness to try to discover the "real" cause. They ask, "Why me?" and finally after ruminating, they begin to accept the fact that their lives may be inexorably altered. This is where uncertainties of identity, self-image, and self-esteem begin to be formulated. This is where ill people struggle to preserve a sense of self. Responsibilities and the identity associated with vocation, profession, or work are stripped from most ill people at this point. They feel that their accomplishments and the cocoon of things that they have done or are interested in are unrecognized or ignored.

> I was a composer and conductor, for heaven's sake. I've conducted in most of the great music venues of the world. They don't know any of that. They treat me like an eccentric old man. They use all these medical terms. I'd like to get them on my turf. I bet they don't know Berlioz from their bum. This whole experience is "Fantastique." Hector would have understood. He was a little crazy, too. They sure don't know who I am. Maybe that's because I'm not anymore.

Arthur Kopit, the playwright who crafted so many successful and critically acclaimed plays, is the author of a powerful play about aphasia, *Wings*. Once, when Jay Rosenbek and I were lecturing at a conference in Dallas where Kopit was the headline speaker, we had the opportunity to spend a long and intriguing night together discussing and exploring the effect of aphasia on identity. Kopit's insights were astonishing. He had done much of his research in preparation for writing *Wings* at the Rusk Rehabilitation Institute. The play was motivated by his tormented experience with his father's severe aphasia. Kopit observed that his father's identity was seriously torqued or twisted by the experience of aphasia. He related that his father would ask him, in convoluted aphasic fashion,

> *Arthur, when am I going to be me again? This is not what I had in mind for "me." After some more rehab will I be me again?*

These are trenchant observations about the effect of aphasia on identity and self and about the struggle people engage in at this stage of the illness experience. The role of identity metamorphosis in neurologic conditions and chronic illness has been a relatively neglected area of attention and clinical research effort.

In stage 3 the family and friends now solidify their commitment to the struggle. They realize that they must "get it together" so that they can be useful. At this stage the family also begins to assume a buffering role and engage in activities that protect the sick person. They hover and attempt to shield the person from concern and worry and the mundane responsibilities of business at home. Sometimes the buffering becomes excessive and this leads to exacerbation of the ill person's sense of loss of identity and responsibility.

This is also a stage where ill persons and their families begin to *renegotiate roles* as recovery progresses. Ill people now start to regain some control over home and work by giving instructions, orders, and issuing decisions even while still hospitalized. Beginning to exert some assertiveness over their outside lives aids them to begin to feel like who they were rather than like anonymous "patients." Morse and Johnson (1991) point out that this is the stage where the ill person attempts to feel useful once again, and even though dependency and roles may have drastically shifted, it is an important time for the family to realize that decision making and tasks can now be relinquished back to the ill person. Morse and Johnson use the metaphor of dance and comment that in this stage the sick person and the well person must learn to lead, follow, change direction, and learn to accept and relinquish a variety of tasks. This is also the important stage where the ill person begins to *set goals*. Planning is an important marker for all sorts of recovery processes and certainly no different in the stages of dealing with neurogenic conditions. Accomplishment of small goals is an important component of this phase, though a risk is that some individuals feel that an all too frequently recurring scene is that a patient is given a goal, struggles to achieve the goal, and finally achieves it, only to have the outcome become another goal that the person feels helpless to achieve. Professionals and family can spend more time and exposure on the successfully achieved objectives at this stage, even though this may slow progression to the next objective. A more crystallized appreciation of progress along with enhanced motivation to continue can be the result of this approach. The family usually engages in *monitoring activities* at this time as well. They express concern that the ill person "not overdo it," and they chaperone, hover, and remain close, ready to intervene whenever they perceive that they are needed.

In this stage of regaining self, the ill person needs much reassurance and experiences much trial-and-error behavior on many tasks of daily living. Lifting heavy objects, making a telephone call, dealing with the checkbook, and regaining sexual activity may be approached with tentativeness.

> *I'm afraid to do too much. Should I or shouldn't I do it? I feel I need to ask someone if I can do these things. Can I do this myself again? Well, let's give it a try. If I'm going to get back driving, I guess I got to start somewhere. The longest journey begins with the smallest step. Is that right?*

The family has an important role at this stage, and Morse and Johnson (1991) note that they usually recognize the uncertainty of the ill person and engage in supporting behavior. They make lifestyle changes, try to second guess needs, read or try to learn about the illness, try not to notice or comment on devastating effects of the condition, and try to remain positive (even though their real feelings may be thinly veiled). This is the stage where family members shower praise and encouragement and try to generate a sense of hope. Professionals can foster the development of this phase in families by their own recognition and support of positive family trends.

In stage 4, regaining wellness, the ill person enters into the rehabilitative phase of a more fully regained sense of self. This stage may or may not necessarily coincide with hospital discharge. Now is the time that rehabilitation continues and, depending on the severity of the residual impairment and disability, the ill person begins to regain more control over his or her life, dependency may be changed, and former relationships may be assumed. Of course, there may be very real limits to how much premorbid normalcy is achieved. Roles and responsibilities may be permanently altered. Patients wants to *take charge* and may feel that they must demonstrate their regained health, altered roles, or regained competencies. Proving themselves to others becomes a frequent process during this stage. Families and friends may *relinquish control* at this stage. Although some degree of hovering and monitoring may be maintained at this point, usually it is covert, as patients increase efforts to demonstrate control over their lives. At this stage, patients learn to trust regained or new abilities and further define and perhaps even accept their limitations. Confidence grows. Days are marked by promotions to higher levels of premorbid functioning and *attaining mastery*. More sorties into the "real world" are attempted, and gradually, the realization that life can go on and in fact be worth living begins to be believed. Comparisons are made either with others or with perceived levels of previous functioning to ensure that objectives

have been achieved or that progress has been made.

This stage can progress for a long time, and unfortunately is incompletely achieved by many, particularly those who fixate on a goal of nothing less than return to "normal" or premorbid functioning. Families may be guarded at this stage and focus on making it through with the concern that there may be setbacks or recurrences. They express the feeling that they do not want to become too enthusiastic about progress "in case something happens." Acceptance of altered lifestyle and making the best of a bad situation is as difficult for some family members at this stage as it is for the patient.

The ultimate place to be in this final stage, and a major task of patients and their families, is that of seeking closure. Getting on with life is a resolution expressed by those who achieve this. Putting the nightmare behind them, continuing to work on rehabilitation or prevention, accepting restrictions, changes, and limitations and planning for the future are healthy markers that signal closure. Some even generate tasks of writing about their experiences, finding ways to help others, or become active with support groups or organizations that deal with their condition or illness.

> *I'm real active with the aphasia newsletter. My writing is slow and not as easy as it once was, but I feel I'm helping others by getting this word out. I also enjoy talking to your class. Teaching those young people what it is like to have aphasia is an important lesson, I think. They always have such good questions. But they need to have the view from under the skin of one. Plus the brownies are always good.*

Adjustments are made. Searches for meaning are launched. New duties, hobbies, and activities are nurtured.

> *This painting is all new to me. Even though I have to do it with only one hand. Let me show you some of my work. This is a watercolor that we are going to use for this year's Christmas cards. I know it's not perfect. But I get a lot of pleasure from it now. You like*

this one of the Model A. I had an old Model A once. Did you ever hear of a rumble seat? Boy, a lot could get done in the rumble seat. I wonder if that's why they named it that? Whatever. My painting means a lot to me now. I probably never would have done this if I hadn't had a stroke.

Sometimes the search for meaning and adjustment is fostered by renewed altruism, less egocentricity, and learning how to become more other-oriented.

I never did much volunteering before. Now I realize that we're not alone on this planet, and there are a lot of people who need help out there. It's nice to just help others. I've been real active in the Special Olympics the last two years. I go there as a volunteer and help out with timing some of the races and stuff. I tell you these kids do a real nice job. It's all relative, I guess. They're not the fastest in the world, but boy that accomplishment of finishing an event is just as meaningful as the big-time Olympics. I guess there's nothing quite like having one of those kids jump into my arms when they finish an event. I'm glad I can help with this. It makes me realize that there's more to life than just sitting at home and stewing over my own problems.

On Being a Patient

One of the most pervasive consumer complaints about health-care delivery is the perception that patients are dehumanized, institutionalized, robotized, and stripped of identity and individualism when control is wrenched from them as they are cloaked in the cape of "patient" (LaPointe, 1996). It is so different on the other side of the fence. The gifted writer-neurologist Oliver Sacks captures the depersonalization of the process remarkably as he relates his own feelings of foreboding and alienation upon becoming a patient (Sacks, 1984).

One's own clothes are replaced by an anonymous white nightgown, one's wrist is clasped by an identification bracelet with a number. One becomes subject to institutional rules and regulations. One is no longer a free agent; one no longer has rights;

one is no longer in the world-at-large. It is strictly analogous to becoming a prisoner, and humiliatingly reminiscent of one's first day at school. One is no longer a person—one is now an inmate. One understands that this is protective, but it is quite dreadful too. And I was seized, overwhelmed, by this dread, this elemental sense and dread of degradation, throughout the dragged-out formalities of admission, until—suddenly, wonderfully—humanity broke in, in the first lovely moment I was addressed as myself, and not merely as an "admission" or "thing." (Sacks, 1984, p. 46)

We, as health-care professionals, must guard against the snare of routineness in our procedures and daily interactions, despite the fact that we may have administered the same test or treatment paradigm dozens of times. "On being a patient" emphasizes affinity with what may be an individual's first experience with a very foreign ordeal. Procedures need to be explained. Rationales need to be revealed and clarified. Questions need to be answered. Fears need to be calmed. Dignity and the uniqueness of the individual need to be preserved. We are compellingly reminded of this when we become patients ourselves and suddenly are thrust into a very different role in the health-care environment. The illness experience can be endured better with the assistance of empathic, compassionate professionals who are in tune with the most efficient ways to nurture adjustment and accommodation.

Adaptation to Chronic Illness

Only in recent years has much attention been directed toward adaptation to chronic illness. The psychological implications of the illness experience can evolve into the need to deal with a chronic condition that may never go away or be significantly improved. Many neurologic conditions fall into this latter category. As mentioned above, that is not to suggest that complete recovery does not occur in some instances, but in far more cases there exist significant residuals that turn out to be a part of a very altered lifestyle. Stroke, for example, is the third leading cause not only of mortality in older persons, but also of chronic long-term disability (Sacco, 1995). Studies of large samples of stroke epidemiology have reported that 70% of stroke survivors are somewhat limited in their activities, and more than 66% were limited in major activities. The Framingham Study of stroke survivors revealed that 31% were dependent in self-care, 20% were dependent in mobility, 71% had decreased vocational function, 62% reported decreased socialization outside the home, and 16% were institutionalized when evaluated at a minimum of 6 months after stroke onset. The figures vary for other causes of neurologic conditions, but for all, the evolution to chronicity is more typical than not (Sacco, 1995).

Chronicity

Chronicity implies long duration. Concepts associated with chronic medical conditions include "irreversible," "enduring," and sometimes "recurring." That being the rather bleak forecast for most with chronic neurologic conditions, it is surprising that more attention has not been paid in the health-care community to strategies designed to help people and families deal with chronicity. Certainly that is part of the enfolded responsibility in the counseling aspects of the job of the speech-language pathologist. As Gregg et al (1989) point out, adjustments to chronic illness must be made over and over, and these adjustments vary across disease processes, age, sources of social support, social mobility, family environment, and internal characteristics of the chronically ill individual. All chronicity, however, may be marked by any number of fears, real or imagined. These include, but are not limited to,

1. Fear of death
2. Fear of incapacitation
3. Fear of pain
4. Fear of abandonment
5. Fear of spreading the disease or condition to others

Stages of Chronicity

Gregg et al (1989) have amplified these apprehensions and have written as well about the stages or emotional reactions associated with chronicity. As with most stages, such as the well-publicized stages of grief, recent research has found that certain caveats are necessary when interpreting them. Not everyone experiences the stages, not everyone experiences all of the stages, and not everyone adheres to the temporal order of them. However, certain identifiable emotional patterns or reactions are more likely to emerge at certain stages than at others. Parallels can also be seen in the general reactions to the illness experience described above. The stages of emotional reaction reported (Gregg et al, 1989) to be associated with chronic conditions include the following:

1. Shock: This stage has been described as a period of "psychic numbness," with muted responses to external stimuli.
2. Realization: Gradual awareness of the reality of the situation and the seriousness of the consequences begin to seep into the individual. Strong feelings of anxiety or depression begin to grow based on the perception that permanent loss of function, unpredictability, or death may lurk on the horizon.
3. Denial: This stage is a defensive retreat from the situation. The ill person simply refuses to acknowledge or accept the existence or seriousness of the situation. It is important to remember that in certain neurologic conditions, as is well chronicled in the chapter on right hemisphere syndrome, the lesion that causes the condition can also affect those portions of the nervous system that are responsible for appropriate emotional reactions. Denial and misperception are an integral part of the sign and symptom complex in right hemisphere syndrome and may not be a reaction to chronicity. Other conditions, such as diffuse neurologic damage in traumatic brain injury, or dementing diseases also

could result in pathologic emotional conditions and reactions. In many cases of chronic illness, however, denial can be a part of the adjustment to the realization of chronicity.

4. Mourning: Grieving the loss of full health is a common reaction. With realization and awareness of the meaning of changed functioning may come a period of mourning and depression. This is also a stage that may be characterized by anger, irritability, frustration, uncooperativeness, and all of the other behavioral accompaniments to depression listed above. Sleep loss, reduced energy level, listlessness, and little interest in worldly events or socialization also can mark this stage.

5. Adaptation: This stage has been referred to as the "acceptance" stage. It is a much more positive stage of the whole experience of chronicity and an end goal, but a stage that not necessarily everyone realizes. The difference between successful, positive rehabilitation and less than optimal rehabilitation can be determined by the degree to which the chronically ill persons and family find acceptance. It is marked by increased ability to work through other emotional reactions to the condition or illness, a realistic acceptance of limitations, and an ability to plan and look forward to the future. It would not be unusual to observe that individuals with chronic conditions may in fact retreat into earlier stages of emotional response with the appearance of complications or recurrence, but the stage is marked by an attitude of accommodation, participation in rehabilitation, and a genuine appreciation of the affirmative assets that remain in life.

Although it has been a goal since the dawn of humankind to attain happiness, and many spiritual, philosophical, and pharmacologic strategies have been proposed and practiced to achieve it, a reality of human existence appears to be that reaching a constant state of nirvana, pleasure, joy, exhilaration, bliss, or contentedness is not probable. But on the balance more pleasure than pain can be achieved, even in the face of chronic medical conditions, and health-care professionals have a responsibility to help patients and their families on the journey to this state of relative equilibrium.

Quality of Life and Coping

Health care in the last decade has crawled and sprung along a path of inevitable change. Escalating health-care costs have resulted in debatable improvements in the overall health of the population. This is coupled with decreased public confidence in the health-care systems of industrialized societies (Snyder, 1999) and a nearly forced incorporation of economic and quality concerns. Emphasis on outcome measures and on quality-of-life issues have permeated the health-care literature and have directed our attention to the psychosocial attributes of illness and wellness. In aphasia and brain damage this has been addressed by a sharper focus on life quality loss and recovery (Blanchard et al, 2001; Code, 1999; Frattali, 1997; Holland, 1998; Lyon, 1998; LaPointe, 1999a,b, 2000, 2001, 2002; Parr et al, 1997; Ross et al, 2002; Worrall & Frattali, 2000).

Coping is a concept that means different things to different people and can be viewed from a multifaceted reflecting globe of perspectives. A definition that encompasses many views is that coping is a response aimed at diminishing the physical, emotional, and psychological burden that is linked to stressful life events and daily hassles (Snyder & Dinoff, 1999).

The concept of *emotional intelligence* has been introduced to help scientists study the nature of coping. Salovey et al (1999) introduced the construct of emotional intelligence and argue that it is this construct that plays a significant role in the coping process. These authors argue that emotional intelligence involves the ability to monitor one's own and others' feelings and emotions, to regulate them, and to use emotion-based information to guide thinking and action. The emotionally intelligent person demonstrates the competencies necessary to facilitate successful coping through several distinctive and identifiable processes (Salovey et al, 1999). The person who can allocate emotional intelligence to regulate mood states can forestall rumination, prompt emotional insight and disclosure, and use social support.

This is an intriguing construct. Much more must be learned about how to measure emotional intelligence, how it interacts with actual coping skill, and whether or not it can be fostered and facilitated. This would appear to be a good path of programmatic clinical research. Emotional intelligence is an independent variable that very clearly should be addressed and clarified as it relates to the variety of coping strategies and skills we see being exhibited by people in quandaries.

One avenue that certainly could be explored in greater depth from both a research and a clinical perspective is the discovery of benefits in adversity. In thinking back on some of the comments put forth by clients and patients who we felt had adequately adjusted to their aphasia, we heard comments such as, "I never knew I could paint until I tried it with my left hand"; "I've focused more on others now instead of myself"; "Slowing down and enjoying the time on the pier lets me see the birds and the sun falling into the water. I love it when the fishing boats come in. I missed all that before."

Benefit finding and *benefit reminding* are concepts advocated by Tennen and Affleck (1999). These authors have linked adversity-related benefit finding to constructs intimately related to adaptation, accommodation, and coping. These concepts include, for example, perceptions of *internal locus of control, dispositional optimism, openness to experience,* and *belief in a just world.* These are all individual and family system concepts that can predict adequate or inadequate coping. Perhaps we can learn more about these concepts. Perhaps we can foster them. Perhaps we should try.

I came across a study years ago from some lost reference source on the topic of benefit finding in adversity. It was conducted in Israel and entitled something like "Finding the Silver Lining in Terminal Medical Conditions," and it revealed the benefits that terminal cancer patients had discovered as they progressed through the stages of their inevitable physical decline. The cited such benefits as the following:

"I can just be myself, now. I don't have to try to impress everyone. What a relief."

"I trivialize the trivial. Thick thighs? Who cares?"

"I notice the elemental things more now. The seasons, coffee flavors, birds, little kids."

"I've mended fences. I'm back with my brother. I hated being on the outs with him."

"You know, when you stop to think about it, it's good to stop to think about it. I can't believe the good life I've had. I have friends and family all over who really love me. So do these two dogs right here. How lucky can you get?"

Family Systems and Caregivers

Much attention has been directed of late to the concept of family systems theory in health and in illness. As mentioned earlier, many conceive of certain neurologic conditions, such as aphasia, as being a family disease (Buck, 1968; Wahrborg, 1991). According to family systems theory, illness in one member affects all family members. Communication patterns, roles, and relationships can be vastly altered within families in the presence of chronic illness. The concepts of the amount of interdependence among family members has been studied recently relative to its relationship to adaptation to chronic illness (Biegel et al, 1991; Gregg et al, 1991). The degree to which a family is *enmeshed* (minimal differentiation among members, with all members overly involved with the ill person and difficulty in determining who is in charge of family decisions) and the degree to which a family may be *disengaged* (rigid subsystem boundaries

Table 1–2. Characteristics of Healthy and Vulnerable Families

Healthy Families	*Vulnerable Families*
Open system	Closed system
Permeable boundary	Tight boundary
Many social institution connections (religious, school, community)	Few social relationships
Well-defined structure	Weak social supports
Access to resources	Restricted access to resources
Receptive to change	Unreceptive to change
Good intrafamily communication	Poor communication

Adapted from Gregg et al (1989), p. 59.

within the group, with members functioning largely autonomously rather than interdependently) have been found to be important predictors of the ease or difficulty of mobilizing families during rehabilitation. Also, families that can be characterized as "open system" (many social relationships and interactions with religious, school, and health institutions) have greater access to social networks and support during attempts to adapt to chronic illness. Families that are more "closed" appear to be more vulnerable during periods of crisis. Table 1–2 lists some of the characteristics of healthy and vulnerable families.

The Raft

The raft that follows the wreck is built from the knowledge, practice, values, and application of rehabilitation science as well as the positive reception and infusion of the important humanistic issues advocated in this chapter. It is clear from the above discussion that family systems and caregivers are key ingredients in adaptation to chronic illness. *Support groups* that offer informational support, emotional buoyancy, and direct training on the enhancement of coping skills are an important part of the adaptation equation, but are elements that are not overly utilized either because of availability or other reasons. The Connect group in the United Kingdom (*www.ukconnect.org*) and other educational

and awareness groups such as the National Aphasia Association and Project Hope in the United States are useful resources. Blanchard describes many of these resources with contact information in the last chapter of this book. Blosser (1996) served as guest editor for a symposium that imparted in-depth discussion of such topics as changes in the American family; suggestions on how people cope; preassessment planning with families; ideas on making time count; reaching families through technology; and forming a therapeutic alliance with older adults. In Blosser's article DePompei offered a list of suggestions from the literature on how people cope (with the underlying assumption that considerable individual and cultural variability may exist). Table 1–3 is an adaptation and expansion of this guide, with the creative help of some of my colleagues and students.

Aristos

Accommodation and acceptance of bad shakes in life and of conditions that may not be able to be changed much is a perilous voyage. In novelist John Fowles's insightful book *The Aristos* (1970), he discusses the necessity of hazard for humankind. What we call suffering, disaster, misfortune, tragedy, or death is the price of living. How we react to these inevitabilities is the measure of how we evaluate and relish our lives. The concept of *Aristos* is taken from the ancient Greek,

Table 1–3. How Do People Cope? A Few Ideas

Psychologically	*Spiritually*
Embrace a cause	Talk to theologian (priest, minister, rabbi, guru)
Get a new interest, craft, hobby	Read spiritual passages
Count blessings or accentuate	Read inspirational stories
the positive	Meditate
List assets	Pray
Proceed one day at a time	Spend time at peaceful places (woods, desert,
Reduce negative thoughts	rivers, seashore, mountains)
Cultivate and maintain humor	Visit house of worship
List strengths of family members	Lunch with a monk
Realize you are not alone	
Dress up	*Cognitively*
Trivialize the trivial	Read a good book
Treasure little gains	Read about the disorder or condition
Keep a journal	Join organizations
Notice elemental things (sunrise, trees,	Talk to other families
coffee flavors)	Attend a workshop
Plot improvements	Listen to an audiotape
	View videotapes or CDs
Physically	Seek information
Continue normal routines	Ask questions
Listen to music, explore new music	Surf the Internet
Play the accordion	Read some poetry
Dance	
Exercise	*Socially*
Fish; catch and release	Interact with old or new friends
Clean house, tidy-up, and organize	Do things with family
Cry	Smoke some meat
Laugh	Grill some eggplant
Rest	Join support groups
Eat cleverly	Get involved in community activities
Walk the wombat	Help others
Take a hike	Take a course
Soak in the Jacuzzi	Tell a joke
Get a massage	Rent a goofy movie
Play pool	Go shopping
Plant a garden and watch it grow	Play with kids
Feed a bird; a chickadee, galah, or roufus-	Visit new places
sided towhee	Adopt a loggerhead turtle
	Save a manatee
	Get a pet

and it means roughly *making the best of a given situation.*

The notion of *Aristos* can aid people on this hazardous voyage. Fowles reminds us that for every wreck there is a raft. Those who have endured neurogenic disorders and conditions and those who help them must never lose sight of the profundity in the rainbow of rehabilitation. If full restoration is not possible, the struggle to improve still is. The process of grappling to optimize and achieve what can be achieved within a given situation is nearly always worth the pain and effort. We have a lot to learn about how to maximize recovery as well as how to attain a state of accommodation and acceptance, but it is extremely important to keep in view the positive end of choosing to get involved with the hardships of others. The Navajo metaphor of dark mist curtains, toil, adversity, frustration, and disappointment can be balanced with equally sanguine images such as those from the Navajo chants (see Preface to the Second Edition) and the Chinese poets (see Preface to the Third Edition).

> *Happily I recover.*
>
> *My eyes regain their power. My head cools.*
>
> *My limbs regain their strength. I hear again.*
>
> *My voice restore for me.*
>
> *In the white of the wings are the footsteps of morning.*
>
> *The sky where dragons were, surely can moisten gardenias and orchids.*

For every wreck there *is* a raft. Recovery. Restoration. Relearning. Renaissance. Surmounting barriers. Adjustment. Acceptance. *Aristos*. All of these are good reasons to get up in the morning. They not only provide solace to the individuals who expend the effort to face these storms, but also provide the balance and fulfillment so necessary for the professionals who choose a life of helping others climb the raft and look for shore.

References

Barrett, A.M. & Gonzalez-Rothi, L.J. (1998). Depression in Patients with Aphasia. *Home HealthCare Consultant, 5,* 18–22.

Biegel, D., Sales, E., Schulz, R. & Rau, M. (1991). *Family Caregiving in Chronic Illness* (pp. 129–146). London: Sage.

Blanchard, A., LaPointe, L.L., Bourgeois, M. & Licht, M. (2001). *Age and Circadian Rhythm Effects on Perceived Quality of Life.* Presented at annual convention of the American Speech-Language-Hearing Association, New Orleans.

Blosser, J. (1996). Working with Families. *ASHA, Winter,* 34–45.

Buck, M. (1968). *Dysphasia: Professional Guidance for Family and Patient.* Englewood Cliffs, NJ: Prentice-Hall.

Code, C. (1996). The Impact of Neurogenic Communication Disorders: Beyond the Impairment. *Disability and Rehabilitation, 18,* 539–591.

Code, C. (1999). Management of Psychosocial Issues in Aphasia. *Seminars in Speech and Language, 20(1),* 1–94.

Code, C., Hemsley, G. & Herrmann, M. (1999). The Emotional Impact of Aphasia. *Seminars in Speech Language, 20,* 19–31.

Code, C. & Müller D. (1989). *Aphasia Therapy* (2nd ed.). London: Cole and Whurr.

Ewing, S. & Pfalzgraf, B. (1990). *Pathways: Moving Beyond Stroke and Aphasia* (p. 167). Detroit: Wayne State University Press.

Fowles, J. (1970). *The Aristos.* Boston: Little, Brown.

Frattali, C. (1997). *Measuring Outcomes in Speech-Language Pathology.* New York: Thieme.

Gregg, C., Robertus, J. & Stone, J. (1989). *The Psychological Aspects of Chronic Illness.* Springfield, IL: Charles C Thomas.

Holland, A. (1998). Functional Outcomes in Aphasia Following Left Hemisphere Stroke. *Seminars in Speech and Language, 19,* 249–260.

Kagan, A. & Gailey, C. (1993). Functional is Not Enough: Training Conversational Partners for Aphasic Adults. In: A. Holland, and M. Forbes (eds), *Aphasia Treatment: World Perspectives* (pp. 199–226). San Diego: Singular Publishing Group.

Kauhanen, M.-L., Korpelainen, J.T., Hiltunen, P., Brusin, E., Mononen, H., Määttä, R., Nieminen, P., Sotaniemi, K.A. & Myllylä, V.V. (1999). Post-Stroke Depression Correlates with Cognitive Impairment and Neurological Deficits. *Stroke, 30,* 1875–1880.

Kennedy, B.S., Kasl, S.V., Brass, L.M., & Vaccarino, V. (2002). Trends in hospitalized stroke for blacks and whites in the United States, 1980–1999. *Neuroepidemiology, 21,* 131–141.

Kopit, A. (1978). *Wings.* New York: Hill and Wang.

LaPointe, L. (1994). Neurogenic Disorders of Communication. In: F. Minifie (Ed.), *Introduction to Communication Sciences and Disorders* (pp. 351–397). San Diego: Singular Publishing Group.

LaPointe, L.L. (1996). On Being a Patient. *Journal of Medical Speech-Language Pathology, 4,* xi–xiii.

LaPointe, L.L. (1999a). Quality of Life with Aphasia. In: C. Code (Ed.), Psychosocial Issues in Aphasia. *Seminars in Speech and Language, 20,* 5–15.

LaPointe, L.L. (1999b). An Enigma: Outcome Measurement in Speech and Language Therapy. *Advances in Speech-Language Pathology, 1,* 57–58.

LaPointe, L.L. (2000). Quality of Life with Brain Damage. *Brain and Language, 71,* 135–137.

LaPointe, L.L. (2001). Darley and the Psychosocial Side. *Aphasiology, 15,* 249–260.

LaPointe, L.L. (2002). The Sociology of Aphasia. *Journal of Medical Speech-Language Pathology, 10,* vii–viii.

LaPointe, L.L. (2003). Functional and Pragmatic Directions in Aphasia Treatment. In: R. de Bleser & I. Papathanasiou (Eds.), *The Sciences of Aphasia (Volume 1): From Theory to Therapy* (pp. 163–172). Oxford: Elsevier Science.

LPAA Project Group (Chapey, R., Duchan, J., Elman, R., Garcia, L., Kagan, A., Lyon, J. & Simmons-Mackie, N.). (2000). Life Participation Approaches to Aphasia: A Statement of Values for the Future. *ASHA Leader, 5,* 4–6.

Lyon, J.G. (1998) *Coping with Aphasia.* San Diego: Singular Publishing Group.

Morse, J. & Johnson, J. (1991). *The Illness Experience: Dimensions of Suffering.* London: Sage.

Parr, S., Byng, S. & Gilpin, S. (1997). *Talking About Aphasia: Living with Loss of Language After Stroke.* Buckingham: Open University.

Ross, K., LaPointe, L. & Katz, R. (2002). *Psychosocial Attitudes of Stroke Survivors and Normal Adults.* Ridgedale, MO: Clinical Aphasiology Conference.

Sacco, R.L. (1995). Risk Factors and Outcomes for Ischemic Stroke. *Neurology, 45,* 10–14.

Sacks, O. (1984). *A Leg to Stand On.* New York: Harper and Row.

Salovey, P., Bedell, B.T., Detweiler, J.B. & Mayer, J.D. (1999). Emotional Intelligence and the Coping Process. In: C.R. Snyder (Ed.), *Coping: The Psychology of What Works* (pp. 141–164). New York: Oxford University Press.

Sarno, M. (1993). Aphasia Rehabilitation: Psychosocial and Ethical Considerations. *Aphasiology 7(4)*, 321–334.

Small, S. (2000). The Future of Aphasia Treatment. *Brain and Language, 71*, 227–232.

Snyder, C.R. (1999). *Coping: The Psychology of What Works*. New York: Oxford University Press.

Snyder, C.R. & Dinoff, B.L. (1999). Coping: Where Have You Been? In: C.R. Snyder (Ed.), *Coping: The Psychology of What Works* (pp. 3–19). New York: Oxford University Press.

Tennen, H. & Affleck, G. (1999). Finding Benefits in Adversity. In: C.R. Snyder (Ed.), *Coping: The Psychology of What Works* (pp. 279–304). New York: Oxford University Press.

Threats, T. (2000). The World Health Organization's Revised Classification: What Does It Mean for Speech-Language Pathology? *Journal of Medical Speech-Language Pathology, 8,* xiii–xviii.

Wahrborg, P. (1991). *Assessment and Management of Emotional and Psychosocial Reactions to Brain Damage and Aphasia*. San Diego: Singular Publishing Group.

WHO (1980). *ICIDH: International Classification of Impairments, Disabilities, and Handicaps*. Geneva, Switzerland: WHO.

Worrall, L. & Frattali, C. (Eds) (2000). *Neurogenic Communication Disorders: A Functional Approach*. New York: Thieme.

2

Functional Neuroimaging: Applications for Studying Aphasia

Cynthia K. Thompson

Recent advances in technology have resulted in methods that can be used to examine the functional neuroanatomy of human sensorimotor and cognitive processes. These functional brain imaging methods include those in which areas of regional cerebral blood flow are correlated with certain behaviors, that is, positron emission tomography (PET) and functional magnetic resonance imaging (fMRI), and those in which event-related potentials (ERPs) are recorded from electroencephalography (EEG) or magnetoencephalography (MEG). The former techniques (PET and fMRI) are the focus of this chapter. The basic neurophsiological principles underlying these methods, their strengths and weakness, and major uses of neuroimaging techniques for aphasia research are addressed. In addition, some guidelines for designing neuroimaging experiments are provided and issues and special considerations relative to neuroimaging aphasic patients are addressed.

Principles of Positron Emission Tomography and Functional Magnetic Resonance Imaging: Some Strengths and Weaknesses

PET and fMRI are useful for visualizing the particular areas of the brain that are involved as individuals perform certain tasks. That is, these techniques have excellent *spatial resolution*. In contrast, neither PET nor fMRI are particularly revealing in terms of the time course of brain activation, that is, they have *poor temporal resolution*. They do not reveal, for example, at what point in time a particular word embedded in an auditory sentence is processed. ERP studies are required for this purpose. While the temporal aspects of language processing are very important, mapping the spatial architecture of language is necessary in order to fully understand the neural underpinnings of language. However, future work examining language processing in both normal and aphasic individuals may benefit from combining spatial and temporal techniques.

Both PET and fMRI take advantage of the physiological principle that changes in the cellular activity of the brain are accompanied by changes in regional blood flow (Buckner & Logan, 2001). This means, for example, that the volume of blood flow in areas of the brain involved in language increases during language comprehension and production activities. This boost in blood flow is accompanied by heightened glucose utilization and oxygen consumption. In PET studies, blood flow changes that occur under certain task conditions are directly measured. Using an intravenous injection of a radioactive isotope (contrast medium), changes in blood flow can be detected. However, in fMRI studies, rather than directly measuring blood flow, a blood oxygen level dependent (BOLD) signal (Ogawa et al., 1990) is detected. The BOLD signal results from the contrast that arises when changes in blood flow exceed changes in tissue oxygen consumption. While the exact relation between blood flow, glucose metabolism and oxygen consumption is not completely understood, changes in blood flow and glucose utilization appear to exceed oxygen consumption (Blomqvist et al., 1994; Fox et al., 1988). Increases in blood flow, therefore, result in a greater concentration of oxygen in the blood (oxyhemoglobin) in the active region than is actually consumed. The net result is a decrease in deoxyhemoglobin concentration in the blood, which conveys a signal that can be detected using MRI.

There are other important difference between PET and fMRI. As pointed out, PET is an invasive procedure, requiring use of a contrast medium. FMRI does not require a contrast medium and is, therefore, completely noninvasive, requiring only that the subject lies still and perform the behavioral tasks presented. Thus, PET may be contraindicated in studies requiring repeat scans because of radiation exposure. For example, studies examining changes in activation patterns occurring over time as is required in studies of language recovery in aphasia may best be accomplished using fMRI. In addition, PET has poorer spatial resolution than fMRI. In PET data analysis, smoothing is required in order to overcome misalignment of activation foci across subjects due to anatomical and functional variability, and to maximize within-subject signal to noise ratio by suppressing high-frequency spatial noise. As a result, the final activity level at a given voxel location is a sum of weighted activation values in the spatial neighborhood, resulting in large neighborhood effects. Finally, compared to PET, fMRI is less expensive and can be performed in hospitals where MRI scanners are usually available.

However, fMRI is not without weaknesses. One problem with fMRI is that it is very sensitive to motion artifact, which poses a problem for data acquisition (Woods et al., 1998). Brain motion, resulting from subject movement, or even from respiratory and cardiac cycles can disrupt the ability to acquire valid fMRI data, even though motion-correction algorithms are part of fMRI data analysis packages, and motion can be reduced using head immobilization techniques. Motion artifact also reduces the feasibility of using fMRI for studying the neural correlates of language production, since overt production involves changes in air volume, as well as movement of the facial muscles and articulators, although some innovative techniques already have been advanced for overcoming this inherent weakness (see, for example, Dogil et al., 2002).

There also are some potential limitations of fMRI in terms of the areas of the brain that can be imaged. Due to the physics of the fMRI signal, regions near the orbital frontal cortex and the anterior temporal lobes are difficult to image. This is thought to be because of the close proximity of the nasal cavity and the middle ear to the sphennoidal sinuses and the auditory canal, respectively. In these regions the air-tissue interfaces cause small, local distortions of the magnetic field and the signal-to-noise ratio is very low. Because of this, a lack of activation in these regions may be seen in certain experiments even when they are involved in the cognitive task under study.

To summarize, PET and fMRI allow examination of regions (spatial areas) of the brain that are active under certain task conditions. While fMRI has better spatial resolution than PET, neither technique is useful for fine-grained analysis of the temporal cascade of activity across areas of the brain (temporal resolution). Also, while the two techniques rely on cerebral blood flow as a basis for the detected signal, the fMRI signal results from a BOLD signal, rather than from direct changes in blood flow volume as in PET. Further, a contrast medium is required for PET in order to visualize blood flow changes, while fMRI is completely noninvasive. However, fMRI is more sensitive to motion artifact than PET and there are certain regions of the brain that cannot be easily imaged using fMRI.

Applying Functional Neuroimaging to the Study of Aphasia

There are several applications of PET and fMRI studies that are relevant to the study of aphasia. Neuroimaging studies are useful for studying the way that language is processed in normal, non-brain-damaged individuals, providing a basis for understanding how the language system is fractionated when brain damage occurs. PET and fMRI studies also are useful for examining the recovery of language in brain-damaged individuals with aphasia, and they can help to evaluate the effects of treatment, providing data relevant to the neurobiology of language recovery.

The Neural Correlates of Language Processing

Understanding the way that language is processed in normal individuals provides a basis for understanding how the language system is compromised with brain damage. Prior to the discovery of neuroimaging technology, study of the brain and language was largely accomplished through investigations of brain-damaged patients, for example in lesion-deficit correlational studies of patients with aphasia and related disorders. While such studies have provided much insight into how language is processed, there are several serious problems that delimit conclusions drawn from them. Patient lesions often involve cortical and subcortical tissue, resulting in complex language deficits involving more than one component of language (e.g., naming and sentence production). In addition, patients are known to develop compensatory strategies to overcome their functional deficits. Thus performance on behavioral tasks, correlated with lesion site, may reflect use of these strategies, obscuring the language problem. One other problem is that the lesioned area of the brain is part of a distributed language network; therefore, it is difficult, if not impossible, to determine from lesion studies whether the noted language function is disrupted due to the tissue lesioned or due to damage to a crucial part of the language network. For example, there are several reports in the literature of patients with lesions in the left frontal opercular area who show disturbances in certain syntactic processes. This observation, however, does not mean that the frontal opercular area is *responsible* for syntactic processing; rather, it can only be inferred that this area is *involved* in syntactic processing. Precisely how it is involved cannot be determined from such data.

Cortical stimulation mapping techniques and the Wada technique also have provided insights into the organization of language in the brain. These techniques are used to guide neurosurgical procedures in patients, prior to surgery, in order to avoid disruption of the language network during surgery. Therefore, one major limitation of these methods is that the subjects under study are neurologically compromised (e.g., the reason for the neurosurgery is to address some neurological problem such as intractable seizures), and therefore, mappings of their language ability may only indirectly elucidate how language operates under normal conditions.

Neuroimaging studies allow inspection of language processing in non-brain-damaged individuals. Unlike lesion studies, in which only the lesioned area of the brain can be investigated, neuroimaging studies examine distributed cortical areas involved in processing language. Indeed, neuroimaging studies already have begun to add to what we know about the neural correlates of language, i.e., regions of the brain not typically associated with language have been identified and components of the language network involved in particular aspects of language processing such as lexical-semantic processes and syntactic processing have begun to be mapped more precisely. While it is beyond the scope of this chapter to provide a complete review of PET and fMRI studies of language, a few are summarized below as examples of such work.

The neural correlates of word production have been investigated by a number of researchers. Moore and colleagues (Moore & Price, 1999; Price et al., 1996, 1997), for example, undertook a series of studies in attempt to isolate brain mechanisms involved in various components of the multi-component task of naming. At a minimum, naming involves conceptual, lexical, phonological and articulatory processes as per models of lexical processing (see Levelt, 1993, 1999). In addition, production of words when naming objects (or pictures) or reading involves visual object or word recognition processes, respectively. Therefore, in their studies, tasks designed in attempt to tease apart these various processes were included. For example, naming pictures was contrasted with viewing nonsense figures and saying "okay" in attempt to control for visual object recognition and articulatory processes (Price et al., 1997); and reading words silently was contrasted with viewing consonant letter strings (Price et al., 1996). Results showed activation of the frontal opercular area for both reading and naming, suggesting that this area is involved in the stage of lexical access in which the phonological form of a word is constructed (i.e., prior to the engagement of articulatory processes). These findings were in accord with those derived from lesion studies, in that patients with frontal opercular infarcts show naming deficits thought to derive from difficulty translating word from representations into articulatory sequences (Mesulam, 1990; Mohr et al., 1978).

In addition to frontal areas, word production also activated the left posterior ventral temporal lobe [Brodmann's area (BA) 37], near the inferior temporal and fusiform gyri. Based on this observation as well as other data indicating that semantic processes involve activation in regions that lie medially and anteriorly to the fusiform gyrus (BA 20), the authors concluded that the posterior ventral temporal region is crucial for lexical retrieval.

AQ1

Temporal lobe regions also have been implicated in several word production studies investigating categories of objects (Damasio et al., 1996; Bookheimer et al., 1995; Martin et al., 1996; Moore & Price, 1999). For example, in a PET study of word naming by semantic class, Damasio et al. (1996) showed increased rCBF in distinct inferior temporal lobe regions associated with certain categories. Summary data from nine normal participants showed significant activation in the left posterolateral inferior temporal lobe when tool naming was contrasted with animal naming, while naming animals contrasted with tools showed stronger activation in medial inferior temporal area. In addition, naming photographs of persons (as compared to naming tools and animals) activated the temporal poles, bilaterally. Similar, although not identical, findings were reported by Martin et al. (1996) and Moore and Price (1999). Martin et al. reported bilateral PET activation in the ventral temporal lobes (and in Broca's area) for naming animals, whereas, naming tools activated the left middle temporal gyrus (as well as the left premotor area). Moore and Price (1999) found that for man-made objects (vehicles and tools) significant activation was found in the left posterior middle temporal cortex; for natural objects (animals and fruits), naming activated bilateral anterior temporal and right posterior middle temporal cortices. These findings indicate that regions within the temporal lobe, beyond Wernicke's and surrounding areas (in both the left and right hemispheres) are involved in naming. While subject to some debate and unclear what the precise function of these regions are in word processing, these and other data indicate that they are part of the language processing network.

Several neuroimaging studies have examined regional brain activity associated with processing language at the sentence level. In general, these studies have noted bilateral recruitment of both anterior (i.e., Broca's and surrounding areas) and posterior (i.e., Wernicke's and surrounding areas) brain sites, although, in the right hemisphere, greater posterior as compared to anterior activation has been found (Bavelier et al., 1997; Friederici, 2000). Bavelier et al. (1997), for example, examined processing of visually presented simple declarative sentences in an fMRI study. Results showed that the sentence task (as compared to a consonant string control task) recruited Broca's area, the superior temporal sulcus, and the angular gyrus in the left hemisphere and the superior temporal sulcus in the right. Friederici (2000) found a similar pattern, although in that study subjects listened to (rather than read) grammatically simple sentences (presented either in normal prose or "syntactic prose", that is, strings of "grammatically correct" pseudowords). They found bilateral recruitment of the superior temporal region in both conditions, and additional bilateral frontal activation for syntactic prose.

Studies concerned with the neural correlates of processing canonical versus noncanonical sentences demonstrate a somewhat different pattern (Caplan et al., 1998, 1999; Just et al., 1996; Ni et al., 2000; Stromswold et al., 1996). These studies largely have shown that Broca's area activation in the left hemisphere is associated with processing complex syntactic constructions. For example, Stromswold et al. (1996) and Caplan et al. (1998) examined complex center-embedded relative clause sentences (e.g., "The juice that the child spilled stained the rug") and simpler ones with a right-branching relative clause (e.g., "The child spilled the juice that stained the rug") in PET studies. Both studies showed significant activation constrained to Broca's area (left pars opercularis) when subjects processed the syntactically more complex sentences Results of these studies suggest that Broca's area is crucial for syntactic processing.

Just et al. (1996), however, found both Broca and Wernicke area activation under complex sentence processing conditions. Specifically, they studied three sentence types, from least to most complex: conjoined (e.g.,

"The reporter attacked the senator and admitted the error"), subject-relatives (e.g., "The reporter that attacked the senator admitted the error"), and object-relatives (e.g., "The reporter that the senator attacked admitted the error"). Results showed that processing of all three sentence types activated both Wernicke's and Broca's area in the left hemisphere, and that the number of voxels activated in these areas increased with sentence complexity. They also reported activation in right hemisphere homologous areas, although to a lesser extent than that seen in the left hemisphere. The lack of agreement across studies likely relates, at least in part, to differences in behavioral tasks used in each, since brain activation varies systematically during language processing as a function of task demands. Notably, Caplan et al. (1998, 1999), Stromswold (1996), and Ni et al. (2000) used anomaly judgment tasks; whereas, Just et al. (1996) required subjects to answer questions about sentences, a task with involved sentence comprehension. Therefore, it is possible that Wernicke's area may be recruited for sentence processing to a greater extent when comprehending sentences is required.

In summary, studies examining the neural correlates of language processing in normal individuals have implicated brain sites in the left hemisphere that have not been previously associated with language processing. In addition, many studies investigating language processing in normals show recruitment of right hemisphere sites as well as left hemisphere areas. These observations indicate that normal language processing recruits tissue in both the left and right brain, albeit most studies show greater leftward activation, and that the language network includes extra-perisylvian mechanisms. The precise function of these areas, as well as more traditional language processing areas, remains largely unclear. Further research is needed to elucidate these functions as well as identify other regions of the brain that might be involved in the language processing network.

Examining the Neural Mechanisms Supporting Recovery of Language in Aphasia

Neuroimaging studies also are useful for investigating the mechanisms underlying recovery of language in aphasia. As in studies of normal language processing, prior to the discovery of functional neuroimaging, studies elucidating the neural tissue recruited to support recovery of language largely involved observations of patients. Behaviorally, there is substantial evidence that individuals with aphasia show recovery of language function despite sustained damage to left hemisphere language areas (Holland et al., 1996). Observations that language recovers to some degree even in individuals with large left hemisphere lesions led researchers to believe that the right hemisphere plays a strong role in recovery of language (Basso et al., 1989; Willmes & Poeck, 1993). Clinical evidence supporting this theory came as early as 1893 when Gowers observed that recovered language function following initial left hemisphere injury deteriorates when a new right hemisphere infart occurs. Studies of language development and restitution in left-hemispherectomized individuals also provide compelling evidence that the right hemisphere has the capacity to subserve language (Dennis & Whitaker, 1976; Wilson, 1970).

There also is clinical evidence that recovery of function involves expanded cortical language regions in the left hemisphere (Kertesz, 1988). For example, individuals with aphasia often show further language decline following a second stroke in the left hemisphere (Basso et al., 1989), suggesting that cortical regions in the left hemisphere, perhaps dedicated to another function in pre-infarction states, were recruited into the language network following the first stroke.

A few neuroimaging studies examining the mechanisms underlying recovery of language in aphasia have been reported. Results of these studies largely corroborate the patient studies. Studies using single photon emission computed tomography (SPECT) or positron emission tomography (PET) show increased glucose metabolism or regional cerebral blood flow (rCBF) in the right hemisphere as well as in undamaged portions of the language network in the left hemisphere (Demeurisse & Capon, 1987; Cappa et al., 1997; Heiss et al., 1993, 1999; Weiller et al., 1995). Weiller et al. (1995), for example, examined rCBF in six normal subjects and six individuals who had putatively recovered from Wernicke's aphasia as they repeated pseudowords and performed a verb generation task. Results showed greater rCBF in the right hemisphere homologues of both

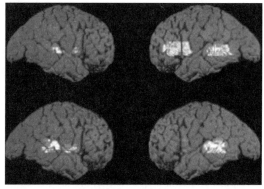

Normal Participants

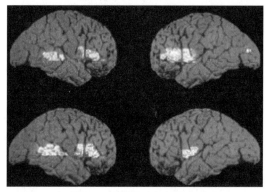

Recovered Wernicke's Patients

Figure 2–1. Activation patterns found by Weiller et al. (1995) in a positron emission tomography (PET) study examining verb generation (top) and pseudoword repetition (bottom) in normal participants and six patients after recovery from Wernicke's aphasia. Lateral left and right hemispheres shown for both tasks for both participant groups. (See Color Plate 2–1.)

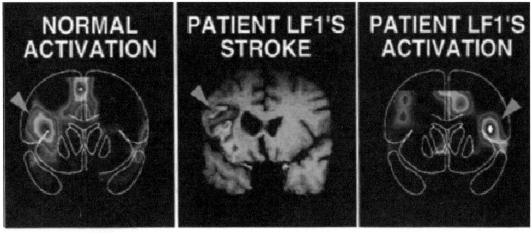

Figure 2–2. PET activation seen in normal participants (left image) and in LF1, a stroke patient with a left anterior lesion (middle image) during a speech production (word-stem completion) task (right image) (Buckner et al., 1996). (See Color Plate 2–2.)

Wernicke's and Broca's areas, that is, in the superior temporal gyrus and the inferior premotor and lateral prefrontal cortices, under both conditions as compared to the normal participants (Fig. 2–1).

Buckner et al. (1996) also reported a shift from the left to right hemisphere in a patient (LF1) with a left frontal lobe lesion and mild nonfluent aphasia resulting from stroke. At 6 months post-stroke, neuropsychological testing showed impairment in verbal fluency across a number of tasks; however, he showed good performance on a word-stem completion task. This task, used in several PET and fMRI studies (Buckner et al., 1995; Ojemann et al., 1998), required generation of a complete word when presented with letter strings comprising the first few letters of target words. For example, "str ___" and "cou___" were presented and the subject was expected to produce the words "string" and "courage". To determine what parts of

the brain were recruited to support this task, a PET study was performed. Results showed that, while normal participants showed robust activation in the left frontal area—precisely the area lesioned in LF1—the patient showed activation in the right frontal area (Fig. 2–2). Similar findings were reported by Cao et al. (1999) in patients who were at least 5 months post-stroke. Using fMRI to examine lexical-semantic processing, Cao et al. found significantly greater right hemisphere activation in the patients as compared to the normal subjects. Data such as these suggest that homologous right hemisphere regions can assume the function of damaged left hemisphere regions.

Several studies also have found partial restitution of damaged functions in the left hemisphere (Cao et al., 1999; Heiss et al., 1997; Weiller et al., 1995). For example, Weiller et al. reported activation in their Wernicke's patients in undamaged areas of the left hemisphere, that is, frontal areas in and around Broca's area, extending to the prefrontal cortex. Alsop et al. (1996) reported a similar pattern in patients with temporal lobe lesions (one patient with an arteriovenous malformation and one with a glioma), that is, both subjects recruited perilesional areas, not observed in the normal subjects, for language processing. Heiss et al. (1997) also demonstrated in a longitudinal study that recovery from aphasia is related to reactivation of areas in the left hemisphere surrounding the infarction. Results of these and other studies largely support early lesion-deficit correlational studies, suggesting that there are two primary candidates for language recovery in aphasic patients with left hemisphere lesions: (1) undamaged portions of the left hemisphere (typically these regions are perilesional); and (2) right hemisphere brain sites.

As discussed above, however, it is important to keep in mind that normals show both right hemisphere activation as well as recruitment of unusual left hemisphere regions during language processing. These observations suggest that the right brain and/or perilesional (or other left brain) activation seen in studies with aphasic patients may reflect, at least in part, the large-scale neural network that subserves language under normal conditions (Mesulam 1990, 1994, 1998). Therefore, it is important to include repeat scans (i.e., scans prior to, during, and/or following recovery) in aphasia recovery studies. Without repeat scans the extent to which activation patterns noted in recovery states reflect recruitment of new neural tissue or premorbid language processing routines is unknown. It also is suggested that such work include careful study of individual subjects rather than, or in addition to, groups of patients (as in Weiller et al., 1995, for example). The degree of right hemisphere recruitment, for example, will likely be influenced by the extent of cell loss (lesion size) in the left hemisphere. Further, because of heterogeneity in site and size of lesion and other patient variables (see below

for more discussion about these issues), peri-lesional recruitment may be difficult to detect in studies examining group trends in the data.

Effects of Treatment on Neural Recruitment

One very important use of functional neuroimaging is to study the effects of treatment. It is now a well known fact that neural plasticity extends into adulthood and that there are strong effects of the environment on neural organization and reorganization of function. Studies have shown, for example, that motor learning and motorically enriched environments, tactile stimulation, and auditory stimulation strongly influence neural organization of the primary motor, somatosensory, and auditory cortex, respectively (Greenough et al., 1985; Jenkins et al., 1990; Nudo et al., 1996; Recanzone et al., 1993; Van Praag et al., 1999). For example, Nudo et al. (1996) found plastic changes in the functional topography of the primary motor cortex in adult squirrel monkeys following motor learning tasks, and Jenkins et al. (1990) reported enlargements of somatosensory areas associated with controlled tactile stimulation in adult owl monkeys.

Studies also have shown that rehabilitative training after injury results in enhancement of representational plasticity (Nudo et al., 1996; Xerri et al., 1998). For example, Nudo et al. (1996) trained monkeys to retrieve pellets from small wells, an activity that requires skilled digital use. Following training, lesions in the motor cortex were induced, following which the monkeys were once again trained to perform the task. Comparison of intracortical micro-stimulation maps of the motor cortex derived before and after lesion revealed substantial rearrangement of representations. Areas of cortical digital representation were expanded, while wrist and forearm representations were contracted.

These findings indicate that experience directly shapes physiological reorganization following brain damage. Thus, it is likely that treatment provided for aphasia influences the extent and manner of reorganizational processes. However, research examining the neural bases of treatment-induced recovery from aphasia is limited. One study examining the effects of short-term auditory comprehension treatment on brain activation was that of Musso et al. (1999). Four patients with Wernicke's aphasia secondary to lesions in the left temporoparietal area underwent a series of 12 consecutive PET scans. During each scan, subjects were required to follow commands to either "point to" or "take" certain objects. Between each of the 12 scans (12-minute intervals), patients' comprehension was tested using a shortened form of the Token Test [the sTT, part of the Aachen Aphasia Bedside Test (Biniek et al., 1992)] and treatment focused on language comprehension was provided. Group results showed activation in two brain sites correlating with improved sTT performance. These included the right hemisphere homologue of Wernicke's area and the posterior part of the precuneus in the left hemisphere.

We also recently undertook an fMRI study to determine neural patterns associated with recovery (Thompson et al., under review). The aim was to examine the neural correlates of treatment-induced improvements in sentence comprehension in patients with agrammatic, Broca's aphasia. Six patients participated in the study. Prior to treatment all participants were administered a series of tests. All showed reduced sentence length and grammaticality in their spontaneous speech; they produced more open-class than close-class words, and more nouns than verbs. Language comprehension was largely intact, although all had impaired ability to comprehend complex, noncanonical sentences. Three of the six patients also were tested under fMRI conditions and then were provided with treatment. One of these patients (O.J.) underwent repeat behavioral

testing and fMRI scans at a 5-month interval prior to treatment. The fMRI task required listening to sentences during active conditions, either simple subject-clefts (e.g., "It was the thief who chased the artist") or complex object-clefts (e.g., "It was the artist who the thief chased"). In the control conditions, subjects heard single animate nouns. In all conditions, pictures were presented together with the auditory sentences or words. When a sentence (or word) matched a picture, the subjects were required to press a button. Thirty-two contiguous 4-mm axial slices (AC-PC) were obtained using whole-brain echo-planar imaging and analyzed using SPM99.

The treatment focused on production and comprehension of noncanonical sentences using a linguistic-specific treatment, that is, Treatment of Underlying Forms (see Thompson, 2001, for details). This treatment uses a series of steps to train (a) verb and verb argument comprehension and production and (b) the movement operations required to form the surface structure of noncaononical sentences. Following treatment, fMRI scans were once again completed for the treated subjects, and all language measures were re-administered to all subjects.

Results showed significant changes in behavioral tests administered pre- and post-treatment for the treated subjects only. Concomitant changes also were noted in fMRI activation patterns for the treated subjects, while no change in activation patterns was seen on repeat pre-treatment fMRI scans for O.J. (Fig. 2–3). On the post-treatment scans, all participants showed recruitment of the right hemisphere homologue of Wernicke's and surrounding areas (BA 22, 21, and 37). Two patients also showed activation of the right hemisphere homologue of Broca's area for sentence conditions as compared to the single word condition, and those with some sparing of left hemisphere language areas showed post-treatment recruitment of perilesional areas (BA 44, 45, 21, 22).

When we compared the post-treatment activation patterns of our aphasic patients to

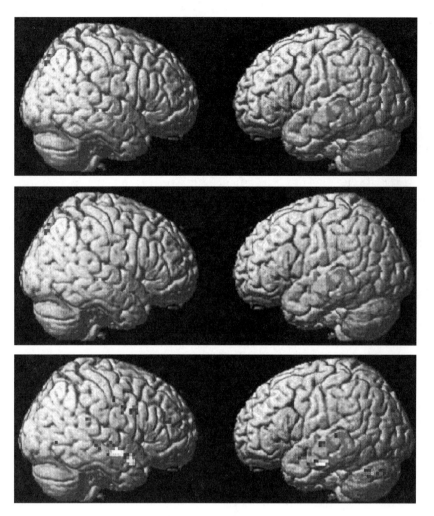

Figure 2–3. FMRI activation [Statistical Parametric Mapping (SPM) images] found on repeat fMRI studies with a nonfluent aphasic patient. Shown are significant activations found during sentence versus single word processing. Pretreatment (top and middle images) activation was constrained to small superior parietal and temperopareital foci; on post-treatment, bilateral activation of the middle temporal cortex, and the right hemisphere homologue of Broca's area as well as dorsolateral prefrontal and intraparietal areas were noted. (See Color Plate 2–3.)

normal participants (see Thompson et al., under review), we found some compelling similarities. As shown in Figure 2–4, our normal participants ($n = 8$), who underwent the same scanner tasks as the aphasic patients, showed bilateral activation of Wernicke's and Broca's area in the left hemisphere for sentences as compared to words. In addition, they showed bilateral dosolateral prefrontal and intraparietal activation, likely reflecting visual attention as well as working memory networks. Comparing O.J.'s recruitment to that of the normals, for example, showed that on his final scan he recruited bilateral temporal lobe regions (BA 22) similar to that of the normal participants

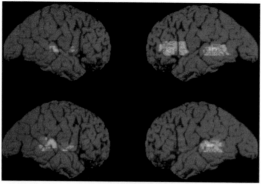

Normal Participants

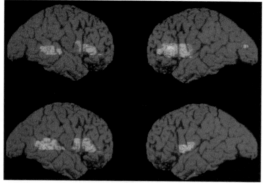

Recovered Wernicke's Patients

Color Plate 2–1. Activation patterns found by Weiller et al. (1995) in a positron emission tomography (PET) study examining verb generation (top) and pseudoword repetition (bottom) in normal participants and six patients after recovery from Wernicke's aphasia. Lateral left and right hemispheres shown for both tasks for both participant groups. (See Figure 2–1, p. 24.)

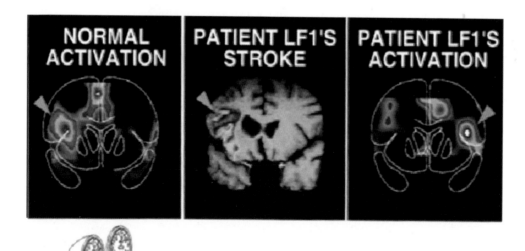

Color Plate 2–2. PET activation seen in normal participants (left image) and in LF1, a stroke patient with a left anterior lesion (middle image) during a speech production (word-stem completion) task (right image) (Buckner et al., 1996). (See Figure 2–2, p. 25.)

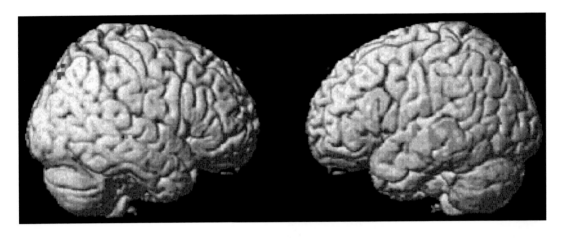

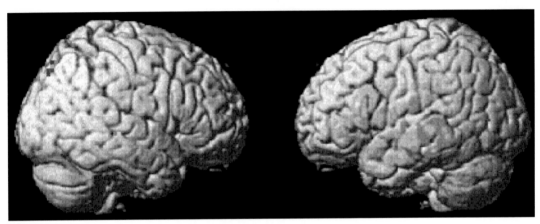

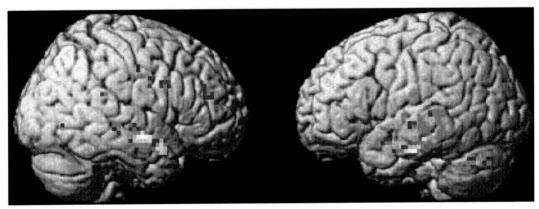

Color Plate 2–3. FMRI activation [Statistical Parametric Mapping (SPM) images] found on repeat fMRI studies with a nonfluent aphasic patient. Shown are significant activations found during sentence versus single word processing. Pre-treatment (top and middle images) activation was constrained to small superior parietal and temperoparietal foci; on post-treatment, bilateral activation of the middle temporal cortex, and the right hemisphere homologue of Broca's area as well as dorsolateral prefrontal and intraparietal areas were noted. (See Figure 2–3, p. 28.)

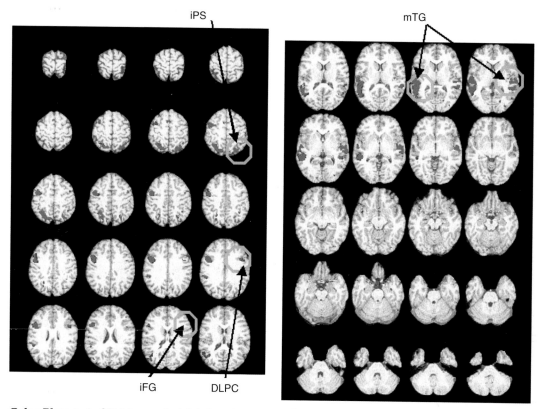

Color Plate 2–4. SPM image (axials) showing areas of significant activation for eight normal participants during sentence as compared to single word conditions in an fMRI study. Slices are 3 mm thick, going from Z = 60 (top left slice) to Z = -9 (bottom right slice). Areas activated by patient O.J., indicated by yellow circles, include bilateral middle temporal gyri (mTG), and right hemisphere Broca's area (iFG), dorsolateral prefrontal cortex (DLPC), and the intraparietal sulcus (iPS). (See Figure 2–4, p. 29.)

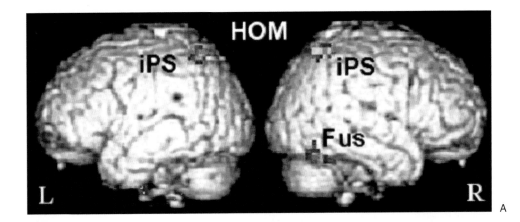

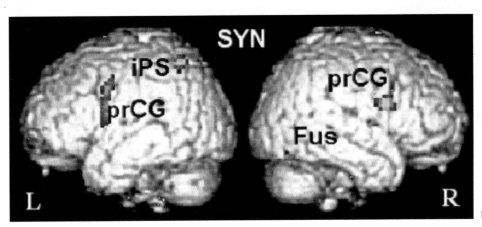

Color Plate 2–6. fMRI Results. Areas of significant activation for primary progressive aphasia (PPA) greater than controls in (A) phonology (HOM) and (B) semantics (SYN). Areas include intra-parietal sulcus (iPS), fusiform gyrus (Fus), precentral gyrus (prCG), and thalamus (not pictured). No areas of significant activation for controls greater than PPA were present for either task. (See Figure 2–6, p. 35.)

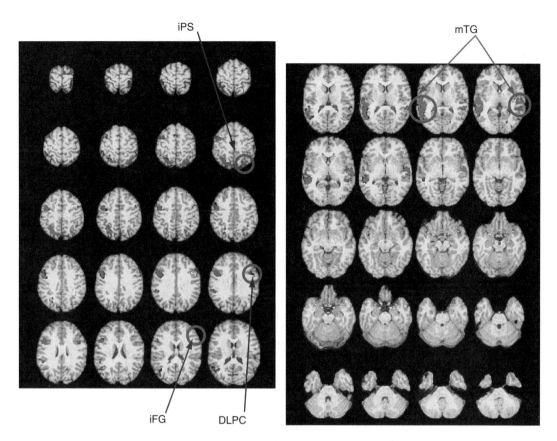

Figure 2–4. SPM image (axials) showing areas of significant activation for eight normal participants during sentence as compared to single word conditions in an fMRI study. Slices are 3 mm thick, going from Z = 60 (top left slice) to Z = −9 (bottom right slice). Areas activated by patient O.J., indicated by yellow circles, include bilateral middle temporal gyri (mTG), and right hemisphere Broca's area (iFG), dorsolateral prefrontal cortex (DLPC), and the intraparietal sulcus (iPS). (See Color Plate 2–4.)

(see circled areas in Fig. 2–4). However, instead of left recruitment of Broca's area, he showed activation of BA 44 in the right hemisphere. Finally, he showed activation of dosolateral prefrontal (BA 9) and intraparietal areas (BA 7) similar to that of the normals, but constrained to the right hemisphere.

The extent to which right hemisphere recruitment reflects "recovery" of function, however, has been questioned. Some researchers suggest that right brain take over of function may reflect inefficient language processing (Selnes, 1999). Belin et al. (1996), for example, investigated rCBF patterns in

seven aphasic patients who received melodic intonation therapy (MIT), a treatment program focused on teaching patients to produce words using song-like prosody (Sparks et al., 1974; Sparks & Holland, 1976). Following treatment, the patients underwent PET studies in which they were required to repeat words under two conditions, (a) when the words were presented with normal intonation, a "usual word" condition, and (b) when the words were "MIT-loaded". Results showed that under the usual word condition, the foci of PET activation was in the right perisylvian region. However, under the "MIT-loaded" condition, activation shifted to the left anterior brain. This and other observations let Selnes (1999) to conclude that "recruitment of right-hemisphere structures for language recovery is a last-resort type of strategy and one that yields a less than satisfactory overall degree of language recovery in most instances. The preferred strategy, and one that yields the greatest functional degree of recovery, is to integrate other left hemisphere structures with remaining functional language areas in the dominant left hemisphere" (p. 419). Grafman (2000) also suggested that homologous right brain adaptation is most likely to occur when lesions completely destroy cortical regions that serve a particular function. Transfer of function is less likely to occur when damage is incomplete because homologous sites are inhibited under normal conditions by connections from contralateral regions. When damage is incomplete inhibitory input is retained, thereby precluding transfer of function. While these theories about the role of the right hemisphere in recovery of function are interesting, there are data suggesting that they may not be completely correct. For example, in our study (Thompson et al., under review) and in that of Heiss et al. (1999), patients with lesions constrained to the left frontal region showed recruitment of Wernicke's area on the right, which correlated with improved language function. Further study of recovery patterns in aphasia with careful attention to lesion site and extent as well as a careful detailing of the patients' pre versus post "recovery" language abilities will help to clarify this issue.

Factors Related to Neuroplastic Processes

There are several factors that may influence the mechanisms recruited to support language processing in aphasic individuals. These can be conceptualized as follows: (a) organism-internal variables, (b) organism-specific variables, and (c) organism-external variables (Table 2–1). Organism internal factors include neurophysiological processes that are at work during spontaneous recovery and thereafter, such as neuronal regeneration and sprouting, changes in neurotransmitter release, and return to pre-stroke levels of blood flow. Organism-specific factors include those related to the neural insult itself, such as the site and extent of lesion as well as subject variables, including age, education, motivation and other related factors that influence recovery. Finally, organism-external factors have to do with the post-stroke linguistic experiences of the patient, for example, the type and extent of treatment received.

Clearly all of these factors have the potential to shape recovery of brain function. While little research has focused on the influence of these variables, a few studies have

Table 2–1. Variables Related to the Neural Tissue Recruited to Support Language Recovery in Aphasia

Variable Type	Environment/Source	Examples
Organism-internal	Intrinsic environment	Axonal regeneration Remyelination Biochemical recovery
Organism-specific	Intrinsic environment	Lesion site Lesion size Aphasia severity Language deficit patterns
Organism-external	External environment	Treatment type Intensity of treatment

investigated organism-specific factors. Thulborn et al. (1999), for example, examined recovery in two patients with different left hemisphere lesion sites. One patient evinced a lesion in Broca's area, and the other had a lesion in Wernicke's area. Recovery of simple sentence (reading) comprehension was tested over time, with results showing a rightward shift in activation in both patients. However, the specific neural tissue recruited differed in the two patients. The Broca's area lesioned patient progressed to strong right hemisphere activation of Broca's area, while he retained the normal pattern of left hemisphere activation in Wernicke's area (at 6 months post-stroke). Conversely, the Wernicke's patient showed (at 9 months post-stroke) strong activation in the right hemisphere homologue of Wernicke's area and a notable, albeit weaker, increase in activation in Broca's area in the left hemisphere. These data suggest that recruitment of neural tissue for language processing following brain damage is influenced by lesion site.

The size of the lesion also will likely impact the neural tissue engaged to support recovery of function. While neuroimaging studies with aphasic patients have not directly examined lesion size, there are animal data suggesting that it is important to consider. Wishaw and colleagues (see Kolb and Wishaw, 2000), for example, have shown that rats trained to use their forepaws to retrieve small pieces of food loose and then regain this ability with small lesions to the motor cortex. However, rats with larger lesions show less improvement, and those with lesions encompassing most of the sensorimotor cortex show little, if any, recovery.

With regard to organism-external variables, as pointed out above, results of neuroimaging recovery studies to date indicate that improvements in language processing ability, induced by treatment, can be mapped onto the brain. Importantly, it also appears that the areas of the brain engaged to support recovery differ depending on the type of treatment provided. Musso et al. (1999)

trained patients to improve language comprehension and concomitant improvement was noted in right hemisphere homologues of Wernicke's area; our treatment (Thompson et al., under review) focused on syntactic processing (both comprehension and production) and resulted in marked changes in activation in right hemisphere homologues of Broca's area as well as Wernicke's area. Further research examining the influence of the type of treatment on reorganizational processes is needed to corroborate these observations. Because of the relation between behavioral change and brain reorganization that has been noted in animals and now in humans, it is likely that different treatments, resulting in differential behavioral outcomes, may differentially affect the neural tissue recruited.

In summary, there are many factors that have potential to influence the neural mechanisms that support recovery of language in aphasia. The precise influence of these factors on recovery, however, is presently unclear and research is needed to clarify the role that they play.

Issues and Considerations

There are a number of issues and considerations relevant to conducting neuroimaging studies with patients with aphasia. These include issues pertinent to subject and task selection, task performance, experimental design and interpretation of the results. Some of these are highlighted below.

Subject Selection

As with any study involving individuals with aphasia, there are a number of participant variables that must be considered in neuroimaging studies. Some of the most important of these variables include age, gender, education, and premorbid language history and ability, because these variables likely impact organization of language in the brain (see D'Esposito et al., 1999).

In addition, as pointed out above lesion site, size, and time post-stroke also are important to consider. Clearly, when examining the neurobiology of language recovery, the site and extent of the lesion will impact the neural tissue recruited to support recovery. Time post stroke also is important, since activation patterns noted during spontaneous recovery may differ, often quite drastically, from those seen in later stages of recovery. Heiss et al. (1999), for example, studied patients at 2 and 8 weeks post-stroke, and reported remarkable changes in activation patterns from one test period to the other. Thulborn et al. (1999) also reported considerable change in activation patterns during early periods of recovery; i.e., they scanned patients at 76 hours post-stroke and several (up to 9) months later and showed shifts in activation patterns over time. While some studies may aim to examine changes occurring during the spontaneous recovery period, in others this variable will need to be controlled; for example, those examining recovery secondary to treatment. Since the period of spontaneous recovery is not completely clear, and likely varies from one patient to another, it is suggested that repeat scans be performed prior to treatment to determine stability of activation.

Task Selection

Developing the experimental tasks for a neuroimaging study is one of the most difficult aspects of this type of research, particularly when the goal is to study higher cognitive processes such as language. Language is a complex functional system comprised of several components (e.g., lexical-semantic, phonological, syntactic components) that make contact with other cognitive systems during normal processing (e.g., attention and working memory). For example, a simple auditory lexical decision task (i.e., deciding if a letter string is a real word or not) is a multicomponent task, involving primary auditory processes, analysis of complex acoustic patterns (i.e., auditory analysis), a search through the auditory input lexicon, and likely semantic processes as well. In addition, lexical decision usually requires a response, requiring decision making processes and a button press involving the voluntary motor system. Because the goal in neuroimaging work in the domain of language is to isolate certain aspects of language processing, for example, semantic processing, it is imperative that the components of the active and control tasks be carefully analyzed such that the resulting data will reflect the process or processes of interest. In development of these conditions it is important to decompose the various tasks, examining their sensory, motor and cognitive demands, such that the tasks differ only on the variable(s) under study. Psycholinguistic and cognitive neuropsychological models of language can guide development of experimental and control tasks for language experiments. These models, largely based on empirical data, can help to pinpoint the components of the active and control tasks selected and assist in determining whether or not the questions of interest.

Another issue relevant to selection of language conditions is that recruitment of neural tissue differs depending on the linguistic task. For example, a number of studies have shown different patterns of activation for normal participants when they perform word production-type tasks versus semantic processing tasks. Similarly, aphasic patients will likely show different patterns of neural recruitment under different conditions. In a study by Calvert et al. (2000), for example, task-specific differences in fMRI activation were found in a 28-year-old woman after partial recovery from a left hemisphere stroke. Performance of a verbal semantic decision task recruited a network of brain areas that excluded the inferior frontal gyrus (in either hemisphere). In contrast, a rhyming task—thought to place a greater demand on production processes and which activated the left inferior frontal gyrus strongly in normal controls—resulted in prominent activation in the right hemisphere homologue of Broca's area. While this finding might not be surprising, one of the major goals of neuroimaging studies with aphasic patients is to understand the neurobiology of recovery. Thus, it is important to keep in mind that a lack of recruitment of certain brain tissue may not mean that this tissue is not part of the post-stroke language network. Rather, it may only mean that this tissue was not crucial to the task performed. Neuroimaging studies of recovery from aphasia may, therefore, benefit from inclusion of several tasks, tapping language performance in several domains, in order to get a full picture of language recovery. Researchers also should consider including non-language, control tasks to confirm normal, reliable activation under these conditions, in contrast to the language conditions selected.

Task Performance

One crucial issue pertaining to studying patients concerns their ability to perform the tasks selected. As is well known, neurologically impaired subjects may not perform language tasks as well or as efficiently as normal controls (i.e., they may show reduced accuracy and/or delayed reaction times on the tasks of interest), which may result in either decreases or increases in activation relative to normal controls. The factors affecting task performance could relate to the patients' language deficits and/or more general impairments in attention or motivation. One solution to these problems is to include several practice sessions in a simulated scanner, prior to collecting the neuroimaging data. During practice sessions, patients are presented with tasks and stimuli that are similar (but not identical) to those to be used in the experiment. Practice in a simulator will not only provide data relevant to the patients ability to perform the task (i.e., accuracy and response time), it also will allow the patient to become accustomed to the scanner environment (e.g., noise, light-

ing, etc.). For patients who have highly inaccurate performance or have very long reaction times even after repeated simulator sessions, the difficulty level of the task may need to be altered, or the patient may need to be excluded from the study.

Vascular Compromises

The BOLD signal in fMRI studies also may be different for individuals with cerebrovascular disease as compared to neurologically normal subjects. In a recent study by Carusone et al. (2002), subjects with moderate to severe vascular disease were found to have a blunted and delayed Hemodynamic Response Function (HRF) (see Fig. 2–5 comparing the HRF in the normal hemisphere to that in the compromised hemisphere in one of their patients). Vascular compromises likely will not affect block design experiments because the exact shape of the response is not important. However, this is especially important for studies using event-related design and a canonical HRF, as the shape change may alter the results. Since single event studies may be desirable for aphasia studies, allowing inspection of responses to particular stimuli, one solution is to define the shape of each individual's hemodynamic response function prior to their taking part in fMRI (event-related) experiments. For example, a long trial (e.g., 16 seconds) event related design could be used to measure the exact response to the stimuli of interest. This resulting response function could then be used during the data analysis phase as described by Aguirre et al. (1997). Furthermore, having the HRF information would provide insight into changes in the vasculature and rule out hemodynamic changes as the cause of activation changes in the functional maps.

Design of the Experiment

The prototypical experimental design used in PET and fMRI studies is a "boxcar" or block design in which the experimental and con-

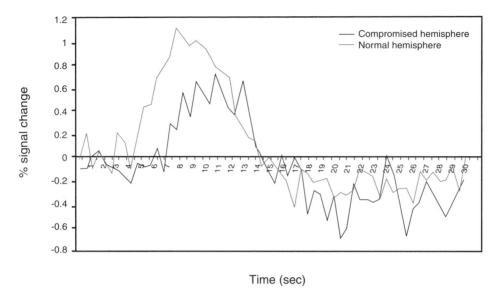

Figure 2–5. Hemodynamic response function (HRF) in the normal hemisphere and the compromised hemisphere in a patient with cerebral vascular disease (Carusone et al., 2002).

trol conditions alternate with one another. Several trials of an active task (A) are presented during a block with the aim being to engage a particular cognitive process; for example, a given block includes a series of pictures to which the subject must make a judgment about its semantic category. These blocks then are alternated with control blocks (B), during which several trials of the control task are presented. The design then is an A-B-A-B design. Blocked designs also can involve more than one active condition (e.g., A and B) and a control task (C) and arranged in a fixed (e.g., A-B-C-A-B-C-A-B-C) or pseudorandomized sequence (A-C-C-B-A-B-C-A-B). Complex factorial designs involving several conditions also can be developed using the block design strategy.

Another option for fMRI studies is the event related design. As is implied by its name, the event related design attempts to model signal changes associated with individual trials (events), rather than blocks of trials occurring in larger units of time. This means that stimuli of different types can (and should) be randomly presented within

an experiment and that separate analysis of the functional responses of a particular type (e.g., correct, incorrect) can be undertaken.

There are some strengths and weaknesses of the two design types. One strength of blocked designs is that they have excellent statistical power (Aguirre et al., 1997). However, behavioral confounds may result from blocking trials. For example, subjects may develop anticipatory behaviors or cognitive strategies for responding to items within a block. Further, when trials are blocked there is no way to separately analyze individual responses within a block. For example, for studies with aphasic individuals, it might be important to examine trials on which the subject responded correctly or incorrectly.

There also are important design issues relevant to validity and reliability. When studying patients, control groups are necessary. In studies examining recovery of language, normal (age-matched) control subjects should be included in order to compare the activation patterns between subject groups. It also is important to perform repeat scans for both the aphasic patients and the control subjects. That is, pre-recovery scans as well as post-recovery scans should be accomplished for the aphasic patients, and for the normals, repeat scans should be included on the same time schedule used with the patients. This will allow inspection of change over time in the patients and stability over time in the normals.

Studies examining the effects of treatment should also include within and between subject controls. Within subjects, at least two scans, should be done prior to treatment to show stability of activation patterns. Treatment then is initiated, and post-treatment neuroimaging data are collected using the same tasks as used in pre-treatment. In addition, a no-treatment control group of aphasic patients, matched for relevant subject variables should be included for experimental control. These control subjects could be entered into treatment once the original subjects' treatment is complete.

Interpretation of Results

One last comment concerns the hypotheses that are generated by the experimenter prior to undertaking experiments examining the

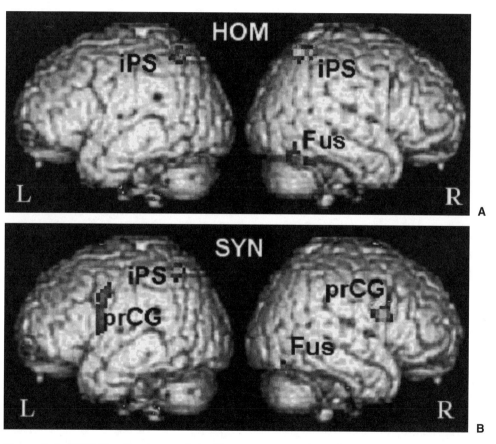

Figure 2–6. fMRI Results. Areas of significant activation for primary progressive aphasia (PPA) greater than controls in (A) phonology (HOM) and (B) semantics (SYN). Areas include intra-parietal sulcus (iPS), fusiform gyrus (Fus), precentral gyrus (prCG), and thalamus (not pictured). No areas of significant activation for controls greater than PPA were present for either task. (See Color Plate 2–6.)

neurobiology of recovery and the interpretation of results. Regions of interest (ROIs) (i.e., defined areas where the experimenter may expect significant signals to be detected, and thereby guide the statistical analyses undertaken), for example, may be defined prior to an experiment, or the experimenter may be open to examining the whole brain for changes in activation correlating with recovery of language. Regardless of which approach is taken, it is important to consider what the particular activation patterns might mean. Intuitively, one might expect increases in activation to show up with recovery; for example, a patient may show little or no activation of a particular area prior to recovery, but once the function returns, activation in that area increases. Another hypothesis might be to expect decreases in activation associated with recovery. While this might seem counterintuitive, abnormally large areas of activation have been noted in patients with dementia. Sonti et al. (2003), for example, recently showed this pattern in patients with primary progressive aphasia (PPA) in two tasks, a homonyms task and a synonyms task as is shown in Figure 2–6. Such data suggest that larger areas of activation may reflect inefficient processing.

Conclusion and Future Directions

This chapter has provided an overview of neuroimaging techniques that can be used for studying language processing in normal individuals and in persons with aphasia. While neuroimaging research is difficult, and there remain many unresolved issues, particularly pertaining to studies with brain-damaged patients, there is much to be gained by applying these techniques to the study of language, aphasia and aphasia recovery. Not only do they hold promise to lead to a more complete understanding of normal language processing, they also will help to inform theories of neuroplasticity and assist with our understanding of the mechanisms that support language recovery. Such research also will likely aid in de-termining the differential effects of certain treatments and may, in turn, influence payor support for aphasia therapy. For example, we may learn that certain treatments trigger a more complete recovery of the language network as compared to other treatments. Neuroimaging may also help us to better understand the potential for certain patients to recover language. Clinical applications such as these are, indeed, exciting and possible. The next decades of neuroimaging research will be crucial ones for helping us to better understand the neural mechanisms of language and its recovery.

References

Aguirre, G., Zarahn, E., D'Esposito, M. (1997). Empirical analysis of BOLD fMRI statistics II. Spatially smoothed data collected under null-hypothesis and experimental conditions. *Neuroimage, 5,* 199–212.

Alsop, D.C., Detre, J.A., D'Esposito, M., Howard, R.S., Maldjian, J.A., Grossman, M., Listerud, J., Flamm, E.S., Judy, K.D., & Atlas, S.W. (1996). Functional activation during an auditory comprehension task in patients with temporal lobe lesions. *Neuroimage, 4,* 55–59.

Basso, A., Gardelli, M., Grassi, M.P., & Mariotti, M. (1989). The role of the right hemisphere in recovery from aphasia: two case studies. *Cortex, 25,* 555–556.

Bavelier, D., Corina, D., Jezzard, P., Padmanabhan, S., Clar, V.P., Karni, A., Prinster, A., Braun, A., Lalwani, A., Rauschecker, J.P., Turner, R., & Neville, H. (1997). Sentence reading: A functional MRI study at 4 Tesla. *Journal of Cognitive Neuroscience, 9,* 664–686.

Belin, P., Van Eeckhout, P., Zilbovicius, M., Remy, P., Francois, C., Guillaume, S., Chain, F., Rancurel, G., & Samson, Y. (1996). Recovery from nonfluent aphasia after melodic intonation therapy: A PET study. *Neurology, 47,* 1504–1511.

Biniek, R., Huber, W., Glindemann, R., Willmes, K., & Klumm, H. (1992). The Aachen Aphasia Bedside Test. Criteria for validity of psychologic tests [German]. *Nervenarzt, 63,* 473–479.

Blomqvist, G., Seitz, R.J., Sjogren, I., Halldin, C., Stone-Elander, S., Widen, L., Solin, O., & Haaparanta, M. (1994). Regional cerebral oxidative and total glucose consumption during rest and activation studied with positron emission tomography. *Acta Physiologica Scandinavica, 151,* 29–43.

Bookheimer, S.Y., Zeffiro, T.A., Blaxton, T., Gaillard, W., & Theodore, W. (1995). Regional cerebral blood flow during object naming and word reading. *Human Brain Mapping, 3,* 93–106.

Buckner, R.L., Corbetta, M., Schatz, J., Raichle, M.E., & Petersen, S.E. (1996). Preserved speech abilities and compensation following prefrontal damage. *Proceedings of the National Academy of Sciences USA, 93,* 274–277.

Buckner, R.L., & Logan, J.M. (2001). Functional neuroimaging methods: PET and fMRI. In: R. Cabeza, & A. Kingstone (Eds.), *Handbook of Functional Neuroimaging of Cognition* (pp. 27–48). Cambridge, MA: The MIT Press.

Buckner, R.L., Raichle, M.E., & Peterson, S.E. (1995). Dissociation of human prefrontal cortical areas across different speech production tasks and gender groups. *Journal of Neurophysiology, 74*, 2163–2173.

Calvert, G.A., Brammer, M.J., Morris, R.G., Williams, S.C.R., King, N., & Matthews, P.M. (2000). Using fMRI to study recovery from acquired dysphasia. *Brain and Language, 71*, 391–399.

Cao, Y., Vikingstad, E., George, K., Johnson, A., & Welch, K. (1999). Cortical language activation in stroke patients recovering from aphasia with functional MRI. *Stroke, 30*, 2331–2340.

Caplan, D., Alpert, N., & Waters, G. (1998). Effects of syntactic structure and propositional number on patterns of regional cerebral blood flow. *Journal of Cognitive Neuroscience, 10*, 541–552.

Caplan, D., Alpert, N., & Waters, G. (1999). PET studies of syntactic processing with auditory sentence presentation. *Neuroimage, 9*, 343–351.

Cappa, S. F., Perani, D., Grassi, F., et al. (1997). A PET follow-up study of recovery after stroke in acute aphasics. *Brain and Language, 56*, 55–67.

Carusone L., Srinivasan, J, Gitelman, D., Mesulam, M-M, & Parrish T. (2002). Hemodynamic response changes in cerebrovascular disease: implications for functional magnetic resonance imaging. *American Journal of Neuroradiology, 23*, 1222–1228.

Damasio, H., Grawbowski, T.J., Trannel, D., Hichwa, R.D., & Damasio, A.R. (1996). A neural basis for lexical retrieval. *Nature, 380*, 499–505.

Demeurisse, G., & Capon, A. (1987). Language recovery in aphasic stroke patients: clinical, CT and CBF studies. *Aphasiology, 1*, 301–315.

Dennis, M., & Whitaker, H.A. (1976). Language acquisition following hemidecortication: Linguistic superiority of the left over the right hemisphere. *Brain and Language, 3*, 404–433.

D'Esposito, M., Zarahn, E., Aguirre, G.K., & Rypma, B. (1999). The effect of normal aging on the coupling of neural activity in to the Bold hemodynamic response. *Neuroimage, 10*, 6–14.

Dogil, G., Ackerman, H., Grodd, W., Haider, H., Kamp, H., Mayer, J., Riecker, A., & Wildgruber, D. (2002). The speaking brain: a tutorial introduction to fMRI experiments in the production of speech, prosody, and syntax. *Journal of Neruolinguistics, 15*, 59–90.

Fox, P.T., Raickle, M.E., Mintun, M.A., & Dence, C. (1988). Nonoxxidative glucose consumption during focal physiologic neural activity. *Science, 241*, 462–464.

Friederici, A.D. (2000). The neural dynamics of auditory language comprehension. In: A. Marantz, Y. Miyashita, & W. O'Neil (Eds.), *Image, Language, Brain* (pp. 127–148). Cambridge, MA: The MIT Press.

Grafman, J. (2000). Conceptualizing functional neuroplasticity. *Journal of Communication Disorders, 33*, 345–355.

Greenough, W.T., Larson, J.R., & Withers, G.S. (1985). Effects of unilateral and bilateral training in a reaching task on dendritic branching of neurons in the rat motor sensory forelimb cortex. *Behavioral Neural Biology, 44*, 301–314.

Growers, W.R. (1893). *A Manual of Diseases of the Nervous System.* London: J & A Churchill.

Heiss, W.D., Karber, H., Weber-Luxenburger, G., Herholz, K., Kessler, J., Pietrzyk, U., & Pawlik, G. (1997). Speech-induced cerebral metabolic activation reflects recovery from aphasia. *Journal of the Neurological Sciences 145*, 213–217.

Heiss, W.D., Kessler, J., Karbe, H., et al. (1993). Cerebral glucose metabolism as a predictor of recovery from aphasia in ischemic stroke. *Archives of Neurology, 50*, 958–964.

Heiss, W.D., Kessler, J., Thiel, A., Ghaemi, M., & Karbe, H. (1999). Differential capacity of left and right hemispheric areas for compensation of poststroke aphasia. *Annals of Neurology, 45*, 430–438.

Holland, A.L., Fromm, V., & DeRuyter, F. (1996). Treatment efficacy for aphasia. *Journal of Speech and Hearing Research. 39*, S27-S36.

Jenkins, W.M., Merzenich, M.M., Ochs, M.T., Allard, T., & Guic-Robles, E. (1990). Functional reorganization of primary somatosensory cortex in adult owl monkeys after behaviorally controlled tactile stimulation. *Journal of Neurophysiology, 63*, 82–104.

Just, M.A., Carpenter, P., Keller, W.F., Eddy, W.F., & Thulborn, K.R. (1996). Brain activation modulated by sentence comprehension. *Science, 274*, 114–116.

Kertesz, A. (1988). What do we learn from recovery from aphasia: In S.G. Waxman (Ed.), *Functional Recovery in Neurological Disease* (vol. 47) (pp. 897–903). New York: Raven Press.

Kinsbourne, M. (1971). The minor hemisphere as a source of aphasic speech. *Trans American Neurological Association, 96*, 141–145.

Kolb, B., & Wishaw , I.Q. (2000). Reorganization of function after cortical lesions in rodents. In: H. S. Levin, & J. Grafman (Eds.), *Cerebral Reorganization After Brain Damage* (pp. 109–129). Oxford: Oxford University Press.

Levelt, W. (1993). Language use in normal speakers and its disorders. In G. Blanken, J. Dittman, H. Grimm, J. C. Marshall, & C.-W. Wallesh (Eds.), *Linguistic Disorders and Pathologies* (pp. 1–15). Berlin: Walter de Gruyter.

Levelt, W. (1999). Producing spoken language: a blueprint of the speaker. In C.M. Brown & P. Hagoort (Eds.), *The Neurocognition of Language* (pp. 83–122). New York: Oxford University Press.

Martin, A., Wiggs, C.L., Ungerleider, L.G., & Haxby, J.V. (1996). Neural correlates of category-specific knowledge. *Nature, 379*, 649–652.

Mesulam, M.-M. (1990). Large-scale neurocognitive networks and selectively distributed processing for attention, language, and memory. *Annals of Neurology, 28*, 597–613.

Mesulam, M.-M. (1994). Neurocognitive networks and selectively distributed processing. *Revue Neurologique, 150*, 564–569.

Mesulam, M.-M. (1998). From sensation to cognition. *Brain, 121*, 1013–1052.

Mohr, J.P., Pessin, M.S., Finkelstein, S., Funkenstein, H.H., Duncan, G.W., & Davis, K.R. (1978). Broca aphasia: Pathologic and clinical. *Neurology, 28*, 311–324

Moore, C.J., & Price, C.J. (1999). Three distinct ventral occipitotemporal regions for reading and object naming. *Neuroimage, 10*, 181–192.

Musso, M., Weiller, C., Kiebel, S., Muller, S., Bulau, P., & Rijntjes, M. (1999). Training-induced brain plasticity in aphasia. *Brain, 122*, 1781–1790.

Ni, W., Constable, R., Mencl, W., Pugh, K., Fulbright, R., Shaywitz, S., Shaywitz, B.K., Gore, J., & Shank-weiler, W. (2000). An event-related neuroimaging study distinguishing form and content in sentence processing. *Journal of Cognitive Neuroscience, 12*, 120–133.

Nudo, R.J., Milliken, G.W., Jenkins, W.M., & Merzenich, M.M. (1996). Neural substrates for the effects of re-habilitate training on motor recovery after ischemic infarct. *Science, 171*, 1791–1794.

Ogawa, S., Lee, T.M., Kay, A.R., & Tank, D.W. (1990). Brain magnetic resonance imaging with contrast de-pendent on blood oxygenation. *Proceedings of the Na-tional Academy of Sciences USA, 87*, 9868–9872.

Ojemann, J.G., Bucker, R.L., Akbudaak, E., Snyder, A.Z., Ollinger, J.M., McKinstry, R. C., Rosen, B.R., Pe-tersen, S.E., Raichle, M.E., & Conturo, T.E. (1998). Functional MRI studies of word stem completion: Reliability across laboratories and comparison to blood flow imaging with PET. *Human Brain Map-ping, 6*, 203–215.

Price, C.J., Moore, C.J., & Friston, K.J. (1997). Subtrac-tion, conjunctions, and interactions in experimental design of activation studies. *Human Brain Mapping, 5*, 264–272.

Price, C.J., Wise, R.J.S., & Frackowiak, R.S.J. (1996). Demonstrating the implicit processing of visually presented words and pseudowords. *Cerebral Cortex, 6*, 62–70.

Recanzone, G.H., Schreiner, C.E., & Merzenich, M.M. (1993). Plasticity in the frequency representation of the primary auditory cortex following discrimina-tion training in adult owl monkeys. *Journal of Neuro-science, 13*, 87–103.

Selnes, O.A. (1999). Recovery from aphasia: Activating the "right" hemisphere. *Annals of Neurology, 45*, 419–420.

Sonti, S.P., Mesulam, M.-M., Thompson, C.K., Johnson, N.A., Weintraub, S., Parrish, T.B., & Gitelman, D.R. (2003). Primary progressive aphasia: PPA and the language network. *Annals of Neurology, 53*, 35–49.

Sparks, R., Helm, N.A., & Albert, M.L. (1974). Aphasia rehabilitation resulting from melodic intonation therapy. *Cortex, 10*, 303–316.

Sparks, R., & Holland, A.L. (1976). Method: melodic in-tonation therapy for aphasia. *Journal of Speech and Hearing Disorders, 41*, 287–297.

Stromswold, K., Caplan, D., Alpert, N., & Rauch, S. (1996). Localization of syntactic comprehension by positron emission tomography. *Brain and Language, 52*, 452–473.

Thompson, C.K. (2001). Treatment of underlying forms: A linguistic specific approach for sentence production deficits in agrammatic aphasia. In: R. Chapey (Ed.), *Language Intervention Strategies in Adult Aphasia* (4th ed.) (pp. 605–628). Baltimore: Williams & Wilkins.

Thompson, C.K., Fix, S.C., Gitelman, D.R., & Mesulam, M.-M. (under review-a). The neurobiology of recov-ered sentence processing ability in aphasia: Recruit-ment of right hemisphere homologues of Broca's and Wernicke's area. *Brain and Language*.

Thulborn, K.R., Carpenter, P.A., & Just, M.A. (1999). Plasticity of language-related brain function during recovery from stroke. *Stroke, 30*, 749–754.

Van Praag, H., Kempermann, G., & Gage, F.H. (1999). Running increases cell proliferation and neurogene-sis in the adult mouse dentate gyrus. *Nature Neuro-science, 2*, 266–270.

Weiller, C., Isensee, C., Rijntjes, R., Huber, W., Muller, S., Bier, D., Dutschka, K., Woods, R.P., Noth, J., & Di-ener, H.C. (1995). Recovery from Wernicke's apha-sia: A positron emission tomographic study. *Annals of Neurology, 37*, 723–732.

Willmes K., & Poeck, K. (1993). To what extent can apha-sic syndrome be localized? *Brain, 116*, 1527–1540.

Wilson, P.J.E., (1970). Cerebral hemispherectomy for in-fantile hemiplegia: A report of 50 cases. *Brain, 93*, 147–180.

Woods, R.P., Grafton, S.T., Holmes, C.J., Cherry, S.R., & Mazziotta, J.C. (1998). Automated image registra-tion: I. General methods and intrasubject, in-tramodality validation. *Journal of Computer Assisted Tomography, 22*, 139–152.

Xerri, C., Merzenich, M.M., Peterson, B.E., & Jenkins, W. (1998). Plasticity of primary somatosensory cortex paralleling sensorimotor skill recovery from stroke in adult monkeys. *Journal of Neurophysiology, 79*, 2119–2148.

3

Social and Life Participation Approaches to Aphasia Intervention

ROBERTA J. ELMAN

An important goal of rehabilitation is to help individuals regain function in order to participate in life as fully as possible. As speech-language pathologists, our scope of practice states: "The overall objective of speech-language pathology services is to optimize individuals' ability to communicate and/or swallow in natural environments, and thus improve their quality of life. This objective is best achieved through the provision of integrated services in meaningful life contexts" (American Speech-Language-Hearing Association, 2001, p. 26).

Models of Health Care

The traditional model in Western medicine has been termed a *medical model*. This paradigm considers problems as personal and residing within each patient. Treatment is given to the patient by an "expert" with the ultimate goal of fixing or curing the disorder. In contrast to the medical model, a *social model* of medicine has evolved. Within this paradigm, the problem is seen as an interaction among personal, physical, environmental, and societal factors. Treatment is collaborative. The individual with the disease or disorder works alongside professionals throughout intervention. The ultimate outcome is to promote positive change even when a cure is not possible.

The World Health Organization (WHO) has recently revised a multipurpose health classification system identified as the International Classification of Functioning, Disability, and Health (ICF), which integrates the medical and social models (WHO, 2001). This classification system offers health-care professionals a framework for describing human functioning and disability. A brief overview of the WHO framework is included in this chapter. The reader is referred to the WHO publication for a complete description of the framework (WHO, 2001).

The ICF framework consists of two parts. The first part is referred to as functioning and disability and has two components: body functions and structures, and activities and participation. Body functions refers to the physiologic or psychological functions of body systems; body structures refers to the anatomic parts of the body and their components. The activities component refers to the performance of a task or action by an individual; participation refers to an individual's involvement in a life situation. The activity and participation components can be modified with performance and capacity qualifiers to account for changes that occur among real-life, standardized, and assisted environments.

The second part of the ICF framework refers to contextual factors with two components: personal and environmental factors. Personal factors include age, race, gender, and lifestyle. Environmental factors are the physical, social, and attitudinal environments in which people live. These may act as facilitators or barriers to an individual's function; qualifiers are available to specify the extent.

Figure 3–1 illustrates the interaction of components within the ICF framework. Each component is expressed as a continuum of function. One end of the continuum indicates intact functioning, and the other end indicates severely reduced function. For example, the component of body functions and structures has a continuum that ranges from intact functioning to complete *impairment*; the activities component ranges from no activity limitation to complete *activity limitation*; and the participation component ranges from no participation restriction to complete *participation restriction*.

Aphasia is a disorder at the body functions and structures level. However, individuals with similar language impairments may have very different activity and participation levels. Let's look at two examples. Mr. G. has a moderate Broca's aphasia. His expressive language is restricted to single words and short phrases with omission of grammatical and functor words. His auditory comprehension is unimpaired for basic information, but Mr. G. has difficulty with more complex instructions and directions. Mr. G.'s activity limitations include not answering the telephone and not engaging in conversation with friends. Mr. G.'s participation restrictions include decreased socializing with friends and loss of his job. Contextual factors that act as barriers to Mr. G. are limited family support and lack of awareness of aphasia among his friends and former colleagues.

Mr. H. has a similar language impairment with a moderate Broca's aphasia. However, Mr. H. has excellent family support and attends an aphasia group program in his community. With instruction from the speech-language pathologist, he has learned to ask for clarification when he does not understand spoken directions. In addition, the aphasia group members suggested that he trigger his telephone answering machine to record lengthy or complex message while talking on the telephone, so that he can listen to the information as many times as needed. His friends and family have read information about aphasia and have attended caregiver and speech-language therapy sessions to learn as much as they can. With this

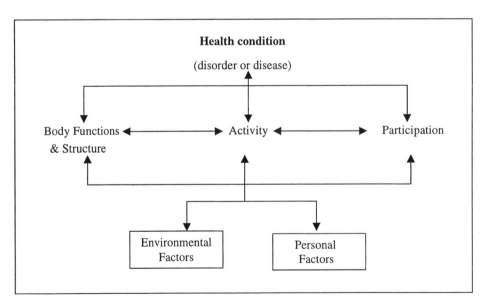

Figure 3–1. Interaction among the components of International Classification of Functioning, Disability, and Health (ICF) (From WHO, 2001.)

education, Mr. H.'s friends and family are able to act as facilitators for his communicative attempts by encouraging him to use alternate ways to communicate, such as writing or drawing when he has word-finding problems. Mr. H. feels comfortable interacting with his friends from before his stroke, and he has made new friends within the aphasia group program. Although he has been unable to return to his former job, he has begun to volunteer at a local Humane Society and feels extremely positive about the contribution he is making to his community.

Mr. G. and Mr. H. illustrate how very similar language impairments can impact individual's lives very differently. In addition to working on impairment level language tasks, a critical role for speech-language pathologists is to take a social approach and work toward increasing environmental facilitators and reducing environmental barriers whenever possible. When contextual factors are facilitating rather than interfering with function, individuals with aphasia are often able to participate more fully with an improved quality of life.

Evolution Toward a Social Approach

The application of a social approach to aphasia intervention has occurred relatively recently. Pioneers such as Sarno and Holland were early and vocal advocates of real life and functional assessments (Sarno, 1969; Holland, 1980) as well as the psychosocial impact of aphasia (Sarno, 1981). However, the majority of clinicians and researchers continued to concentrate on impairment-level linguistic treatment tasks. Little consideration was given to real-life activities or life participation issues, and aphasia treatment remained focused on stimulus-response linguistic tasks. Therapy was typically provided in a nondescript therapy room within a medical setting. Given the office setting, individuals with aphasia rarely had the opportunity to meet others who were dealing with similar challenges, and important psychosocial issues related to coping with aphasia were unlikely to be addressed.

Beginning in the 1990s, a focus on the social factors of aphasia began to emerge in earnest. During this time, a number of researchers and clinicians focused on real-life communicative contexts and quality of life or other psychosocial issues that are often associated with aphasia (Armstrong, 1993; Brumfitt, 1993; Byng et al., 2000; Code & Müller, 1992; Elman, 1998; Hoen et al., 1997; Holland, 1991; Jordan & Kaiser, 1996; Kagan & Gailey, 1993; LaFond et al., 1993; LaPointe, 1996; LeDorze & Brassard, 1995; Lyon, 1992, 1996, 1997a,b, 1998, 2000; Parr, 1994; Parr et al., 1997; Sarno, 1993; Simmons-Mackie, 1998; Walker-Batson et al., 1999; Worrall, 1992). Incorporating a social approach into aphasia intervention and research is by no means complete, but momentum continues to build. LaPointe (2002) suggests that an important next step is to articulate a "sociology of aphasia" that could integrate the psychosocial ramifications of aphasia with the neurolinguistic knowledge.

One social approach to aphasia intervention is the life participation approach to aphasia (LPAA). LPAA is a philosophy that emphasizes reengagement in life for all those affected by aphasia (LPAA Project Group, 2000, 2001). LPAA unites various approaches to assessment, intervention, research, and advocacy with five core components in its framework: (1) The explicit goal is enhancement of life participation. (2) All those affected by aphasia are entitled to service. (3) Both personal and environmental factors are targets of assessment and intervention. (4) Success is measured via documented life enhancement changes. (5) Emphasis is placed on availability of services as needed at all stages of life with aphasia. LPAA suggests that advocacy efforts should be targeted to those components that are not available in our current healthcare systems.

Emphasis on Wellness and Quality of Life

The social approach to medical and communicative disorders is also being influenced by an increasing focus on wellness and quality of life. Ryff (1989) and Ryff and Singer (1998, 2000) suggest that positive health should not be looked at as the absence of disease, but rather as the presence of such important factors as leading a purposeful life (Markus & Nurius, 1986) and having quality connections to others. Ryff and Singer's work has particular implications for individuals who face aphasia due to the isolation that often results from the disorder (Sarno, 2004). A body of research, from various fields, indicates that social connection is highly correlated with longevity (Ryff & Singer, 2000). As aphasiologists, we have a responsibility to help connect people with aphasia with friends and family in order to help them maintain interpersonal connections (Elman, 2002; Kagan, 1995; Kagan & Gailey, 1993; Lyon, 1992, 2000; Lyon & Shadden, 2001; Sarno, 1991).

Focus on Conversation

Conversation is all around us. These days, it is actually difficult to find a place where people aren't conversing, especially as cell phones have increased conversational opportunities. Environments that were formerly quiet are now commonly filled with one-sided cell phone conversations! Conversations are important for a variety of reasons. First, they are the means by which humans both create and maintain social relationships (Kagan & Gailey, 1993). Conversation is the "cement" that holds together family relationships and friendships. The everyday talk that we engage in helps to connect us to one another. Brown and Yule (1983) categorize language use into two basic functions: transactional language, which is the exchange of content or information, and interactional language, which is used to affiliate with others (Brown & Yule, 1983; Simmons-Mackie, 2001). Second, conversation is the way in which most of us interface with the various communities to which we belong, as well as with our society at large (Kagan & Gailey, 1993; Pound et al., 2000). Whether we need help from an elected city official or desire library privileges at the local library, we usually start the process with a conversation. A social approach to communication disorders addresses the importance of conversation in language use.

A social approach to aphasia rehabilitation is critical because people are social beings who interact with others within a context of various environments and communities. Language is used primarily to communicate with others, regardless of the modality used. We cannot, and should not, divorce language from the communicative contexts or the communicative purposes for which it is used. In fact, the most important goal of aphasia rehabilitation may be to help people maintain and create interpersonal relationships and social contacts.

The Insider's Perspective

A social approach to aphasia intervention recognizes that the viewpoint of the language user is paramount. The person living with a communication disorder has an insider's perspective that no one else has (Parr, 1994; Parr et al., 1997). It is vital to acknowledge and incorporate the language user's input and goals during all phases of intervention. The speech-language pathologist is an important member of the collaborative team, but the person with aphasia or other language disorder is the team captain. People with severe language impairments should not be eliminated from this collaboration because of their restricted language use. Instead, environmental facilitators, including such techniques as written choices, drawing, pictorial representations, and number lines have been used successfully to gain input from those with severe aphasia (Bernstein-Ellis & Elman, 1999; Garrett & Beukelman, 1992; Kagan, 1998; Kagan & Kimelman, 1995).

Evaluation

A social approach demands that *authentic* language use is captured during the evaluation process (Simmons-Mackie & Damico, 1996). Standardized testing and language batteries are an important part of this process, but additional information is typically needed to capture language use in the individual's natural environment. Evaluation should be able to determine the strengths and weaknesses at impairment, activity, and participation levels of functioning (LeDorze & Brassard, 1995; Rogers et al., 1999; WHO, 2001). As previously mentioned, the language user's input and perspective is a critical piece of the evaluation process. Other sources of potential input include interviews or questionnaires regarding language use with family/friends as well as observation in the individual's natural environments (Garrett, 1999; Murray & Chapey, 2001; Simmons-Mackie, 2001; Simmons-Mackie & Damico, 1996; Worrall & Frattali, 2000). A multimethod approach, incorporating both quantitative and qualitative evaluation measures, provides the clinician with information that is most likely to be representative of the individual's actual language use (Brewer & Hunter, 1989; Elman, 1995). This triangulation of information has the potential to provide the most accurate snapshot of an individual's language strengths and weaknesses in order to determine the treatment plan.

Treatment

A social approach to treatment requires that each individual's language impairment be viewed within the context of the individual's entire life. Depending on the needs and preferences of the person with aphasia, family members, time post-onset, and numerous other variables, the speech-language pathologist recommends a treatment plan. Attempts are made to incorporate the daily activities and life participation events of that individual into the treatment plan from the very beginning. For example, an impairment-level word retrieval task for a carpenter may emphasize naming of various tools needed on his job rather than randomly selected photographs. An avid bridge player may be given pictographs to enable her resumed participation in her weekly bridge game.

The local paramedics may be given specific props and training in supported conversation techniques so that they can identify the critical medical needs of those with aphasia (Kagan, 1995, 1998). These examples are consistent with ICF and LPAA frameworks (WHO, 2001; LPAA Project Group, 2000, 2001). Treatment targets include impairment, activity, and participation levels as well as removing environmental barriers and increasing environmental facilitators. The ultimate goal of the speech-language pathologist is not on increasing language skills in the therapy room, but on bridging language skills and adaptations into the real-life needs of the person with aphasia (Elman, 2004). In addition, tasks aimed at language recovery as well as those that target compensation for language deficits are both appropriate aspects of the treatment plan. The ultimate treatment focus is determined by the needs and potentialities of each individual (Elman, 1995).

Specific Treatment Approaches

Group Treatment

Group treatment is currently enjoying a renaissance. Originally provided during World War II as a practical way to serve the many injured soldiers, interest has been rekindled in recent years (Kearns & Elman, 2001). Aphasia group treatment has demonstrated efficacy and effectiveness (Aten et al., 1982; Bollinger et al. 1993; Elman & Bernstein-Ellis, 1999a,b; Wertz et al., 1981), and when groups are conducted in a collaborative fashion, they are a prime example of a social approach to intervention. Elman and Bernstein-Ellis (1999a) propose several advantages to group treatment as compared to individual treatment: groups increase the variety of communicative functions or speech acts used among group members; groups provides a wider array of communicative partners, which may increase generalization; groups have the potential to improve psychosocial function both directly or indirectly; and groups can be a cost-effective method of providing service. Groups also provide an excellent environment for language improvisation, which is important for novel and creative language use (Elman, 2004). In addition, groups provide members with a sense of community. Membership in communities fosters interpersonal flourishing and has been shown to impact overall health and well-being (Elman, 2002; Ryff & Singer, 1998, 2000).

It is also possible that groups may have a "preventive" benefit if started early on in an individual's rehabilitation. By reducing the isolation that commonly occurs with aphasia (Sarno, 1986, 2004), negative psychosocial reactions such as depression or frustration may be avoided. Research into this possible preventative impact of group treatment is certainly warranted.

The stated purposes of aphasia groups differ: some target specific speech and language skills, whereas others focus on psychosocial functioning or family support (Kearns & Elman, 2001). Some groups address the issue of personal identity and a need for moving forward in life with aphasia (Elman, 1999a; Elman & Bernstein-Ellis, 1999b; Pound et al., 2000). The most common purpose of most aphasia groups is actually a hybrid—speech-language skills as well as counseling/psychosocial factors are addressed within group sessions (Kearns & Elman, 2001).

Several texts provide detailed information regarding aphasia group methods and techniques (Avent, 1997; Elman, 1999a, 2000; Kearns & Elman, 2001; Marshall, 1999a,b; Pound et al., 2000; Vickers, 1998). Group treatment should not be undertaken without specific clinical education and training. Unfortunately, few clinicians report any specific training in group methods or techniques (Kearns & Simmons, 1985). Group therapy presents significant challenges for clinicians because group members' strengths and weaknesses must be considered. Aphasia group facilitation has been compared to conducting a symphony orchestra, except that the exact "language score" is unknown until it is produced (Elman, 1999a, 2004). At a min-

imum, therapists who provide aphasia group treatment should be familiar with the theory and clinical techniques associated with group process and group dynamics from such disciplines as psychology and social work (Bertcher, 1994; Elman, 2000; Ewing, 1999; Luterman, 1996; Yalom, 1985).

Roger Ross, a stroke survivor with aphasia, who himself conducted self-help groups, eloquently summarizes the importance of aphasia groups: "I have a sense that, after my stroke, I did not get better until I met other people with the same problem. My colleagues and I believe that joining a group is the most important thing that a stroke survivor can do for himself or herself" (Holland & Ross, 1999, p. 116).

Communicative Partners and Volunteers

Communicative partners are volunteers who have been trained to communicate with individuals having aphasia (Lyon, 1989, 1996, 1997b; Lyon et al., 1997). The speech-language pathologist provides training on successful strategies and methods of communicating with the individual who has aphasia. Once the dyad is communicating effectively within the therapy setting, the individual with aphasia and his/her communicative partner begin independent participation in community activities of choice. A communicative partner provides individuals with aphasia with added interpersonal support as well as increased participation in the community. A communicative partner program is an innovative application of a social approach to aphasia intervention.

Couples/Family Training

Couples and family training is another social approach to treatment. Alarcon et al. (1997) videotape communication sessions between family members and individuals with aphasia. They provide structured viewing with specific therapist feedback of successful and unsuccessful interactions. In this way, family members are taught to use those communicative approaches that are most effective. Lyon (1996, 1997a, 1999, 2000) provides couples training in which both the individual with aphasia and his/her spouse are provided treatment. Pre- and poststroke activities are reviewed with each member of the couple choosing one or more activities to resume poststroke. The therapist provides counseling and training to support resumption of these activities. Boles and Lewis (2000) describe solution-focused aphasia therapy with couples, one of which has aphasia. In this approach, couples are guided to find effective strategies and solutions for post-stroke issues.

Self-Advocacy Training

Coles and Eales (1999) describe a system of self-help support groups available to people with aphasia in the United Kingdom. These groups are started with the organizational support and guidance of a speech-language therapist. Following the initial stages of group development, the speech-language therapist "retreats" and group members hold their own group meetings. Each local group sets its own agenda, with community and political advocacy projects often undertaken (Coles & Eales, 1999). Additional reports of successful self-advocacy training have also been described (Kagan & Cohen-Schneider, 1999; Pound et al., 2000).

Work Environment

Targeting the work environment can be an effective approach to intervention. Although common in traumatic brain injury rehabilitation for years, work environment treatment has been used much less frequently in aphasia intervention. Employers and colleagues should be given general education regarding aphasia in addition to being provided with those communication strategies that are most successful for the individual with aphasia. Because aphasia awareness is so limited (Elman et al., 2000; Simmons-Mackie et al., 2002), speech-language pathologists should anticipate that coworkers and employers will have many misconceptions about the disorder. Providing aphasia training can serve to reduce environmental barriers that

a person with aphasia would otherwise encounter when returning to work (Garcia et al., 2000; Lyon & Shadden, 2001).

Conversational Coaching

Conversational coaching utilizes scripted conversation, practice, and therapist feedback to develop conversations for specific situations (Holland, 1991). For example, an individual with aphasia may want to work on a scripted scenario for making conversation with someone new at a party, or being able to order a favorite cocktail at a restaurant or bar (Holland, 2002). In a collaborative fashion, the therapist works with the client to develop a suitable script while providing feedback regarding the effectiveness of the communication. Depending on the strengths and challenges of the individual, scripts can be written out or created using key words and pictures. Videotapes of treatment sessions are useful to foster discussion and learning. In addition, family members and friends can be recruited into the conversational coaching process.

Augmentative and Alternative Communication

Even with intensive speech-language therapy, full recovery of language is often not possible for people with aphasia. Depending on the severity and type of language impairment, many people with aphasia can benefit from various augmentative and alternative communication (AAC) techniques that help them compensate for their language disorder. Using AAC fits well into a social approach because an individual's perspective, his/her communicative strengths and challenges, and various communicative environments are taken into consideration when creating the treatment plan (Hux et al., 2001).

Clinical techniques that are used in aphasia treatment have not always been considered AAC, but they are consistent with an AAC philosophy as they replace, supplement, or scaffold natural speech (Hux et al., 2001). Such treatment techniques include communicative drawing (Lyon, 1995), written choice communication (Garrett & Beukelman, 1992), gestural training (Coelho, 1991; Skelly, 1979), electronic devices, supported conversation for adults with aphasia (Kagan, 1998), communication books, and rating scales (Garrett & Ellis, 1999). In addition, family members, friends, and colleagues of people with aphasia can be instructed in the use of one or more of these techniques in order to assist both interactional and transactional communication in a variety of real-life situations and environments.

Internet Training

As Elman (2001) has indicated, the increasing role of the Internet in our daily lives has created a digital divide for many individuals with aphasia. People who do not have Internet skills will increasingly encounter participation restrictions in areas such as communication, health care, and government access (Elman, 2001). Several treatment programs have recently incorporated Internet training for individuals with aphasia in an attempt to bridge this digital divide (Egan et al., 2004; Elman et al., 2003; Sohlberg et al., 2002). These programs indicate that individuals with aphasia can learn to use e-mail, search engines, and e-commerce when given specialized training, and for some, continued support. In addition, suggestions for improving Web site accessibility, including page layout, language use, and navigation techniques have been proposed (Egan et al., 2004; Elman et al., 2003). As computer technology and the Internet continue to gain dominance in our daily living, training and advocacy for those with aphasia become increasingly important (Elman, 2001).

Discharge Issues

Decisions about discharge planning and discharge criteria are typically made by healthcare professionals as part of the intervention process (Hersh, 1998). Within a social model, discharge planning is viewed as collaborative, with the individual who is receiving the service having an equal say in the discharge

decision. Elman and Bernstein-Ellis (1995) reported that individuals with aphasia were receiving fewer authorized sessions from third-party payers. They noted that the term *functional* was being used by payers to describe those individuals who could communicate basic wants and needs; continued treatment for language skills beyond this basic level was typically denied. In these cases, discharge was payer determined without any input from the client, and little from the therapist.

Chronicity of Aphasia

Sarno (1991) reminds us that aphasia is often a chronic disorder. Although individuals improve following speech-language treatment, a residual, chronic aphasia often remains. Individuals with chronic aphasia can benefit from continued communicative support and treatment (Elman, 1998; Elman & Bernstein-Ellis, 1999a,b; Kagan & Gailey, 1993; Simmons-Mackie, 1998). Given limitations in available treatment, as well as a focus on wellness and the desire to provide programs for individuals with chronic aphasia, interest is currently growing in organizations and services that operate "outside the box" of traditional healthcare reimbursement (Elman, 1998, 1999b). Not-for-profit organizations such as the Aphasia Center of California in the United States and the Aphasia Institute in Canada offer community-based programs with values consistent with a LPAA philosophy and a social approach to intervention.

Advocacy and Raising Awareness

Elman et al. (2000) reviewed the usage of the word *aphasia* in 50 newspapers with the largest circulations in the United States. They reported that *aphasia* was rarely used especially when compared to names of other neurologic disorders with similar or lower incidence rates. These authors asserted that low media attention correlates with low awareness and results in a negative impact on available services, psychosocial adjustment of individuals who had the disorder, and funded research. Elman et al. (2000) proposed a multifaceted campaign of advocacy, political activism, and judicial action to increase awareness and media attention. Simmons-Mackie et al. (2002) surveyed members of the general public in Australia, the United Kingdom, and different regions of the United States to determine public awareness of aphasia. Their findings confirmed that awareness of aphasia was quite low—approximately 5% of the people surveyed were able to provide a general definition. Organizations such as the National Aphasia Association and Aphasia Hope Organization in the United States, Speakability in the United Kingdom, and organizational counterparts in other nations provide a start in raising awareness. However, a targeted media and political campaign is vital in order to reach the vast majority of the populace (Elman et al., 2000; Simmons-Mackie et al., 2002).

Conclusion

Social and life participation approaches focus on reestablishing both desired activities and social contacts for people living with aphasia. The speech-language pathologist has a vital role to play in both optimizing communication skills and improving the quality of life for those with aphasia. Intervention should incorporate meaningful life contexts as well as the perspective of each individual. In addition, speech-language pathologists must join voices with all those impacted by aphasia to raise awareness, increase funding, and reduce isolation.

References

Alarcon, N., Hickey, E., Rogers, M. & Olswang, L. (1997, March). Family Based Intervention for Chronic Aphasia. Paper presented at the Nontraditional Approaches to Aphasia Conference, Yountville, CA.

American Speech-Language-Hearing Association. (2001). *Scope of Practice in Speech-Language Pathology.* Rockville, MD: Author.

Armstrong, E. (1993). Aphasia Rehabilitation: A Sociolinguistic Perspective. In: A. Holland (Ed.), *Aphasia Treatment: World Perspectives* (pp. 263–290). San Diego, CA: Singular Publishing.

Aten, J., Caliguri, M. & Holland, A. (1982). The Efficacy of Functional Communication Therapy for Chronic Aphasic Patients. *Journal of Speech and Hearing Disorders, 47,* 93–96.

Avent, J. (1997). *Manual of Cooperative Group Treatment for Aphasia.* Boston: Butterworth-Heinemann.

Bernstein-Ellis, E. & Elman, R. (1999). Group Communication Treatment for Individuals with Aphasia: The Aphasia Center of California approach. In: R. Elman (Ed.), *Group Treatment of Neurogenic Communication Disorders: The Expert Clinician's Approach* (pp. 47–56). Boston: Butterworth-Heinemann (*www.harcourthealth.com*).

Bertcher, H. (1994). *Group Participation: Techniques for Leaders and Members* (2nd ed.). Thousand Oaks, CA: Sage Publications.

Boles, L. & Lewis, M. (2000). Solution-Focused Co-Therapy for a Couple with Aphasia. *Asia Pacific Journal of Speech, Language and Hearing, 5,* 73–78.

Bollinger, R., Musson, N. & Holland, A. (1993). A Study of Group Communication Intervention with Chronically Aphasic Persons. *Aphasiology, 7,* 301–313.

Brewer, J. & Hunter, A. (1989). *Multimethod Research: A Synthesis of Styles.* Thousand Oaks, CA: Sage.

Brown, G. & Yule, G. (1983). *Discourse Analysis.* Cambridge: Cambridge University Press.

Brumfitt, S. (1993). Losing Your Sense of Self: What Aphasia Can Do. *Aphasiology, 7,* 569–591.

Byng, S., Pound, C. & Parr, S. (2000). Living with Aphasia: A Framework for Therapy Interventions. In: I. Papathanasiou (Ed.), *Acquired Neurological Communication Disorders: A Clinical Perspective* (pp. 49–75). London: Whurr.

Code, C. & Müller, D. (1992). *The Code-Müller Protocols: Assessing Perceptions of Psychosocial Adjustment to Aphasia and Related Disorders.* London: Whurr.

Coelho, C. (1991). Manual Sign Acquisition and Use in Two Aphasic Subjects. In: T. Prescott (Ed.), *Clinical Aphasiology Conference Proceedings* (Vol. 19, pp. 209–218). Austin, TX: Pro-Ed.

Coles, R. & Eales, C. (1999). The Aphasia Self-Help Movement in Britain: A Challenge and an Opportunity. In: R. Elman (Ed.), *Group Treatment of Neurogenic Communication Disorders: The Expert Clinician's Approach* (pp. 107–114). Boston: Butterworth-Heinemann.

Egan, J., Worrall, L., & Oxenham, D. (2004). Accessible Internet Training Package Helps People with Aphasia Cross the Digital Divide. *Aphasiology, 18,* 265–280.

Elman, R. (1995). Multimethod Research: A Search for Understanding. In: M. Lemme (Ed.), *Clinical Aphasiology* (Vol. 23, pp. 77–81), Austin, TX: Pro-Ed.

Elman, R. (1998). Memories of the "Plateau": Health Care Changes Provide an Opportunity to Redefine Aphasia Treatment and Discharge. *Aphasiology, 12,* 227–231.

Elman, R. (Ed.). (1999a). *Group Treatment of Neurogenic Communication Disorders: The Expert Clinician's Approach.* Boston: Butterworth-Heinemann (*www.harcourthealth.com*).

Elman, R. (1999b). Practicing Outside the Box. *ASHA, 41,* 38–42.

Elman, R. (2000). Working with Groups: Neurogenic Communication Disorders and the Managed Care Challenge. [Videotape.] Rockville, MD: American Speech-Language Hearing Association.

Elman, R. (2001). The Internet and Aphasia: Crossing the Digital Divide. *Aphasiology, 15,* 895–899.

Elman, R. (July, 2002). Aphasia Groups: Healing Through Community. Keynote address presented to the International Aphasia Rehabilitation Conference, Brisbane, Australia.

Elman, R. (2004). Group Treatment and Jazz: Some Lessons Learned. In: J. Duchan, & S. Byng (Eds.), *Challenging Aphasia Therapies: Broadening the Discourse and Extending the Boundaries* (pp. 130–133). London: Psychology Press.

Elman, R., Parr, S., & Moss, B. (2003). The Internet and Aphasia: Crossing the Digital Divide. In: S. Parr, J. Duchan, & C. Pound (Eds.), *Aphasia Inside Out* (pp. 103–116). Buckingham, UK: Open University Press.

Elman, R. & Bernstein-Ellis, E. (1995). What is functional? *American Journal of Speech-Language Pathology*, 4, 115–117.

Elman, R. & Bernstein-Ellis, E. (1999a). The Efficacy of Group Communication Treatment in Adults with Chronic Aphasia. *Journal of Speech, Language, and Hearing Research*, 42, 411–419.

Elman, R. & Bernstein-Ellis, E. (1999b). Psychosocial Aspects of Group Communication Treatment: Preliminary Findings. *Seminars in Speech and Language*, 20, 65–72.

Elman, R., Ogar, J. & Elman, S. (2000). Aphasia: Awareness, Advocacy, and Activism. *Aphasiology, 14*, 455–459.

Ewing, S. (1999). Group Process, Group Dynamics, and Group Techniques with Neurogenic Communication Disorders. In: R. Elman (Ed.), *Group Treatment of Neurogenic Communication Disorders: The Expert Clinician's Approach* (pp. 9–16). Boston: Butterworth-Heinemann.

Garcia, L.J., Barrette, J. & Laroche, C. (2000). Perceptions of the Obstacles to Work Reintegration for Persons with Aphasia. *Aphasiology, 14*, 269–290.

Garrett, K. (1999). Measuring Outcomes of Group Therapy. In: R. Elman (Ed.), *Group Treatment of Neurogenic Communication Disorders: The Expert Clinician's Approach* (pp. 17–30). Boston: Butterworth-Heinemann.

Garrett, K. & Beukelman, D. (1992). Severe Aphasia. In: K. Yorkston (Ed.). *Augmentative Communication in the Medical Setting* (pp. 245–321). Tucson: Communication Skill Builders.

Garrett, K. & Ellis, G. (1999). Group Communication Therapy for People with Long-Term Aphasia: Scaffolded Thematic Discourse Activities. In: R. Elman (Ed.), *Group Treatment of Neurogenic Communication Disorders: The Expert Clinician's Approach* (pp. 85–96). Boston: Butterworth-Heinemann.

Hersh, D. (1998). Beyond the "Plateau": Discharge Dilemmas in Chronic Aphasia. *Aphasiology, 12*, 207–218.

Hoen, B., Thelander, M. & Worsley, J. (1997). Improvement in Psychological Well-Being of People with Aphasia and Their Families: Evaluation of a Community-Based Programme. *Aphasiology, 11*, 681–691.

Holland, A. (1980). *Communication Activities of Daily Living*. Austin, TX: Pro-Ed.

Holland, A. (1991). Pragmatic Aspects of Intervention in Aphasia. *Journal of Neurolinguistics*, 6, 197–211.

Holland, A. (July, 2002). Aphasia and Learning: A Contemporary Overview. Keynote address presented to the International Aphasia Rehabilitation Conference, Brisbane, Australia.

Holland, A. & Ross, R. (1999). The Power of Aphasia Groups. In: R. Elman (Ed.), *Group Treatment of Neurogenic Communication Disorders: The Expert Clinician's Approach* (pp. 115–117). Boston: Butterworth-Heinemann.

Hux, K., Manasse, N., Weiss, A. & Beukelman, D. (2001). Augmentative and Alternative Communication for Persons with Aphasia. In: R. Chapey (Ed.), *Language Intervention Strategies in Aphasia and Related Neurogenic Communication Disorders* (4th ed., pp. 675–687). Baltimore: Lippincott, Williams & Wilkins.

Jordan, L. & Kaiser, W. (1996). *Aphasia—A Social Approach*. London: Chapman & Hall.

Kagan, A. (1995). Revealing the Competence of Aphasic Adults Through Conversation: A Challenge to Health Professionals. *Topics in Stroke Rehabilitation, 2*, 15–28.

Kagan, A. (1998). Supported Conversation for Adults with Aphasia: Methods and Resources for Training Conversation Partners. *Aphasiology, 12*(9), 816–830.

Kagan, A. & Cohen-Schneider, R. (1999). Groups in the Introductory Program at the Pat Arato Aphasia Centre. In: R. Elman (Ed.), *Group Treatment of Neurogenic Communication Disorders: The Expert Clinician's Approach* (pp. 97–106). Boston: Butterworth-Heinemann (*www.harcourthealth.com*).

Kagan, A. & Gailey, G. (1993). Functional Is Not Enough: Training Conversation Partners for Aphasic Adults. In: A.L. Holland and M.M. Forbes (Eds.), *Aphasia Treatment: World Perspectives* (pp. 199–225). San Diego: Singular Publishing Group.

Kagan, A. & Kimelman, M. (1995). Informed Consent in Aphasia Research: Myth or Reality? In: M. Lemme (Ed.), *Clinical Aphasiology* (Vol. 23, pp. 65–76). Austin, TX: Pro-Ed.

Kearns, K. & Elman, R. (2001). Group Therapy for Aphasia: Theoretical and Practical Considerations. In: R. Chapey (Ed.), *Language Intervention Strategies in Aphasia and Related Neurogenic Communication Disorders* (4th ed., pp. 316–337). Baltimore: Lippincott, Williams & Wilkins.

Kearns, K. & Simmons, N. (1985). Group Therapy for Aphasia: A Survey of Veterans Administration Medical Centers. In: R.H. Brookshire (Ed.), *Clinical Aphasiology Conference Proceedings* (pp. 176–183). Minneapolis: BRK.

LaFond, D., DeGiovani, R., Joannette, Y., Ponzio, J. & Sarno, M. (Eds.). (1993). *Living with Aphasia: Psychosocial Issues*. San Diego, CA: Singular Publishing.

LaPointe, L. (1996). Adaptation, Accommodation, Aristos. In: L. LaPointe (Ed.), *Aphasia and Related Neurogenic Disorders* (2nd ed.). New York: Thieme.

LaPointe, L. (2002). The Sociology of Aphasia. *Journal of Medical Speech-Language Pathology, 10*, vii–viii.

LeDorze, G. & Brassard, C. (1995). A Description of the Consequences of Aphasia or Aphasic Persons and Their Relatives and Friends, Based on the WHO Model of Chronic Diseases. *Aphasiology, 9*, 239–255.

LPAA Project Group. (2000). Life Participation Approach to Aphasia: A Statement of Values for the Future. *ASHA Leader*, 5, 4–6. (*www.asha.org/publications/ashalinks.htm*).

LPAA Project Group. (2001). Life Participation Approach to Aphasia: A Statement of Values for the Future. In: R. Chapey (Ed.), *Language Intervention Strategies in Aphasia and Related Neurogenic Communication Disorders* (4th ed., pp. 235–245). Baltimore: Lippincott, Williams & Wilkins.

Luterman, D. (1996). *Counseling Persons with Communication Disorders and Their Families* (3rd ed.). Austin, TX: Pro-Ed.

Lyon, J. (1989). Communication Partners: Their Value in Reestablishing Communication with Aphasic Adults. In: T. Prescott (Ed.), *Clinical Aphasiology Conference Proceedings* (Vol. 18, pp. 11–17). Boston: College-Hill.

Lyon, J. (1992). Communicative Use and Participation in Life for Aphasic Adults in Natural Settings: The Scope of the Problem. *American Journal of Speech and Language Pathology, 1*, 7–14.

Lyon, J. (1995). Drawing: Its Value as a Communication Aid for Adults with Aphasia. *Aphasiology, 9*, 33–94.

Lyon, J. (1996). Optimizing Communication and Participation in Life for Aphasic Adults and Their Prime Caregivers in Natural Settings: A Use Model for Treatment. In: G. Wallace (Ed.), *Adult Aphasia Rehabilitation* (pp. 137–160). Newton, MA: Butterworth Heinemann.

Lyon, J. (1997a). Treating Real-Life Functionality in a Couple Coping with Severe Aphasia. In: N. Helm-Estabrooks & A. Holland (Eds.), *Approaches to the Treatment of Aphasia* (pp. 203–239). San Diego, CA: Singular Publishing.

Lyon, J. (1997b). Volunteers and Partners: Moving Intervention Outside the Treatment Room. In: B. Shadden & M. Toner (Eds.), *Communication and aging* (pp. 299–324). Austin, TX: Pro-Ed.

Lyon, J. (1998). *Coping with Aphasia*. San Diego, CA: Singular Publishing.

Lyon, J. (1999). Service Delivery for People Confronting Aphasia: Some Thoughts and Practical Suggestions in Troubled Times. In: R. Elman (Ed.). *ASHA Special Interest Division 2 Newsletter: Neurophysiology and Neurogenic Speech and Language Disorders, 9*, 18–23.

Lyon, J. (2000). Finding, Defining, and Refining Functionality in Real-Life for People Confronting Aphasia. In: L. Worrall & C. Frattali (Eds.), *Neurogenic Communication Disorders: A Functional Approach*. New York: Thieme.

Lyon, J., Cariski, D., Keisler, L., Rosenbek, J., Levine, R. & Kumpula, J. (1997). Communication Partners: Enhancing Participation in Life and Communication for Adults with Aphasia in Natural Settings. *Aphasiology, 11*, 693–708.

Lyon, J. & Shadden, B. (2001). Treating Life Consequences of Aphasia's Chronicity. In: R. Chapey (Ed.), *Language Intervention Strategies in Aphasia and Related Neurogenic Communication Disorders* (4th ed., pp. 297–315). Baltimore: Lippincott Williams & Wilkins.

Marshall, R. (1999a). A Problem-Focused Group Treatment Program for Clients with Mild Aphasia. In: R. Elman (Ed.), *Group Treatment of Neurogenic Communication Disorders: The Expert Clinician's Approach* (pp. 57–65). Boston: Butterworth-Heinemann.

Marshall, R. (1999b). *Introduction to Group Treatment for Aphasia*. Boston: Butterworth-Heinemann.

Markus, H. & Nurius, P. (1986). Possible Selves. *American Psychologist, 41*, 954–969.

Murray, L. & Chapey, R. (2001). Assessment of Language Disorders in Adults. In: R. Chapey (Ed.), *Language Intervention Strategies in Aphasia and Related Neurogenic Communication Disorders* (4th ed., pp. 55–126). Baltimore: Lippincott Williams & Wilkins.

Parr, S. (1994). Coping with Aphasia: Conversations with 20 Aphasic People. *Aphasiology, 8*, 457–466.

Parr, S., Byng, S., Gilpin, S. & Ireland, S. (1997). *Talking About Aphasia: Living with Loss of Language After Stroke*. Buckingham, UK: Open University Press.

Pound, C., Parr, S., Lindsay, J. & Woolf, C. (2000). *Beyond Aphasia: Therapies for Living with Communication Disability*. Oxon, UK: Winslow Press.

Rogers, M., Alarcon, N. & Olswang, L. (1999). Aphasia Management Considered in the Context of the WHO Model of Disablements. In: I.R. Odderson & E. Halar (Eds.), *Physical Medicine and Rehabilitation Clinics of North America on Stroke*. Philadelphia: WB Saunders.

Ryff, C. (1989). Happiness Is Everything, or Is It? Explorations on the Meaning of Psychological Well-Being. *Journal of Personality and Social Psychology, 57*, 1069–1081.

Ryff, C. & Singer, B. (1998). The Contours of Positive Human Health. *Psychological Inquiry, 9*, 1–29.

Ryff, C., & Singer, B. (2000). Interpersonal Flourishing: A Positive Health Agenda for the New Millennium. *Personality and Social Psychology Review, 4*, 30–44.

Sarno, J. (1991). The Psychological and Social Sequelae of Aphasia. In: M. Sarno (Ed.), *Acquired Aphasia* (2nd ed., pp. 499–519). San Diego: Academic Press.

Sarno, M.T. (1969). *Functional Communication Profile*. New York: Institute for Rehabilitation Medicine, NYU Medical Center.

Sarno, M.T. (1981). *Acquired Aphasia* (1st ed.) New York: Academic Press.

Sarno, M.T. (1986). The Silent Minority: The Patient with Aphasia. *The 1986 Hemphill Lecture*, Rehabilitation Institute of Chicago.

Sarno, M.T. (1993). Aphasia Rehabilitation: Psychosocial and Ethical Considerations. *Aphasiology, 7*, 321–334.

Sarno, M.T. (2004). Keynote Presentation, Connect Launch Conference. In: J. Duchan & S. Byng (Eds.), *Challenging Aphasia Therapies: Broadening the Discourse and Extending the Boundaries* (pp. 19–31). London: Psychology Press.

Simmons-Mackie, N. (1998). A Solution to the Discharge Dilemma in Aphasia: Social Approaches to Aphasia Management. *Aphasiology, 12*, 231–239.

Simmons-Mackie, N. (2001). Social Approaches to Aphasia Intervention. In: R. Chapey (Ed.), *Language Intervention Strategies in Aphasia and Related Neurogenic Communication Disorders* (4th ed., pp. 246–268). Baltimore: Lippincott Williams & Wilkins.

Simmons-Mackie, N., Code, C., Armstrong, E., Stiegler, L. & Elman, R. (2002). What Is Aphasia? Results of an International Survey. *Aphasiology, 16*, 837–848.

Simmons-Mackie, N. & Damico, J. (1996). Accounting for Handicaps in Aphasia: Communicative Assessment from an Authentic Social Perspective. *Disability and Rehabilitation, 18*, 540–549.

Skelly, M. (1979). *Amer-Ind Gestural Code Based on Universal American Indian Hand Talk*. New York: Elsevier.

Sohlberg, M., Fickas, S. & Todis, B. (2002). Think & Link: E-Mail for Individuals with Cognitive Disabilities. *http://www.think-and-link.org*.

Vickers, C. (1998). *Communication Recovery: Group Conversation Activities for Adults*. San Antonio, TX: Communication Skill Builders.

Walker-Batson, D., Curtis, S., Smith, P. & Ford, J. (1999). An Alternative Model for the Treatment of Aphasia: The Lifelink Approach. In: R. Elman (Ed.), *Group Treatment of Neurogenic Communication Disorders: The Expert Clinician's Approach* (pp. 67–75). Boston: Butterworth-Heinemann (*www.harcourthealth.com*).

Wertz, R., Collins, M., Weiss, D., Kurtzke, J., Friden, R., Brookshire, R., Pierce, J., Holtzapple, P., Hubbard, D., Porch, B., West, J., Davis, L., Matovitch, V., Morley, G. & Resurreccion, E. (1981). Veterans Administration Cooperative Study on Aphasia: A Comparison of Individual and Group Treatment. *Journal of Speech and Hearing Research, 24*, 580–594.

World Health Organization. (2001). *International Classification of Functioning, Disability and Health, ICF.* Geneva, Switzerland: WHO.

Worrall, L. (1992). Functional Communication Assessment: An Australian Perspective. *Aphasiology, 6*, 105–111.

Worrall, L. & Frattali, C. (Eds.). (2000). *Neurogenic Communication Disorders: A Functional Approach.* New York: Thieme.

Yalom, I. (1985). *The Theory and Practice of Group Psychotherapy,* (3rd ed.). New York: Basic Books.

4

Language and Discourse Deficits Following Prefrontal Cortex Damage

Carol Frattali[†] and Jordan Grafman

Damage to the prefrontal cortex (PFC) can result in subtle yet pervasive language disturbances that differ from the classic characteristics of aphasia. Atypical in symptomatology are the syntactic impairments of agrammatism or paragrammatism, receptive impairments of auditory recognition or comprehension, or lexical errors of semantic and phonemic paraphasias. More typical are degradations in the finer-grain features of language processing and production as they occur in communicative contexts; for example, misinterpreted or missed contextual cues, faulty anaphoric reference, selection of nondominant meanings of ambiguous words, violations of discourse topic rules, misorderings of the temporal sequence of events filed in working memory that guide current discourse paths during social interactions, inflexibility in shifts of focus during change of topic and varying perspective-taking on an issue, insensitivity to adjusting communication style to connect with the listener (having theory of mind), and the summative lack of awareness of these differences. Often considered either elusive in their clinical identification, or subclinical or mild in their isolated severity, these language deficits can have profound effects on communication in its on-line and natural environments.

While conversing with persons who have sustained focal damage to prefrontal areas, the communication partner often perceives communicative missteps. These perceptions lead to doubt as to whether the communicative problem lies with the person or partner. The communication partner initiates, queries, or remarks; the person with PFC damage responds in characteristically well-produced syntax, lexicon, and phonology. Yet the response may fall short of what is considered expected, acceptable, or sufficient from pragmatic, propositional, or contextual points of view during the course of conversation.

This chapter describes the neuroanatomical features and neural pathways of the prefrontal cortex, identifies the language/discourse and related cognitive/affective deficits commonly associated with prefrontal damage, details the clinical evaluation procedures within a framework of prevailing prefrontal theories, and discusses treatment options.

Pathophysiology

The prefrontal cortex occupies 29% or roughly one third of the human cortex, a proportion greater than those of most other primates. Believed to explain why humans have comparatively superior cognitive capabilities, this claim has only recently been disputed on the basis of overall relative size of the frontal lobe during evolution (Semendeferi et al., 2002). Rather than size, the specialized cognitive

[†]Dr. Frattali passed away in July 2004. This chapter is dedicated to an outstanding colleague and good friend whose insights into the language functions of the prefrontal cortex greatly influenced my own thinking on the topic—Jordan Grafman.

abilities attributed to the so-called frontal advantage in humans is thought to be due to individual cortical area differences and richer neural interconnectivity.

The prefrontal cortex is so called (*pre-* is an imprecise prefix) because it characterizes the portion of the frontal lobe anterior to classical motor areas. Table 4–1 and Figure 4–1 detail its dorsolateral, orbitofrontal, and medial frontal/cingulate areas, corresponding Brodmann's areas (BAs), fronto-subcortical circuitry, and associated neurobehavioral deficits. Of note is that the major cortical connections of the head of the caudate nucleus and the mediodorsal nucleus of the thalamus come from prefrontal cortex. These two structures are considered the subcortical components of the prefrontal network (Mesulam, 2000). Mesulum divides the frontal lobes into three functional sectors:

- Motor-premotor sector: includes BA 4 and 6, the supplementary motor area (medial aspect of BA 6), the frontal eye fields (BA 8/6), and parts of Broca's area (BA 44).
- Paralimbic sector: located in the ventral and medial part of the frontal lobe and contains cortex of anterior cingulate complex (BA 23, 32), the parolfactory gyrus (gyrus rectus, BA 25), and posterior orbitofrontal regions (BA 11–13).
- Heteromodal sector: contains BA 9 and 10, anterior BA 11 and 12, and BA 45–47.

Depending on lesion location, damage to the motor-premotor sector can result in weakness, alteration of muscle tone, release of grasp reflexes, incontinence, akinesia, mutism, aprosody, apraxia, and some motor components of unilateral neglect and Broca's aphasia. The terms *prefrontal cortex* and *frontal lobe syndrome* often exclude the motor-premotor sector and refer typically to the paralimbic and heteromodal sectors of the frontal lobe. Lesions in the orbitofrontal and medial frontal areas (containing the paralimbic sector) are associated with *disinhibition syndrome* (impulsivity with loss of judgment, insight, and foresight); lesions in the dorsolateral frontal lobe (containing the heteromodal sector) are more likely to cause the *abulic syndrome* (loss

of creativity, initiative, and curiosity, with apathy and emotional blunting) (Mesulum, 2000).

Nature and Differentiating Features

The case of Phineas Gage, which dates to 1848 as originally described by his physician, John Harlow, is illustrative of how the behavioral deficits of prefrontal damage are classically described (Macmillan, 2000). Gage was injured when a tamping rod, accidentally projected by an explosion, penetrated his face obliquely from below and through the left orbit, traversing the base of the skull and inflicting massive damage to his frontal lobes, destroying principally the left orbito-medial area. The injury caused a cluster of behavioral deficits that led his friends to say that Gage was "no longer Gage" (Macmillan, 2000, p. 13). Unlike his premorbid personality, Gage now exhibited inordinate profanity with loss of moral judgment, indecision, capriciousness, unpredictability of action, poor planning, and uncontrolled impulsivity (Ferrier, 1878; Harlow, 1868). This detailed account of the profound behavioral changes that occurred from the injury and inflicted massive damage to prefrontal regions (Gage lived for more than a decade after his injury) contributed fundamentally to our understanding of localized brain function.

Classic Behavioral Sequelae

Frontal syndrome is an umbrella term for the range of behavioral manifestations of PFC damage, with each patient showing different distributions of deficits as dictated by size, site, laterality, and nature of the lesion among other neurophysiologic and psychological factors. Mesulum (2000) conceptualizes the PFC as a site for the confluence of two functional axes: one for working memory-executive function-attention (heteromodal sector); the other for comportment or proper behavior (paralimbic sector). Fuster (1997) details three cognitive functions represented in the PFC: short-term working memory, preparatory set, and inhibitory control. Cummings (1995) identifies at least

Table 4–1. Prefrontal Neuroanatomic Areas, Brodmann's Areas, Fronto-Subcortical Circuitry, and Associated Neuropsychological Behaviors

Prefrontal Area	Brodmann's Areas	Fronto-Subcortical Circuitry	Neuropsychological Behaviors
Dorsolateral	BA 8, 9, 10, and 46	Begins on the lateral convexity of the frontal lobe anterior to the premotor area (BA 6). Includes the dorsolateral portion of the caudate nucleus, areas of the globus pallidus and substantia nigra, and ventral anterior and medial dorsal nuclei of the thalamus. Circuit originates in the association cortex of the frontal lobe, receiving input from and providing efferent output to posterior temporal, parietal, and occipital association areas. Posterior cortical input reaches the frontal lobe via the superior longitudinal fasciculus from the parietal lobe and via the inferior longitudinal fasciculus or inferior occipitofrontal bundle from the occipital lobe.	Mediates executive function: retrieval deficit (poor recall, intact recognition), reduced verbal and nonverbal fluency, perseveration, difficulty shifting set, reduced mental control, poor abstraction, impaired response inhibition. May have dynamic aphasia.
Orbitofrontal	BA 10, 11–13, 47	Begins in the orbital cortex on the inferior surface of the frontal lobe anterior to the premotor cortex. Circuit includes the ventral portion of the caudate nucleus, the globus pallidus, and substantia nigra, and the ventral anterior and dorsal medial nuclei of the thalamus. It projects from the orbitofrontal cortex to the ventral portion of the caudate nucleus.	Mediates socially modulated civil behavior: disinhibition, tactlessness, impulsivity. May have difficulty with set shifting; may be drawn to use objects in the environment (utilization behavior). May have limited personal direction of one's behavior. Also may have obsessive-compulsive disorders.
Medial/anterior cingulate (medial frontal)	6 (supplementary motor); 8–10, 12; 23, 24, 32 (anterior cingulate)	Begins in the cortex of the anterior cingulate, including the nucleus accumbens (ventromedial or limbic striatum), globus pallidus and substantia nigra, and medial dorsal nucleus of the thalamus.	Mediates motivation; disorders include apathy with reduced interest, motivation, engagement, and activity maintenance. Impaired inhibition in go-no-go tests may be present. May manifest catatonia with reduced spontaneous behavior. Left lesions may produce transcortical motor aphasia (reduced spontaneous output with retained ability to repeat what is heard). Damage to anterior cingulate and supplementary motor area may produce akinetic mutism.

Sources: Cummings (1995), Fuster (1997), Grafman (1995), and Mesulum (2000).

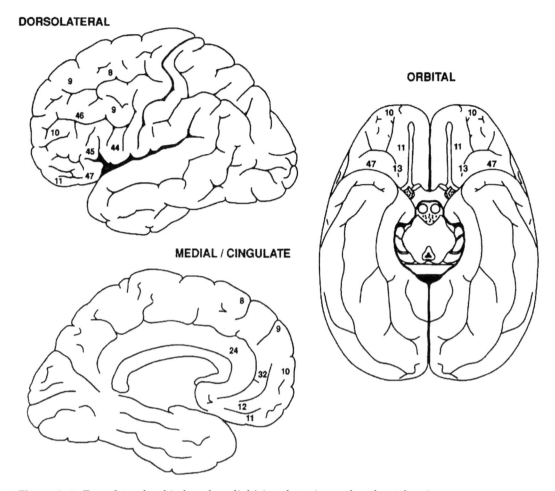

Figure 4–1. Dorsolateral, orbital, and medial/cingulate views of prefrontal regions.

one principal behavior for each prefrontal-subcortical circuit—the dorsolateral frontal-subcortical circuit mediating executive behavior, the orbitofrontal-subcortical circuit mediating socially modulated civil behavior, and the medial frontal-subcortical circuit mediating motivation.

DORSOLATERAL FRONTAL-SUBCORTICAL CIRCUIT

Called the "dorsolateral," "dysexecutive," or "frontal abulia" syndrome, behavioral features include lack of drive, apathy, lack of interest in self and surrounding world, deficit in selective attention with the inability to direct or focus on a particular sense, and difficulty initiating spontaneous and deliberate action. Mesulum (2000) uses descriptors of

loss of creativity, initiative, and curiosity, with presence of apathy and emotional blunting.

Depression may be present, especially in patients with left-hemisphere lesions. Abulia may be misinterpreted as a sign of depression.

ORBITOFRONTAL-SUBCORTICAL CIRCUIT

Called the "orbitomedial" or "frontal disinhibition" syndrome, behavioral features include excessive energy and drive; impulsivity with loss of judgment, hindsight, insight, and foresight; deficit in exclusionary attention (inability to suppress interference from external stimuli or internal states); imitation of others and utilization behavior (compulsion to use objects and tools simply by their presence; lack of interference control); and impaired moral judgment, disinhibition, and disregard for ethical principles.

The disinhibition may be misdiagnosed as mania.

MEDIAL FRONTAL-SUBCORTICAL CIRCUIT

Damage to the anterior cingulate and supplementary motor area located in the mesial cerebral surface of the left hemisphere can lead to akinetic mutism. These areas play an important role in initiation and maintenance of speech. Damage does not cause aphasia but varied degrees of akinesia (difficulty with initiation of movement), and mutism (complete absence of speech). Much rarer is that damage to the supplementary motor area can present as transcortical motor aphasia.

Language and Discourse Deficits

Luria (1970) suggested that the special position of language in the organization of behavior is compromised following PFC damage. Accordingly, the prefrontal syndrome is caused largely by disruption of the regulatory role of language on general behavior (Luria, 1970; Luria & Homskaya, 1964). Behavior, in Luria's view, suffers from a lack of the internalized linguistic schema that normally precede and guide any purposeful action and depend on the integrity of the prefrontal cortex. Translated in daily life terms, patients know what they should do and can verbalize it, but cannot always do as they should. Therefore, there is a dissociation of word and deed. This notion suggests that language is impaired not at a strict linguistic level but at a cognitive level of complex, goal-directed, and intentionally regulated behavior. Even the language impairments of dynamic aphasia and discourse impairment have been described as action planning deficits, but as specific to language use (Alexander, 2002). It is hypothesized that language deficits following PFC damage are a consequence or a symptom of primary cognitive deficits involving, along with action planning, the cognitive processes of memory and attention (Ferstl et al., 1999). Arguably, a growing corpus of neuroimaging and lesion studies is beginning to weaken the above claims as being all-inclusive of the nature of language disturbances following PFD damage. Particularly implicated, as detailed below, is the special role of the PFC in context-sensitive semantic processing and selection.

DYNAMIC APHASIA

Lesions in dorsolateral areas (BA 9, 10, and 46) can produce what is called dynamic aphasia, characterized by the cardinal features of (1) reduction in spontaneous speech with lack of initiation, (2) limitations in the amount and range of narrative expression, and (3) loss of verbal fluency (Benton, 1968). Although articulation and speech motor programming remain intact, language is impoverished with decreases in propositions and length and complexity of responses. Embedded or dependent clauses are seldom used in either verbal or graphic form. Dynamic aphasia has been described singly as a disturbance of complex, open-ended sentence assembly (Alexander, 2002).

Dynamic aphasia (sometimes called prefrontal aphasia) can result in right as well as left hemisphere lesions, although it is most severe in left and bilateral lesions (Barbizet et al., 1975). Hughlings Jackson (1915) was perhaps the first to suggest that prefrontal lesions resulted in impoverished language. Kleist (1934) placed particular emphasis on the posterior portion of the second frontal convolution (BA 9) in relation to deficits of verbal thought, including loss of speech spontaneity in absence of articulatory disorder, simplification of grammar, and (in some cases) impairment of verbal thought processes. The condition has also been variably termed central motor aphasia (Goldstein, 1948), minimal grade of verbal aphasia (Zangwill, 1966), and frontal dynamic aphasia (Luria, 1970). Zangwill (1966) extended the description of deficits, remarking on the disinclination to engage in tasks that call for sustained verbal effort. Although conversational speech may appear normal and tested naming deficit is absent, the patient complains of real difficulty in evoking appropriate words and phrases.

TRANSCORTICAL MOTOR APHASIA

Transcortical motor aphasia can sometimes occur following prefrontal cortex damage. It is most often described as occurring from lesions in the left lateral frontal lobe, variably anterior and superior to Broca's area (Alexander, 1997, 2002; Goldstein, 1948; Goodglass, 1993), to a lesser degree following damage to portions of Broca's area, and an even lesser degree following damage to the left supplementary motor area (Brun, 1987). Transcortical motor aphasia is characterized by nonfluent output, relatively spared auditory comprehension, and intact auditory-verbal repetition. The nonfluency differs fundamentally from the agrammatic output following Broca's aphasia. It is described as simplified, repetitive, and delayed with variable severity of dysnomia (Alexander, 2002). Response may be echolalic, with failure to inhibit repetition possibly causing this behavioral feature.

AKINETIC MUTISM

Mutism without overt language deficits can be caused by damage to the ascending dopaminergic systems originating in the ventral tegmental area of the upper midbrain and terminating in the supplementary motor area and anterior cingulate. When lesions of these pathways or their terminal cortical areas are bilateral, complete akinetic mutism results (Alexander, 2002). When unilateral, impoverishment of speech is less dramatic and there is presence of contralateral akinesia. The akinetic mute patient fails to communicate both by word and gesture/facial expression. The drive to communicate is absent. Although the will to speak (and thus initiation) may be absent, if these patients are asked direct questions, they may be able to write their responses, which are often short and cryptic. Nevertheless, with the ability to communicate in the graphic mode, patients may be candidates both for family counseling in ways to prompt/optimize response and for assessment/training of augmentative communication systems.

DISCOURSE IMPAIRMENTS

The term *discourse* can be defined as language in use, or linguistic forms designed to serve purposes or functions of human affairs (Brown & Yule, 1983). It is also described as the level of language that relates each item and proposition to what has gone before (Caplan, 1999). On the side of discourse *production*, one form of discourse describes the expression of content (i.e., transactional); another describes the expression of social relations and personal attitudes (i.e., interactional) (Brown & Yule, 1983). On the side of discourse *processing*, discourse can be considered the ability to make connections within and between sentences and using context as the basis of understanding (Caplan, 1999).

Descriptions of language disturbances in patients with PFC damage come mostly from studies on discourse production. They classically include reduced or enhanced speech output, failure to structure, failure to stay within a given topic, verbosity, tangentiality, lack of cohesion, and difficulties with temporal sequencing (Ferstl et al., 1999). Less studied are language disturbances stemming from faulty discourse processing. According to theories of discourse comprehension (Kintsch, 1994), the processes (e.g., selection of information, reduction, generalization, retrieval strategies, sequential ordering, structuring, and planning processes) are needed to derive higher-level representations from the surface structure (i.e., the exact wording of the text). These representations (the macrostructure or situation model) encode the structure of the text and its gist in relation to the comprehender's prior knowledge about the topic.

Forms of discourse can be considered rule-bound (e.g., pleading a court case, writing a scientific paper) or free (e.g., describing a vacation, writing a personal letter). They also require some knowledge about listener expectations, limitations, and internal states (Alexander, 2002). Therefore, the narrator must have a "theory of mind," making the necessary adjustments to connect with the listener.

STORY COMPREHENSION

In our research, we have been accruing discourse processing data from adults with focal prefrontal damage stemming primarily from penetrating head injury. One of our tasks requires generation of thematic aspects of stories (Craig & Frattali, 2000). After reading stories that carry moralistic themes, modified from a set of international children's stories (Arbuthnot, 1976), we recorded and analyzed responses to the question, "What was the general theme or main point of the story?" The clinical characteristics identified by analysis of thematic statements included faulty anaphoric reference and links (overuse of nonreferential pronouns), embellishment (exaggeration of facts), confabulation (fabricated facts), failure to structure with tangentiality of points and irrelevant detail, vague statements open to various interpretations, only partial or narrow ability to capture thematic aspects of stories (gist), faulty temporal sequencing of events and cause/effect relations, and reduced ability to synthesize details into a holistic story conceptualization. When compared with a control group, significant between-group differences were found in response accuracy to story comprehension questions and identification of thematic aspects of stories. The discourse dimensions of unity and informativeness were rated significantly lower than that of controls by three independent judges. Results suggest that discourse impairment following PFC damage represents a breakdown of both semantic networks that link propositional information into a connected memory structure (required to recall story details). This interpretation coincides with Grafman's (1995) framework of structured event complexes (summarized below), suggesting that information processing components are represented in units weighted toward sequential rather than singular aspects of events. In particular, the discourse feature of unity, which requires temporal serialization and integration of details and conceptualization of the story as a whole, was a differentiating feature of patients with PFC damage.

In related studies of thematic knowledge (Maguire et al., 1999; Nichelli et al., 1995; Partiot et al., 1996; Sirigu et al., 1998; Zalla et al., 2002), the prefrontal cortex is found to play a major role in story processing. In the Nichelli et al. study, right and left prefrontal cortices were consistently but selectively activated across grammatical, semantic, and moral conditions. In the Zalla et al. study, patients with PFC damage had difficulty in processing figurative moralistic meaning, syntactic features, and inference generation. Further, patients with PFC had difficulty recalling narrative components of a story, reconstructing the sequence of events, and correctly answering inferential questions.

PROCESSING AMBIGUITY IN TEXT

Other tasks included in our research probe on-line processing of ambiguities in text. In a recent study of processing lexical ambiguities (Frattali et al., 2001), we tested the hypothesis that the prefrontal cortex mediates suppression of context-inappropriate meanings of lexical ambiguities, with both left and right regions serving complementary functions in suppression and text comprehension. Using a noun-verb homograph contextual judgment task, response times and response accuracies to test words appearing in immediate and delayed (1500 ms later) time intervals were recorded in a group of patients with PFC damage (PFCD) and a control group. Significant between-group differences in response times were found, with correspondingly higher error rates related to context-inappropriate meanings in the PFCD group. Results revealed inverse patterns of suppression between groups, with the appearance of decreased interference over time in the PFCD group. However, measures of enhancement and suppression separated group response tendencies, with higher enhancement correlating with lower response accuracy for context-inappropriate meanings in the PFCD group and higher suppression correlating with higher response accuracy in the control group. These results suggest a loss of the control aspects of inhibitory processes in lexical ambiguity resolution following PFCD. By side of lesion, the worst response accuracies were found in the left- and bilateral-lesion groups, suggesting the dominance of the left hemisphere in lexical ambiguity resolution. In the comprehension task, suppression measures correlated significantly with both re-sponse times and error rates in the left-lesion group only. These findings support Beeman's (1998) model of semantic coding cooperatively engaging both cerebral hemisphere but with the left prefrontal cortex dominating in context-sensitive semantic selection. The find-ings further support the pivotal function of suppression and enhancement (Gernsbacher, 1990) as integral to on-line management of se-mantic information and subsequent discourse comprehension skill.

SUPPORTING RESEARCH FINDINGS

Since the 1980s, there have been some 50 studies published in the research literature focused on language processes in study of the human prefrontal cortex (Binder et al., 1997; Buckner et al., 1995; Chee et al., 2000; Crozier et al., 1999; Demb et al., 1995; Gabrieli et al., 1996; Kapur et al., 1994; Nichelli et al., 1995; Petersen et al., 1988, 1990; Poldrack et al., 1999; Price et al., 1994; Robertson et al., 2000; Thompson-Schill et al., 1997; Zalla et al., 2002). Two review articles from the literature offer a compendium of converging evidence that the prefrontal cortex does indeed play a role in important aspects of semantic process-ing (Gabrieli et al., 1998; Thompson-Schill et al., 1997). The review by Gabrieli and col-leagues attempted to characterize and map mental operations mediated by the left infe-rior frontal cortex, especially the anterior and ventral portion of the gyrus (BA 11, 45, 47) with positron emission tomography (PET) and magnetic resonance imaging (MRI). Many of these studies unexpectedly identi-fied this prefrontal area as being involved in the analysis of word meaning.

The landmark study by Petersen and col-leagues (1988) was the first study of its kind implicating the left prefrontal area in seman-tic analysis of words. This PET study com-pared neural activations when participants generated a verb (e.g., "eat") to a presented noun (e.g., "cake"), or simply read the noun. Verb generation relative to reading resulted in three main activations: left inferior frontal gyrus, cingulate, and right cerebellum (which

provided evidence that the cerebellum plays a role in cognition and beyond that of motor control). Gabrieli and colleagues (1996) con-ducted a functional MRI (fMRI) study, requir-ing subjects to make semantic judgments about whether words referred to concrete (e.g., "table") or abstract (e.g., "truth") enti-ties. This was compared to a task that re-quired nonsemantic judgments about whether words appeared in upper- or lower-case let-ters. Semantic relative to nonsemantic judg-ments resulted in greater activations in the left inferior prefrontal gyrus. Kapur and col-leagues (1994) conducted a PET study requir-ing participants to decide whether words referred to living (e.g., "dog") or nonliving (e.g., "table") entities. The comparison task required participants to decide whether a word contained a certain letter. Once again, greater left prefrontal activations were found in semantic, relative to nonsemantic, deci-sions. The above studies provided converg-ing evidence that the left prefrontal cortex mediates semantic judgment. A limitation that called these convergent findings into question, however, related to the consistently less diffi-cult comparison tasks. So, did left prefrontal activations reflect semantic analysis per se or simply the extended processing of words?

An answer to the above question is found in two separate study findings that con-trolled for task difficulty. Demb et al. (1995) conducted an fMRI study by adding a third condition requiring minimal semantic analy-sis but even more extended processing than the semantic task (i.e., to decide whether the first and last letters of a word were ascend-ing or descending alphabetically, which be-come the difficult nonsemantic task). With the first condition (semantic task) requiring abstract versus concrete word classifications and the second condition (easy nonsemantic task) requiring upper- versus lower-case let-ter classifications, two analyses (semantic compared with difficult nonsemantic task; semantic compared with easy nonsemantic task) resulted in identical left prefrontal acti-vations, with greater activation for the seman-tic relative to easy or difficult nonsemantic task. Further support is found in the study by Spitzer et al. (1995). In this fMRI study, two tasks were matched in difficulty: a semantic (word pairs related in meaning) and nonsemantic task (rows of asterisks with same or different colors). Left prefrontal activations again were found for the semantic relative to nonsemantic task. Left prefrontal activations, therefore, reflected semantic processing rather than task difficulty.

Although some of the above studies are addressed in the Thompson-Schill et al. (1997) article, the authors stated that conclusions regarding prefrontal mediation of semantic retrieval remained uncertain. They set out to test an explanation, based on the argument by Cohen and Servan-Schreiber (1992) that the prefrontal cortex enables flexible and context-sensitive responses, particularly in tasks for which a response other than the prepotent one must be selected. Thus, they tested a hypothesis of semantic selection rather than semantic retrieval. Their fMRI study was designed to manipulate selection demands of semantic tasks [task A: generation task (verb generation to presented nouns with high- and low-selection demands); task B: classification task (classification of common objects with high- and low-selection demands); task C: comparison task (comparison of probe words to target word with high- and low-selection demands)]. For each task, direct comparison of high versus low selection yielded activation of several regions of significant differences. There were greater activations in the left inferior frontal gyrus (IFG) (clustered in BA 44, 45, or Broca's area; BA 8, 9) during the high selection conditions. These findings led the investigators to conclude that these prefrontal regions (with left IFG predominating) mediate semantic selection among competing alternatives in working memory, rather than mere retrieval of semantic knowledge.

Evaluation

The subtle or fleeting nature of certain prefrontal deficits may escape detection by conventional clinical tests. In these cases, experimental assessment may be the preferred mode of evaluation; see Grafman (1999) for further discussion). Clinical evaluation also gains in sensitivity and specificity if framed by prevailing theories of prefrontal function. In this way, an investigational approach to assessment is taken, thus leading to testable hypotheses related to the nature of language and discourse deficits, and effective rehabilitative methods.

Prevailing Theories of Prefrontal Cortex Functions

Grafman (1995) offers a comparative and critical review of prevailing models of prefrontal cortex functions, drawing similarities and distinctions across these models. Among these models, and of particular interest here are Grafman's (1995) structured event complex (SEC) model, Damasio's (1996) somatic marker theory, and Norman and Shallice's (1986) model of attentional control.

THE STRUCTURED EVENT COMPLEX

Grafman (1995) suggests that the prefrontal cortex stores a specific kind of symbolic representation, which predicts that single units of memory would be capable of storing an SEC that varies in the number of single events it encapsulates. In other words, the SEC is defined as a set of events, structured in a particular sequence, which as a "complex" composes an integrated and serial activity that often is goal oriented (Grafman, 2002). A goal of restaurant dining with a friend offers an example. This activity comprises a structured set of events that includes selecting an appropriate restaurant, making a reservation, leaving the house, driving to the restaurant, parking the car, being seated, ordering, eating, etc. The SEC contains macrostructure-level information relevant to the consequences of past and current behavior by virtue of its storing events that have occurred in the past and will occur in the future. Thus, in the restaurant example, restaurant selection involves weeding out those establishments that have been found to have poor service, difficult parking, and bad food;

it also takes into consideration the type of "friend" being taken, with selection made on the basis of cuisine, ambience, etc. Finally, the SEC can occur at many levels of cognition, from word-level recognition of a set of speech sounds to a set of action events.

Specific to discourse, the SEC can serve as the underlying representation for knowledge acquired from following a set of directions, understanding a narrative, or absorbing a conversation if cast within the domain of discourse processing; and for knowledge imparted from giving directions, telling a story, and making a "wish list" if cast within the domain of discourse production.

SOMATIC MARKER THEORY

This framework, proposed by Damasio (1996), is thought to explain the failure of patients with prefrontal lesions to select appropriate social behaviors and act accordingly. Patients are considered to have a defect in activation of somatic markers. The hypothesis is that somatic signals bind to social behaviors, thus ensuring relevance by providing a modulating signal when a social decision must be made. This "tag" could be self-perceived as a sensation mediated by the autonomic nervous system. These tags may be helpful both in selecting appropriate behaviors and in inhibiting inappropriate behaviors. The explanation of failures to make social decisions is the lack of somatic marker intervention during social interactions. Quantitative estimates of these markers can be made via psychophysiologic recordings during task performances (e.g., galvanic skin response).

MODEL OF ATTENTIONAL CONTROL

In the model proposed by Norman and Shallice (1986), two control mechanisms are thought to determine how individuals monitor their activities. The contention scheduler (CS) operates via automatic or direct priming of stored knowledge either by environmental stimuli or conceptual thought; the supervisory attention system (SAS) reflects conscious awareness (within working memory limitations) of internal knowledge states that

prioritize action despite conflicting or absent environmental stimuli. Whereas the CS is automatic, the SAS is controlled. The latter (SAS), therefore, can override the former (CS) control mechanism. An example of the SAS overriding the CS is found in deferring answering the telephone when it rings in another person's office or helping oneself to food served to another person. Patients with prefrontal damage may be hyperresponsive to the automatic demands of the environment (captured in prehension and go-no-go tasks), consequently resulting in impulsivity and disinhibition.

Clinical Tests

Table 4–2 summarizes a set of selected clinical tests and measures either specifically validated for assessment of prefrontal function or applicable to the language/discourse deficits that can be present. Key to diagnostic precision in assessing prefrontal function is comprehensive measurement of the full range of behaviors that may be impaired. This principle applies to assessment of both executive function and language/discourse domains in order to understand their interrelationships and thus the underlying nature of the deficits. A second important principle of comprehensive assessment of prefrontal function is collaboration with clinical neuropsychologists. These are the professionals most highly qualified to assess dysexecutive function. A third and final principle is to extend assessment beyond the confines of the examination room. The keen diagnostician systematically observes and documents behavior in different settings, as some of the most useful information related to prefrontal function comes from the patient's interactions in natural environments (e.g., using the elevator, eating in the cafeteria, interacting with and reacting to staff/other patients).

Treatment

Effective rehabilitation of frontal lobe dysfunction hinges wholly on our knowledge about frontal lobe function. To date, we have

Table 4–2. Characteristics of Selected Clinical Tests of Frontal Lobe Function

Test (Reference)	Purpose/ Assessment Domains	Assessment/ Scoring Method	Time Require-ments	Psychometric Features
Executive Functions:				
Adden-brooke's Cognitive Examina-tion (Math-uranath et al., 2002)	Tests orientation, atten-tion, memory (episodic and semantic memory), language (naming, com-prehension repeating words and sentences, reading regular and ir-regular words, writing), visuospatial ability (copying, drawing clock face), verbal fluency (let-ter "P" and category flu-ency for animals).	Maximum score of 100 weighted as follows: ori-entation (10), attention (8), memory (35), verbal fluency (14), language (28), visuospatial ability (5). Component raw scores, except for verbal fluency (scaled scores), and composite score.	15–20 min.	Study evaluated 266 sub-jects (clinic group = 139; control group = 127). Subjects with frontotem-poral dementia (FTD) = 29; Alzheimer's disease (AD) = 69. High reliabil-ity, construct validity, and sensitivity (93%, using 88 as cut-off). Differentiates AD from FTD using ratio score [verbal fluency + language]/ [orientation + memory] of <2.2 for FTS and >3.2 for AD.
Behavioral Assessment of the Dy-sexecutive Syndrome (BADS) (Wilson et al., 1996)	Designed to predict every-day problems caused by dysexecutive syndrome: rule shifting, action pro-gram, key search, tempo-ral judgment, map use, Modified Six Elements Test [subjects do three tasks (dictation, arith-metic, picture naming) of which each divided into two parts], the Dysexecu-tive Questionnaire (DEX)(changes in emotion or personality, motivation, behavior, cognition).	Profile score, ranging from 0 to 4, is calculated for each test (on basis of how controls perform). DEX comprises 20 items scored in 5-point Likert scale (separate forms for patient, caregiver).	60 min.	Performance norms on basis of 216 control sub-jects and 78 patients with range of neurologic dis-orders (59% closed head injury). High interrater reliability 0.88–1.00); test-retest reliability data unclear (low to moderate correlations).
Delis-Kaplan Executive Function System (D-K EFS) (Delis et al., 2001)	Designed to measure dif-ferent aspects of execu-tive functions in children and adults. Measures set shifting (Trail-Making Test), verbal and design fluency, inhibition (Color Word Interference Test), concept formation (Sort-ing Test), reasoning (20-Questions Test), word context, verbal reasoning (proverbs), and planning (tower task).	Scores are given for alter-nate forms of each test. Multiple measures are available for each test with scoring instructions available in the booklet. Age-corrected, contrast, and composite scores based on factors are also available.	180 min.	Performance norms based on a stratified sample of 1750 children, adolescents, and adults, ages 8–89 years of age. Sparse data available for patients. Age corrected scores are available. Cor-relations between alter-nate forms of a test and test-retest reliability with same test version are modest. Just published.
CLOX (executive clock drawing task)	Designed to discriminate executive impairment from nonexecutive con-structional impairment; unprompted drawing task sensitive to execu-	1- to 2-point values as-signed to 15 organiza-tional elements for CLOX 1 and CLOX 2.	10–15 min.	Validated in study of 90 elderly subjects (45 from retirement community; 45 with probable AD). Scores correlated highly *(continued)*

Table 4–2. Characteristics of Selected Clinical Tests of Frontal Lobe Function (continued)

Test (Reference)	Purpose/ Assessment Domains	Assessment/ Scoring Method	Time Require- ments	Psychometric Features
(Royall et al., 1998)	tive control (CLOX1) and copied version that is not (CLOX2).			with cognitive severity ($r = .85$ with mini-mental status examination). CLOX subscales discriminated between AD and normal aging (83.1% of cases correctly classified, and between AD subgroups with and without constructional impairment (91.9% of cases correctly classified). High interrater reliability [$r = .94$ (CLOX1); $r = .93$ (CLOX2)].
Frontal Assessment Battery (FAB) (Dubois et al., 2000)	Bedside cognitive and behavioral battery comprising six subtests: conceptualization, mental flexibility, motor programming, sensitivity to interference, inhibitory control, and environmental autonomy.	Four-point scoring system (scores of 0 to 3) for each subtest; subtest scores added for total score.	10 min.	Validated in study of 42 normal subjects and 121 patients with frontal lobe dysfunction. Correlated with Mattis Dementia Rating Scale ($r = .82$) and aspects of Wisconsin Card Sorting Test ($r = .77$, $r = .68$). High interrater reliability ($k = .87$), internal consistency (Cronbach's $\mu = .78$), and discriminant validity (89.1% of cases correctly identified in discriminant analysis).
Stroop Color and Word Test (Golden, 1978)	Assesses the ability to sort information from the environment and selectively react to this information. Associated with cognitive flexibility. Patient is asked to alternately read words, name color that word is printed in.	Two scoring methods: time to complete 100 items, and number of items that can be completed in a set time period. Yields Word Score, Color Score, and Color-Word Score.	15 min.	Reliability highly consistent across different versions of the test. Test-retest reliabilities range from 0.71–0.88 for the three raw scores. Normative data are available. All Stroop scores can be converted into t-scores (mean of 50; SD of 10). Age correction are applied if patients are over 45 or under 17 years.
Test of veryday Attention (TEA) (Robertson et al., 1994)	Tests selective attention, sustained attention, attentional switching, divided attention. Eight subtests (three parallel versions) include map search, elevator counting, elevator counting with distraction, visual elevator, elevator count-	Norm-referenced scores, including subtest scaled-scores and percentile ranges	45–60 min.	Normative sample was 154 normal volunteers ranging from 18–80 years, stratified into four age bands/two levels of education. Validation study also included 80 unilateral stroke patients. Test-retest reliability ($r = .68$–$.90$), low

Table 4–2. Characteristics of Selected Clinical Tests of Frontal Lobe Function (continued)

Test (Reference)	Purpose/ Assessment Domains	Assessment/ Scoring Method	Time Requirements	Psychometric Features
	ing with reversal, telephone search, telephone search while counting, lottery.			reliability in dual task decrement ($r = .41–.61$). Principal components analysis identified four factors explaining 62.4% of variance.
Wisconsin Card Sorting Test (WCST) (Heaton et al., 1981)	Tests abstract reasoning and ability to shift cognitive sets, by sorting cards with changing sorting principles (by color, form, number) that force patient to develop new sorting strategy.	Normalized and percentile scores can be yielded for major WCST scores. Scores are assigned by three dimensions: correct-incorrect, ambiguous-unambiguous, perseverative-nonperseverative. Raw scores are converted into standard, T, and percentile scores.	30 min.	Normative data derived from 899 normal subjects, 6 1/2–89 years, corrected for education. In various studies, high interscorer ($r = .89–1.00$, with exception of Learning to Learn score) and intrascorer reliability ($r = .91–.96$). Has good construct validity.

Language/Discourse:

Test (Reference)	Purpose/ Assessment Domains	Assessment/ Scoring Method	Time Requirements	Psychometric Features
An Object and Action Naming Battery (Druks & Masterson, 2000)	Assesses and differentiates ability to name actions and objects. Stimuli were matched on psycholinguistic variables of printed word frequency, rated age-of-acquisition, and rated familiarity. Also provided are phoneme and syllable lengths and ratings for imageability and visual complexity (important predictors of naming performance).	Set includes 100 verbs and 162 nouns. First response is recorded, with notations for latency, prompt, and subsequent response. Patient's performance can be compared with normative data.	Up to 60 min.	Normative data collected from non-brain-damaged elderly participants (23 adults between ages of 61 and 70; 22 between ages of 71 and 80). Psychometric data currently not available.
Assessment of the Pragmatic Aspects of Language (Prutting & Kirchner, 1987)	Assesses verbal aspects (speech acts, topic, turn taking, lexical selection/use, stylistic variation), paralinguistic aspects (intelligibility and prosodics), and nonverbal aspects (kenesics and proxemics).	Pragmatic aspects rated as appropriate, inappropriate, no opportunity to observe, with notation of examples and comments. Language sample videotaped and transcribed for discourse analysis.	30 min. (for language sample)	None available.
Communication Activities of Daily Living, 2nd edition (CADL-2) (Holland et al., 1999)	Tests functional communication across dimensions of reading, writing, using numbers; social interactions, divergent communication; contextual communication; nonverbal communication; sequential relationships; humor/	Three-point scoring system (correct, adequate, incorrect); total raw score converted to percentiles and stanine scores.	30 min.	Standardized on sample of 175 adults with neurologically based communication disorders. Test-retest coefficient = .89, with stanine score coefficient = .92. Interrater coefficient for stanine score = .99. Moderately high correlation of *(continued)*

Table 4–2. Characteristics of Selected Clinical Tests of Frontal Lobe Function (continued)

Test (Reference)	Purpose/ Assessment Domains	Assessment/ Scoring Method	Time Require- ments	Psychometric Features
	metaphor/absurdity.			stanine score with WAB AQ (see below) (r = .66).
Discourse Compre- hension Test (Brookshire & Nicholas, 1993)	Assesses comprehension and retention of spoken or written narrative dis- course—stated and im- plied details and main ideas. Stimuli include two practice stories and 10 stories (five stories/ sets A & B; of ~200 words in length).	Yields category scores (up to 20) for stated main idea, implied main idea, stated detail, implied de- tail; overall score (up to 80).	30 min. /each set	Validation study (listen- ing comprehension) in- cluded 40 adults with no brain damage, 20 adults with aphasia, 20 nonapha- sic adults with RHBD, 20 adults with TBI. Cutoff scores for normal perfor- mance. Moderate correla- tions with SPICA, BDAE AUD, Test-retest for RBD: r = .95; for aphasia: r = .87.
RIC Evalu- ation of Communi- cation Problems in Right Hemi- sphere Dys- function – revised (Halper et al., 1996)	Assesses cognitive as- pects of communication attributed to right cere- bral hemispheric func- tion. Subtests of particu- lar interest include Behavioral Observation Profile, Rating Scale of Pragmatic Aspects of Communication, Metaphorical Language.	Pragmatic aspects of com- munication rated on a 4- point ordinal scale across dimensions of nonverbal communication (intona- tion, facial expression, eye contact, gestures and proxemics), verbal com- munication (conversation initiation, turn taking, topic maintenance, re- sponse length, presuppo- sition, referencing skills), and narrative discourse- completeness. Metaphori- cal interpretation rated on a two-point scale taking into account literal and personal interpretation, repeats, and no response.	60 min.	Study sample included 40 subjects with unilateral right hemisphere stroke and 36 normal subjects. Interrater reliability (among trained raters) ranged from r = .98–1.00. For Rating Scale of Prag- matic Communication, point-biserial correla- tions ranged from .70 to .85 for seven areas (facial expression, intonation, gestures and proxemics, conversational initiation, eye contact, turn taking, and topic maintenance) indicating correlations with total subtest score.
Western Aphasia Battery (WAB) (Kertesz, 1982)	Evaluates main clinical aspects of language func- tion. Oral subtests of par- ticular interest include Spontaneous Speech and Naming Sections; de- signed to elicit conversa- tional speech (i.e., con- tent and fluency).	Calculation of Aphasia Quotient (AQ) (up to 100) if all subtests of oral portion of assessment are administered. Arbitrary cutoff AQ of 93.8 set limit of aphasia.	60 min.	Extensively standardized in its previous version. New version: 20 patients (stable chronic infarcts; one head injury) assessed on old and new WAB. All subtest correlations sig- nificant (p = .01); t-test showed no significance between subtotal means, except in repetition task (lower mean on new test). No substantial dif- ference between old and new version.

BDAE, Boston Diagnostic Aphasia Examination; RBD, right brain damage; RHBD, right hemisphere brain damage; TBI, traumatic brain injury.

yet to succeed in fully solving the mysteries of the frontal lobes and their specialization in human behavior, particularly as they relate to language and discourse. Effective and empirically tested rehabilitative treatment strategies, therefore, remain only in formative stages. Nevertheless, progress has been made on the basis of prevailing theory and testable hypotheses that have direct implications for medical rehabilitation.

Burgess and Robertson (2002) offer a practical set of six principles that may direct methods of rehabilitation on the basis of prevailing theory: (1) Consider the use of feedback systems to modify dysexecutive behavior, especially symptoms of disinhibition and distractibility (i.e., loss of goals). (2) Consider the use of simple interrupts when patients fail to carry out intended tasks despite good recall. (3) Keep instructions simple and unambiguous. (4) Use simple reinforcement and reward techniques. (5) Include assessment of competence in a wide range of situations for pre- and posttreatment evaluation. (6) Do not necessarily start rehabilitation by treating the most troublesome dysexecutive problem; rather, consider which problems may benefit by initial groundwork elsewhere.

Because many of the deficits surrounding the use of language relate to communication in context, language treatment strategies should be directed toward use of communication in natural environments. These strategies, based on individual patterns of strengths and weaknesses, should address a set of the following goals: increased structure and salience of topic-driven communication, use of referential pronouns (or repeats of proper names) when referring to persons and their actions, appreciation of multiple meanings of ambiguous words and the structured/purposeful use of context to aid in correct meaning selection, improvement in understanding cause-and-effect relationships in narrative comprehension, story telling along serial events that adhere to before/after relationships, "think before doing" approach to response, paired verbal/graphic responses to reduce perseverative graphic errors, chunking of information and associative strategies to reduce working memory demands, answering wh-questions (who, what, where, when, why) in comprehending story-level material, turn-taking strategies to increase initiation of communication, family instruction to provide structure to conversation, and use of questions (e.g., direct vs. indirect, forced choice vs. free choice, simple vs. complex or compound questions) to aid in successful communicative attempts. Once strategies are developed, individual treatment can proceed to interpersonal interaction group treatment, with assignment for selecting and elaborating on topics (while adhering to a defined set of discourse rules as agreed to by the group) rotated among group members. Finally, we suggest that the SEC framework (Grafman, 1995, 2002) can be applied to rehabilitation in treatment of order and timing of events, and integration of these serial-order events into a thematic representation. Such an approach to treatment in the discourse domain would aim to improve the processing, analysis, and use of narrative information to result in outcomes of coherent and cohesive narratives that improve functional communication in its on-line management and real-time demands.

Conclusion

Language and discourse deficits following prefrontal damage can be enigmatic in their clinical identification, yet have profound effect on functional communication in daily life contexts. From a rehabilitative perspective, a useful conceptualization that can guide treatment options relates principally to addressing the temporal integration of contextual knowledge. Central to successful rehabilitation is the on-line management of contextual information using a theoretical framework, such as the SEC, that allows guided formation of testable hypotheses and the systematic exploration of intervention strategies. By virtue of advances in theory and neuroimaging technologies, knowledge about the specialized role of the prefrontal cortex in language and discourse will continue to be uncovered. The speech-language pathologist, then, can anticipate a richer rehabilitation science base, and the attainment of more consistent and favorable outcomes that permit the fulfillment of life goals for this patient population.

References

Alexander, M.P. (1997). Aphasia: Clinical and Anatomic Aspects. In: T.E. Feinberg & J.J. Farah (Eds.), *Behavioral Neurology and Neuropsychology* (pp. 133–149). New York: McGraw-Hill.

Alexander, M.P. (2002). Disorders of Language after Frontal Lobe Injury: Evidence for the Neural Mechanisms of Assembling Language. In: D.T. Stuss & R.T. Knight (Eds.), *Principles of Frontal Lobe Function* (pp. 292–310). New York: Oxford University Press.

Arbuthnot, M.H. (1976). *The Arbuthnot Anthology of Children's Literature.* New York: Lothrop, Lee, & Shephard.

Barbizet, J., Duizabo, P. & Flavigny, R. (1975). Role des Lôbes Frontaux dans le Langage. *Revue Neurologique, 131,* 525–544.

Beeman, M. (1998). Course Semantic Coding and Discourse Comprehension. In: M. Beeman & C. Chiarello (Eds.), *Right Hemisphere Language Comprehension* (pp. 255–284). Mahway, NJ: Lawrence Erlbaum.

Benton, A.L. (1968). Differential Behavioral Effects in Frontal Lobe Disease. *Neuropsychologia, 6,* 53–60.

Binder, J.R., Frost, J.A., Hammeke, T.A., Cox, R.W., Rao, S.M. & Prieto, T. (1997). Human Brain Language Areas Identified by Functional Magnetic Resonance Imaging. *Journal of Neuroscience, 17,* 353–362.

Brookshire, R.H. & Nicholas, L.E. (1993). *Discourse Comprehension Test.* Tucson, AZ: Communication Skill Builders.

Brown, G. & Yule, G. (1983). *Discourse Analysis.* Cambridge, MA: Cambridge University Press.

Brun, A. (1987). Frontal Lobe Degeneration of Non-Alzheimer Type I. Neuropathology. *Archives of Gerontology and Geriatrics, 6,* 193–208.

Buckner, R.L., Raichle, M.E. & Petersen, S.E. (1995). Dissociation of Human Prefrontal Cortical Areas Across Different Speech Production Tasks and Gender Groups. *Journal of Neurophysiology, 74,* 2163–2173.

Burgess, B.W. & Robertson, I.H. (2002). Principles of the Rehabilitation of Frontal Lobe Function. D.T. Stuss & R.T. Knight (Eds.), *Principles of Frontal Lobe Function* (pp. 557–572). New York: Oxford University Press.

Caplan, D. (1999). *Language: Structure, Processing, and Disorders.* Cambridge, MA: MIT Press.

Chee, M.W.L., Sriram, N., Soon, C.S. & Lee, K.M. (2000). Dorsolateral Prefrontal Cortex and the Implicit Association of Concepts and Attributes. *NeuroReport, 11,* 135–140.

Cohen, J.D. & Servan-Schreiber, D. (1992). Content, Cortex and Dopamine: A Connectionist Approach to Behavior and Biology in Schizophrenia. *Psychological Review, 99,* 45–77.

Craig, G. & Frattali, C.M. (2000). "Getting the Gist" of Stories: Effects of Prefrontal Cortex Damage. *ASHA Leader, 5,* 219.

Crozier, S., Sirigu, A., Lehericy, S., van de Moortele, P.F., Pillon, B., Grafman, J., Agid, Y., Dubois, B. & LeBihan, D. (1999). Distinct Prefrontal Activations in Processing Sequence at the Sentence and Script Level: An fMRI Study. *Neuropsychologia, 37,* 1469–1476.

Cummings, J. (1995). Anatomic and Behavioral Aspects of Frontal-Subcortical Circuits. In: J. Grafman, K.J. Holyok & F. Boller (Eds.), *Structure and Functions of the Human Prefrontal Cortex* (vol. 769, pp. 1–13). Annals of the New York Academy of Sciences. New York: New York Academy of Sciences.

Damasio, A.R. (1996). The Somatic Marker Hypothesis and the Possible Functions of the Prefrontal Cortex. *Philosophical Transactions of the Royal Society of London, Series B: Biological Sciences, 351,* 1413–1420.

Delis, D., Kaplan, E. & Kramer, J. (2001). *Delis-Kaplan Executive Function System (D-K EFS).* San Antonio, TX: Psychological Corporation.

Demb, J.B., Desmond, J.E., Wagner, A.D., Vaidya, C.J., Glover, G.H. & Gabrieli, J.D. (1995). Semantic Encoding and Retrieval in the Left Inferior Prefrontal Cortex: A Functional MRI Study of Task Difficulty and Process Specificity. *Journal of Neuroscience, 15,* 5870–5878.

Druks, J. & Masterson, J. (2000). *An Object and Action Naming Battery.* East Sussex, UK: Psychology Press.

Dubois, B., Slachevsky, A., Litvan, I. & Pillon, B. (2000). The FAB: A Frontal Assessment Battery at Bedside. *Neurology, 55,* 1621–1626.

Ferrier, D. (1878). The Goulstonion Lectures of the Localisation of Cerebral Disease. *British Medical Journal, 397–402,* 443–447.

Ferstl, E.C., Guthke, T. & van Cramon, D.Y. (1999). Change of Perspective in Discourse Comprehension: Encoding and Retrieval Processes after Brain Injury. *Brain and Language, 70,* 385–420.

Frattali, C., Wesley, R. & Grafman, J. (2001). Suppressing Inappropriate Meanings of Lexical Ambiguities: Effect of Prefrontal Cortex Damage. In: *Clinical Aphasiology Conference Program Manual* (p. 8).

Fuster, J.M. (1997). *The Prefrontal Cortex: Anatomy, Physiology, and Neuropsychology of the Frontal Lobe* (3rd ed). Philadelphia: Lippincott-Raven.

Gabrieli, J.D., Desmond, J.E., Demb, J.B. & Wagner, A.D. (1996). Functional Magnetic Resonance Imaging of Semantic Memory Processes in the Frontal Lobes. *Psychological Science, 7,* 278–283.

Gabrieli, J.D., Poldrack, R.A. and Desmond, J.E. (1998). The Role of the Left Prefrontal Cortex in Language and Memory. *Proceedings of the National Academy of Sciences, 95,* 906–913.

Gernsbacher, M.A. (1990). *Language Comprehension as Structure Building.* Hillsdale, NJ: Erlbaum.

Golden, C.J. (1978). *Stroop Color and Word Test.* Wood Dale, IL: Stoelting.

Goldstein, K. (1948). *Language and Language Disturbances.* New York: Grune & Stratton.

Goodglass, H. (1993). *Understanding Aphasia.* San Diego: Academic Press.

Grafman, J. (1995). Similarities and Distinctions Among Current Models of Prefrontal Cortical Functions. *Annals of the New York Academy of Sciences, 769,* 337–368.

Grafman, J. (1999). Experimental Assessment of Adult Frontal Lobe Function. In: B.L. Miller & J. Cummings (Eds.), *The Human Frontal Lobes: Function and Disorders* (pp. 321–344). New York: Guilford.

Grafman, J. (2002). The Structured Event Complex and the Human Prefrontal Cortex. In: D.T. Stuss & R.T. Knight (Eds.), *Principles of Frontal Lobe Function* (pp. 292–310). New York: Oxford University Press.

Halper, A.S., Cherney, L.R. & Burns, M. (1996). *Clinical Management of Right Hemisphere Dysfunction* (2nd ed). Gaithersburg, MD: Aspen.

Harlow, J.M. (1868). Recovery from the Passage of an Iron Bar Through the Head. *Publications of the Massachusetts Medical Society, Boston, 2*, 327–347.

Heaton, R.K., Chelune, G.J., Talley, J., et al. (1981). *Wisconsin Card Sorting Test*. Odessa, FL: Psychological Assessment Resources.

Holland, A., Frattali, C. & Fromm, D. (1999). *Communication Activities of Daily Living* (2nd ed). Austin, TX: Pro-Ed.

Jackson, J.H. (1915). On Affections of Speech from Disease of the Brain. *Brain, 38*, 107–174.

Kapur, S., Rose, R., Liddle, P.F., Zipursky, R.B., Brown, G.M., Stuss, D., Houle, S. & Tulving, E. (1994). The Role of the Left Prefrontal Cortex in Verbal Processing: Semantic Processing or Willed Action? *NeuroReport, 5*, 2193–2196.

Kertesz, A. (1982). *Western Aphasia Battery*. San Antonio, TX: The Psychological Corporation.

Kintsch, W. (1994). The Psychology of Discourse Processing. In: M.A. Gernsbacher (Ed.), *Handbook of Psycholinguistics* (pp. 721–736). San Diego, CA: Academic Press.

Kleist, K. (1934). *Gehirnpathologie*. Leipzig: Barth.

Luria, A.R. (1970). *Traumatic Aphasia*. The Hague: Mouton.

Luria, A.R. & Homskaya, E.D. (1964). Disturbance in the Regulative Role of Speech with Frontal Lobe Lesions. In: J.M. Warren & K. Akert (Eds.), *The Frontal Granular Cortex and Behavior* (pp. 353–371). New York: McGraw-Hill.

Macmillan, M. (2000). *An Odd Kind of Fame: Stories of Phineas Gage*. Cambridge, MA: MIT Press.

Maguire, E.A., Frith, C.D. & Morris, R.G.M. (1999). The Functional Neuroanatomy of Comprehension and Memory: The Importance of Prior Knowledge. *Brain, 122*, 1839–1850.

Mathuranath, P.S., Nestor, P.J., Berrios, G.E., et al. (2002). A Brief Cognitive Test Battery to Differentiate Alzheimer's Disease and Frontotemporal Dementia. *Neurology, 55*, 1613–1620.

Mesulam, M.M. (2000). *Principles of Behavioral and Cognitive Neurology* (2nd ed). New York: Oxford University Press.

Nichelli, P., Grafman, J., Pietrini, P., Clark, K., Lee, K.Y. & Miletich, R. (1995). Where the Brain Appreciates the Moral of a Story. *NeuroReport, 6*, 2309–2313.

Norman, D.A. & Shallice, T. (1986). Attention to Action: Willed and Automatic Control of Behavior. In: R.J. Davidson, G.E. Schwartz & D. Shapiro (Eds.), *Consciousness and Self-Regulation* (vol 4, pp. 1–18). New York: Plenum Press.

Partiot, A., Grafman, J., Sadato, N., Flitman, S. & Wild, K. (1996). Brain Activation During Script Event Processing. *NeuroReport, 7*, 761–766.

Petersen, S.E., Fox, R.T., Posner, M.I., Mintun, M. & Raichle, M.E. (1988). Positron Emission Tomographic Studies of the Cortical Anatomy of Single-Word Processing. *Nature, 331*, 585–589.

Petersen, S.E., Fox, R.T., Snyder, A.Z. & Raichle, M.E. (1990). Activation of Extrastriate and Frontal Cortical Areas by Visual Words and Word-Like Stimuli. *Science, 249*, 1041–1044.

Poldrack, R.A., Wagner, A.D., Prull, M.W., Desmond, J.E., Glover, G.H. & Gabrieli, J.D.E. (1999). Functional Specialization for Semantic and Phonological Processing in the Left Inferior Prefrontal Cortex. *Neuroimage, 10*, 15–35.

Price, C.J., Wise, R.J.S., Watson, J.D.G., Patterson, K., Howard, D. & Fackowiak, S.J. (1994). Brain Activity During Reading: The Effects of Exposure Duration and Task. *Brain, 117*, 1255–1269.

Prutting, C.A. & Kirchner, D.M. (1987). A Clinical Appraisal of the Pragmatic Aspects of Language. *Journal of Speech and Hearing Disorders, 52*, 117–119.

Robertson, D.A., Gernsbacher, M.A., Guidotti, S.J., Robertson, R.R.W., Irwin, W., Mock, B.J. & Campana, S.J. (2000). Functional Neuroanatomy of the Cognitive Process of Mapping During Discourse Comprehension. *Psychological Science, 11*, 255–260.

Robertson, I.H., Ward, T., Ridgeway, V., et al. (1994). *The Test of Everyday Attention*. Bury St. Edmunds, England: Thames Valley Test Company.

Royall, D.R., Cordes, J.A. & Polk, M. (1998). CLOX: An Executive Clock Drawing Task. *Journal of Neurology, Neurosurgery, and Psychiatry. 64*, 588–594.

Semendeferi, K., Lu, A., Schenker, N. & Damasio, H. (2002). Humans and Great Apes Share a Large Frontal Cortex. *Nature Neuroscience, 5*, 272–276.

Sirigu, A., Cohen, L., Zalla, T., Pradat-Diehl, P., Van Eeckhout, P., Grafman, J. & Agid, Y. (1998). Distinct Frontal Regions for Processing Sentence Syntax and Story Grammar. *Cortex, 34*, 771–778.

Spitzer, M., Kwong, K.K., Kennedy, W., Rosen, B.R. & Belliveau, J.W. (1995). Category-Specific Brain Activation in fMRI During Picture Naming. *NeuroReport, 6*, 2109–2112.

Thompson-Schill, S.L., D'Esposito, M., Aguirre, G.K. & Farah, M. (1997). Role of Left Inferior Prefrontal Cortex in Retrieval of Semantic Knowledge: A Reevaluation. *Proceedings of the National Academy of Sciences, 94*, 14792–14797.

Wilson, B., Alderman, N., Burgess, P.W., et al. (1996). *Behavioural Assessment of the Dysexecutive Syndrome (BADS)*. Bury St. Edmunds, England: Thames Valley Test Company.

Zalla, T., Phipps, M. & Grafman, J. (2002). Story Recall in Patients with Damage to the Prefrontal Cortex. *Cortex, 38*, 215–231.

Zangwill, O.L. (1966). Psychological Deficits Associated with Frontal Lobe Lesions. *International Journal of Neurology, 5*, 395–402.

5

Naming and Word-Retrieval Problems

ANASTASIA M. RAYMER

Among individuals with aphasia, one of the most common and persistent symptoms is word-retrieval difficulty or anomia (Goodglass & Wingfield, 1997). Although functionally anomia is evidenced by disruptions in word retrieval during the flow of conversation, its presence is evaluated most commonly in picture confrontation naming tasks. Thus the terms *word retrieval* and *naming* are frequently interchanged, as will be the case in this chapter. A review of the large body of literature in aphasia indicates that naming impairments vary substantially in their cognitive and neural underpinnings among individuals with aphasia. The clinician's goal in working with individuals with anomia is to disentangle the distinct patterns of naming failure through a thorough naming assessment and then to implement appropriate treatments to address the individual's naming dysfunction.

Pathophysiology of Naming Impairments

Cognitive Mechanisms of Naming

An appreciation of the complex cognitive system implemented in word retrieval is integral to understanding the disorders of naming observed in aphasia (Fig. 5–1). Although details of the lexical model are the subject of debate, at least two lexical stages, semantic and phonologic, are critical to the process of word retrieval (Caramazza, 2000; Nickels, 2001). The lexical stages are initially activated by modality-specific input mechanisms storing representations for familiar, previously learned spoken and written words and viewed objects and actions. In the case of confrontation picture naming, the primary input mechanism involves the visual object recognition system. Input representations then activate the semantic system, the store of meanings and information we have learned about words, objects, or actions. In confrontation naming, the semantic system applies meaning to viewed objects or actions. Semantic representations then activate modality-specific output lexicons for spoken and written words. In the case of oral picture naming, we focus on the store of familiar spoken words, the phonologic output lexicon. Words appear to be stored in phonologically similar groupings and are distinguished at this level by word class (i.e., nouns and verbs) (Caramazza & Hillis, 1991). Subsequent to the semantic and phonologic lexical retrieval stages, postlexical phonologic and articulatory processes allow for planning and executing verbal responses. Acquired brain damage that disrupts the activity of this complex system can lead to naming impairments.

Neural Substrates of Naming Impairments

The fact that naming impairments arise in almost all aphasia syndromes suggests that the naming system is mediated by a complex

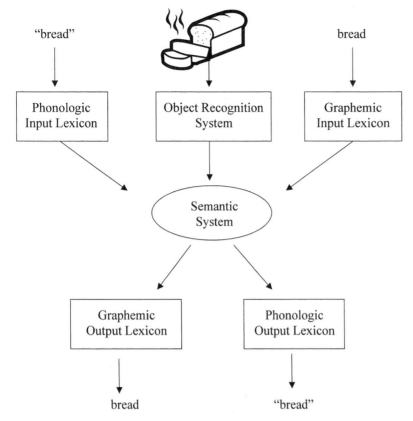

Figure 5–1. Model of lexical processes involved in word retrieval.

neural network, particularly involving the left cerebral hemisphere. Studies from brain-damaged individuals with different forms of aphasia have provided one form of evidence for the neural instantiation of the semantic and phonologic lexical stages engaged during naming (Table 5–1). (Discussion of other forms of evidence, such as the extensive literature on the functional neuroimaging of word retrieval, is beyond the scope of this chapter; see Damasio et al., 2001; Murtha et al., 1999.)

Left hemisphere temporoparietal cortex appears to play a critical role in the representation of semantic knowledge (Goodglass & Wingfield, 1997). This region is implicated in individuals with degenerative dementias leading to semantic dysfunction and naming difficulties (Kertesz et al., 1998). Although semantic impairment has been reported in individuals with large left hemisphere lesions and global aphasia (Hillis et al., 1990), discrete vascular lesions affecting the left

Table 5–1. General Cognitive and Neural Correlates of Naming Impairments Across Aphasia Syndromes

Cognitive Mechanism	Neural Correlate	Aphasia Syndrome
Semantic system	Left temporoparietal	Transcortical sensory, global
Semantic-phonologic access	Left posterior inferior temporal	Anomic
Phonologic output lexicon	Left posterior superior temporal	Wernicke's, conduction
Lexical-syntactic interface	Left frontal operculum	Broca's, transcortical motor

temporo-occipito-parietal junction have been reported to lead to semantically based naming impairments in individuals with aphasia (Hart & Gordon, 1990; Tranel et al., 1997). Lesions in this region often lead to transcortical sensory aphasia, consistent with the notion that naming impairments in these individuals relate to semantic breakdown (Alexander et al., 1989).

Acquired brain damage at times leads to naming impairments restricted to specific semantic categories such as fruits, vegetables, animals, or tools (see Best, 2000, for a review). Tranel et al. (1997) mapped the lesions of individuals with aphasia and naming impairments for different semantic categories. Naming difficulty occurred for animals with left inferior temporal lesions and tools with temporoparieto-occipital lesions. These observations suggest that localized left temporo-occipito-parietal brain regions mediate specific aspects of semantic knowledge.

The neural correlate of the phonologic output lexicon is thought to encompass Wernicke's area in the posterior portion of the left superior temporal gyrus (Goodglass & Wingfield, 1997). Acute lesions in this region lead to profound naming impairments as in Wernicke's aphasia, in which neologisms and semantic paraphasias abound. Following recovery from milder Wernicke's area lesions, however, the naming pattern can evolve to one of phonemic errors in naming as in some individuals with conduction aphasia (Dronkers & Ludy, 1998), suggesting that this region in fact plays a critical role in a lexical-phonologic stage in naming.

Analyses of naming disruption in some individuals with aphasia implicate a disconnection at the interface between semantic and phonologic naming processes. These are individuals whose pattern of language dysfunction relates primarily to naming or anomic aphasia. Whereas they can comprehend words, they are unable to retrieve names of words, whether in speech or in writing. Acute onset of anomic aphasia has been described in individuals with inferior

temporal lobe lesions (Foundas et al., 1998; Raymer et al., 1997a; Tranel et al., 1997) and left thalamic lesions (Raymer et al., 1997b). A number of investigations have reported that lesions of the inferior temporal cortex are associated with naming impairments that preferentially affect the category of nouns (Damasio & Tranel, 1993; Hillis et al., 2002; Tranel et al., 1997), in keeping with the observation that individuals with anomic aphasia have greater difficulty with nouns than with other grammatical categories (Goodglass & Wingfield, 1997).

This classification scheme has focused on left temporoparieto-occipital regions and fluent aphasias implicated in the semantic and phonologic lexical processes of naming. However, individuals with nonfluent aphasias, including Broca's and transcortical motor aphasia, also may present with profound naming impairments (Goodglass & Wingfield, 1997). Lesions of the left frontal operculum have been associated with deficits in naming, often greater for verbs than for nouns (Damasio & Tranel, 1993; Hillis et al., 2002; Tranel et al., 1997). Wilshire and Coslett (2000) proposed that naming impairment in the nonfluent aphasias probably relates to processes other than the semantic and phonologic aspects of naming, potentially involving the interface between syntactic processing and word retrieval.

Nature and Differentiating Features of Naming Impairments

The pattern of naming difficulty, type of errors produced, and accompanying lexical impairments vary depending on which stage in the naming system, semantic or phonologic, is disrupted by brain injury. Impairments related to the object recognition system can disrupt naming abilities, but these impairments are discussed in the realm of visual agnosias, which are beyond the scope of this chapter.

Semantically based naming impairments are associated with difficulty in all lexical tasks that require semantic mediation. That is, impairment is evident for all types of naming tasks regardless of input modality (e.g., picture naming, naming to spoken definitions) or output mode (oral and written naming). In addition, the individual has co-occurring difficulty in spoken and written word comprehension and in interpreting the meanings of viewed objects and gestures, as all of those tasks require semantic mediation for successful performance. Impairment is likely to be quantitatively and qualitatively similar across lexical tasks, that is, with similar proportions and type of errors (e.g., Hillis et al., 1990). Naming errors may take a number of forms including semantically related responses (e.g., "hammer" for screwdriver), semantically empty naming errors ("a thing you use"), or perseverations (e.g., repeated use of the word "eggs" for all naming attempts). Confusions also are evident in comprehension tasks, as these individuals mis-select semantically related foils and even unrelated foils if the semantic impairment is severe enough. Performance in oral word reading and writing to dictation may not be affected, as these tasks also can be accomplished through alternative sublexical or lexical-nonsemantic processes (Raymer & Berndt, 1996).

Researchers have also described individuals with aphasia whose naming and comprehension impairments fractionate according to specific semantic categories such as living and nonliving things, fruits and vegetables, tools and animals (see Best, 2000, for a review). Semantic level breakdown is indicated when these individuals experience difficulties in both comprehension and naming tasks for the specific semantic category, and probably relates to the loss of specific neural networks that mediate critical aspects of semantic information shared by several members of a given semantic category (Caramazza & Shelton, 1998).

A final syndrome often discussed in the realm of semantic impairments is optic aphasia, in which patients experience modality-specific naming failure for viewed objects and pictures. These individuals can name the object when described verbally, and can describe the function of the viewed object, or sort pictures according to semantic categories,

arguing against a visual agnosia in which meaning is not appreciated for viewed objects (Farah, 1990). In the cognitive scheme we have espoused, Hillis and Caramazza (1995a) attributed optic aphasia to an impairment of visual object-to-semantic activation. That is, visual object representations are unable to activate the full semantic representations for viewed objects. Presumably, the incompletely activated semantic information is sufficient to accomplish only some semantic tasks, such as sorting, but not others, such as picture naming.

Impairments affecting the phonologic output lexicon lead to difficulty in all tasks requiring the use of stored phonologic representations. Comprehension abilities are typically preserved. Difficulty is evident in all oral naming tasks (e.g., oral picture naming, oral naming to spoken definitions) and in oral word reading, particularly for words with exceptional spellings (e.g., "choir," "yacht") whose pronunciations cannot be derived correctly through sublexical grapheme-to-phoneme translation processes. Verbal production errors in naming and oral reading may take a variety of forms (Hillis, 2001). Individuals with difficulty activating the output lexicon can make semantic or no response errors. Others with a disturbance affecting the internal structure of phonologic representations may produce neologistic responses if severely impaired (e.g., Kohn et al., 1996), or phonemic paraphasias if representations are partially preserved. Patients with selective impairment for phonologic output may have retained performance in written word production (Caramazza & Hillis, 1990).

Some individuals present with a pattern of impaired performance in all naming tasks, whether for spoken or written output. Comprehension abilities, however, are intact, suggesting the integrity of semantic processing. Although a pattern of impaired oral and written naming may represent concurrent dysfunction of both phonologic and orthographic output lexicons in some individuals (Miceli et al., 1991), other researchers have construed such a pattern as an access failure from semantic to phonologic (and orthographic) lexical stages of naming (Raymer et al., 1997a). Although this distinction is difficult to make, one line of evidence can be oral reading abilities, which can be intact in individuals with semantic-phonologic impairments (Raymer & Berndt, 1996). Naming errors may include circumlocutions, semantically related paraphasias, or no response at all, depending on the amount of information that can be activated in the output lexicon.

Of course, brain damage does not respect the cognitive distinctions among visual object recognition, semantic, and phonologic lexical mechanisms of naming. Therefore, naming impairment can be the result of disruption at multiple stages in the word-retrieval process, leading to severely compromised naming abilities. Moreover, apart from the lexical systems critical to the process of naming, Murray (2000) demonstrated that naming difficulties can be exacerbated by attentional demands at play in the course of cognitive activities.

Assessment of Naming

Although subtests for naming assessment are incorporated in virtually all standardized aphasia test batteries, clinical decision making is enhanced through the use of specialized tools for naming assessment. Standardized tests available to assess naming abilities include the Boston Naming Test (Kaplan et al., 2000), and An Object and Action Naming Battery (Druks & Masterson, 1999). A systematic assessment of lexical processing abilities (i.e., naming and comprehension) is necessary to distinguish the different patterns that naming impairments may take. Clinicians need to consider a number of variables when assessing the integrity of the naming system.

Lexical Task Comparisons

The naming assessment should include a variety of single word processing tasks in which the clinician systematically varies input and output modalities, and analyzes patterns of performance across tasks sharing processing modalities (Table 5–2) (Raymer & Rothi, 2001). Published psycholinguistic tests [e.g., Psycholinguistic Assessment of Language Processing Abilities (Kay et al., 1992); Pyramids and Palm Trees (Howard & Patterson, 1992)] and informal tests such as the Florida Semantics Battery (Raymer & Rothi, 2001) can guide cross-modality assessment of lexical and naming abilities.

Although word-retrieval difficulties can be noted in conversation tasks, systematic naming assessment most likely will be accomplished in structured tasks requiring naming responses to viewed pictures, pantomimes, and spoken and written definitions. Naming to pictures versus definitions can be contrasted to evaluate contributions of visual-semantic access dysfunction to naming failure. To distinguish semantic versus phonologic bases of naming breakdown, performance can be examined in semantic processing tasks, which are also impaired in the case of semantic breakdown. Semantic

Table 5–2. Example of Lexical Assessment Tasks that Vary in Input and Output Modality

Output Modality	Input Modality	
	Speech	Viewed Object
Speech	Oral name to definition	Oral picture name
Writing	Written name to definition	Written picture name
Gesture/pointing	Pantomime to named object Word-to-picture matching Word-to-picture yes/no verification Associated pictures match Category sort Picture rhyme judgment	Pantomime to viewed picture

tasks may include category sorting for closely related semantic categories (e.g., summer vs. winter clothing), and matching associated pictures according to semantic relationships (e.g., rabbit: carrot).

To distinguish impairments that preferentially affect the phonologic output lexicon, performance can be contrasted across modalities of naming as performance may be more impaired for oral than written naming. To further evaluate the integrity of the phonologic output lexicon, it may be necessary to administer tasks that tax phonologic lexical processing such as rhyme judgments for picture pairs (e.g., Do the names of these pictures rhyme?: whale-nail). The rhyming task proves difficult for individuals who fail to activate a full lexical-phonologic representation for the pictures.

Stimulus Characteristics

A large body of literature has shown that a number of stimulus characteristics affect success in naming (see Nickels, 1997, for a review). These factors are an important consideration in naming assessment, as performance is influenced by the choice of stimulus materials. Grammatical categories (e.g., nouns vs. verbs) and semantic categories (e.g., living vs. nonliving items) need to be systematically evaluated, as some individuals are more impaired for one category of words over another. Within standard aphasia tests currently available, an astute examiner may notice either impaired or spared performance related to selective grammatical or semantic categories and then explore category distinctions with additional relevant informal test materials.

A number of other psycholinguistic variables also affect the ability to retrieve words. Researchers who have discussed the effect of word frequency in naming have often reported that higher frequency words are named better than lower frequency words (Raymer et al., 1997a; Zingeser & Berndt, 1988). However, carefully controlled studies have demonstrated that factors such as imageability, length, familiarity, and especially age of acquisition have a more potent effect on noun and verb naming abilities than word frequency (Hirsh & Ellis, 1994; Kemmerer & Tranel, 2000; Nickels & Howard, 1995). Imageable, familiar, and shorter words, and particularly words learned earlier in life are easier to name under conditions of brain damage. Argument structure complexity also plays a critical in the ability to name verbs (Thompson et al., 1997). Naming assessment tasks need to incorporate stimulus materials varying in these important psycholinguistic variables that can influence naming performance. Results of testing that identifies selective categories of difficulty for a patient may allow the clinician to streamline efforts in rehabilitation.

Error Analyses

Another key concept to consider in naming assessment is the pattern of errors produced across tasks. A number of response analysis systems have been described (e.g., Mitchum et al., 1990). The types of verbal errors may provide important clues as to the mechanism underlying a patient's naming impairment. Comparison of performance in tasks that engage the same lexical mechanism should show a qualitatively similar error pattern across tasks. For example, a severe deficit of semantic processing may lead to unrelated response errors in all comprehension and naming tasks. A phonologic output lexicon dysfunction may result in parallel patterns of phonemic paraphasias in oral picture naming and oral reading, especially for words with exceptional spellings.

Examination of the type of error itself within one lexical task is not sufficient to distinguish the level of lexical impairment responsible for the naming error (Hillis & Caramazza, 1995b). Semantic errors in picture naming are a case in point. On the surface, one might assume that these errors represent semantic system dysfunction. Semantic errors may arise from impairment arising at a number of stages in the naming process: semantic system (Hillis et al., 1990), visual-semantic access as in optic aphasia

(Hillis & Caramazza, 1995a), semantic activation of the phonologic output lexicon (Raymer et al., 1997a), and phonologic output lexicon itself (Caramazza & Hillis, 1990). These observations underscore the need to analyze error patterns across lexical tasks to develop an accurate diagnosis regarding the source of the naming errors in an individual with aphasia (Raymer & Rothi, 2001).

The purpose of naming assessment is to specify the mechanisms that are responsible for naming impairment as well as those that are spared. This information may be especially beneficial as the clinician turns toward devising treatments for each patient, as treatments can be tailored either to address specific levels of impairment or to implement spared abilities to enhance naming and communication abilities.

Treatment

Clinicians can select from a number of different treatment approaches to address the communication impairment posed by word-retrieval difficulties. Some naming treatments are restitutive in nature, as they are devised to focus on the specific level of naming impairment and restore functioning in that mechanism (Rothi, 1995). Through naming practice in an enriched lexical environment the ultimate aim is to improve naming abilities in a manner compatible with the normal process of word retrieval. That is, patients participate in tasks that require them to act upon the semantic or phonologic characteristics of words, with the goal of altering levels of activation or interaction among lexical representations implemented in the process of word retrieval. To be effective and have long-term consequences for naming abilities, this type of approach requires intensive practice on a set of selected stimuli (Hinckley & Craig, 1998).

Some other naming treatments tend to be vicariative approaches (Rothi, 1995). They are meant to engage intact cognitive mechanisms to support the process of word retrieval in a manner that differs from the normal process, perhaps leading to fundamental

alterations in the word-retrieval process over time. So, for example, individuals may be taught to use gesture, reading, or writing during the process of word retrieval to improve access to intended words. With practice, individuals may ultimately improve word retrieval in the absence of the facilitating cognitive support, though others may need to rely on the supportive process for the long term.

Finally, some naming treatment approaches are intended to help the patient circumvent the impaired naming system and use compensatory strategies to communicate an intended message in whatever manner is possible. Clinicians encourage patients to use such methods as circumlocution, gesture, drawing, or writing to convey ideas when words fail them. Some treatment approaches are implemented specifically to encourage the use of communication strategies as conversation takes place in a functional context.

Decisions as to the specific approach to take are influenced by factors such as the severity of naming impairment, timing of treatment relative to the onset of injury, the amount of time available to participate in treatment, and personal characteristics and demands for language use. Naming treatment requires an individualized approach to developing treatment goals that are realistic and personally meaningful. A number of specific treatment approaches have been investigated in their effects for word retrieval. For the purposes of this chapter, we limit the discussion to approaches useful in individuals with mild-to-moderate word-retrieval impairments for nouns and verbs, as the severe word-production difficulties implicated in global aphasia, for example, may warrant different types of techniques to improve verbal production (Collins, 1997).

Specific Treatment Approaches

Restitutive Naming Treatments

CUING HIERARCHIES

In working with individuals with aphasia, it becomes immediately evident that breaks in the conversation that arise from an instance of word-retrieval failure can often be overcome with a simple cue provided by the listener. A number of different types of cues can be helpful for unblocking a moment of anomia, including an initial sound, a sentence completion context, an associated word, the written word, or a gesture. However, the problem with all of these cues is that their effects are typically only fleeting. Clinicians instead have turned to cuing hierarchies in an attempt to promote long-term changes in the process of word retrieval. In cuing hierarchy training, when an instance of word-retrieval failure occurs, the clinician systematically provides a series of cues that are more and more potent in their ability to elicit the intended target word, usually the name of a picture (Table 5–3) (Linebaugh, 1997). At the step where the target word is named, the clinician may either rehearse the target word multiple times, or move the patient back up the cuing hierarchy, providing each cue in reverse direction until the patient once again simply looks at the target picture and produces the intended word upon command. Cuing hierarchies are constructed after preliminary probing to determine which are the more and less effective cues for that individual. Although cuing hierarchies typically incorporate both semantic and phonologic information, consistent with the course of word retrieval, some studies have used cues that involve only semantic or phonologic information (Raymer et al., 1993). Patterson (2001) reviewed the evidence for the effectiveness of cuing hierarchies in approximately 10 published studies and reported that

Table 5–3. Example of a Cuing Hierarchy for Naming Treatment

Target picture: blouse

1. "It's clothing."

2. "You can button it."

3. "It starts with /bl/"

4. "It sounds like mouse."

5. Written word: "Here is the word." blouse

6. "Say blouse."

the technique is useful across individuals with a variety of naming impairments. Hillis (1998) described the effects of different types of naming treatments in one woman and found that cuing hierarchy training, although effective for improving naming abilities, was not as potent as another naming treatment devised to specifically address the semantic impairment responsible for the patient's naming impairment.

Semantic Treatments

Recognizing the common role the semantic system plays in both word comprehension and word retrieval, some researchers have developed comprehension treatments to facilitate word-retrieval abilities (Marshall et al., 1990; Nickels & Best, 1996). In these comprehension treatments, patients complete a series of semantic processing tasks such as sorting pictures into categories of increasingly related semantic distinctions, auditory and written word-picture matching with increasingly difficult semantic distractors, and yes/no question verification about semantic characteristics of a target picture. Typically the patients also are allowed to rehearse the names of target pictures in the context of comprehension training, thereby adding a phonologic component to the semantic training. As patients complete the semantic tasks across multiple sessions, naming improvements emerge in a variety of individuals with naming impairments related to either semantic or phonologic dysfunction (see Ennis, 2001, for a recent review).

Drew and Thompson (1999) investigated the importance of the production of target names in the context of semantic comprehension training. They found that subjects benefited maximally during training in which the comprehension tasks were combined with the word-production component of training as compared to comprehension training in isolation. Hence, the comprehension training is most effective when semantic plus phonologic processing is incorporated in the training protocol, in keeping with the normal process of word retrieval.

Some patients with semantic dysfunction seem to lack specific details of semantic representations, and thereby produce many semantic errors in naming. A treatment devised for this type of patient is a semantic distinctions treatment (Hillis, 1998; Ochipa et al., 1998). The clinician provides patients with semantic information about target pictures they are unable to name, and contrasts those features with the semantic features of a closely related object. Both Hillis and Ochipa et al. reported that this technique was effective in their patients with semantically based naming impairments, leading to naming improvements in trained pictures as well as generalization to untrained pictures and untrained lexical tasks incorporating semantic processing (e.g., written naming). Hillis also reported that the semantic distinctions treatment was more effective than a cuing hierarchy treatment in her patient.

Another type of semantic treatment, developed on the basis of cognitive theories of how semantic representations are structured, is semantic feature analysis (SFA) training (see Boyle, 2001, for a recent review). In SFA, clinicians teach patients to use a viewed matrix of printed cue words (e.g., function, properties, category, etc.) displayed in front of them to assist in retrieving semantic information about a target picture along with its name. Boyle (2001) reviewed four studies employing the SFA treatment and reported that SFA training implemented over a number of sessions leads to improved naming of trained pictures and generalization of the semantic feature strategy to improve retrieval of names of some untrained pictures as well.

PHONOLOGIC TREATMENTS

The same phonologic output representation is activated in the course of oral reading, word repetition, and oral picture naming. Capitalizing on this phonologic relationship, some naming treatment studies have used repeated practice with oral word reading or word repetition to improve word retrieval abilities (Miceli et al., 1996; Mitchum &

Berndt, 1994). The effects of word repetition treatment, however, may not be as great or as lasting as other comprehension or cuing hierarchy treatments for individuals with naming impairments (Greenwald et al., 1995; Raymer & Ellsworth, 2002).

Robson et al. (1998) used a phonologic training scheme that paralleled the procedures applied in semantic comprehension treatment. In their phonologic treatment, they required their patient to make judgments about phonologic information for target words corresponding to pictures or descriptions, including the number of syllables in the word and the initial phoneme of the word. Their subject demonstrated improvement in retrieving words trained with this strategy and showed some generalization of the process when naming untrained pictures.

Finally, Spencer and colleagues (2000) described a treatment that incorporates both semantic and phonologic information during the course of training. In their semantic category rhyme therapy (SCRT), the patient looked at a target picture and was given the name of the appropriate semantic category and a rhyming word. Additional phonemic and graphemic cues were provided as necessary to elicit the correct naming response. Once the correct word was elicited, the patient practiced writing and pronouncing the name of the word. Their treatment was effective for improving word retrieval for trained words, and, as training proceeded across several categories, led to improvements for untrained words as well.

Some investigations have directly contrasted the effects of different restitutive treatments within individuals to determine the most effective strategy. Howard et al. (1985) compared the effects of semantic and phonologic comprehension treatments in a group of individuals with naming impairments and reported an advantage of semantic over phonologic treatment. Ennis (1999), using single subject experimental studies, also contrasted semantic and phonologic treatments for noun retrieval in the same individuals and reported that effects of semantic treatment surpassed phonologic treatment in two subjects with primarily phonologic word-retrieval impairments, whereas the reverse pattern of effects, phonologic greater than semantic training, was evident in a third patient with semantic and phonologic impairment. Raymer and Ellsworth (2002) used a similar single subject paradigm in which they contrasted phonologic and semantic training for one subject with selective verb-retrieval impairment and reported that both treatments led to improvements for trained verbs and increases in the use of grammatical sentences incorporating those trained verbs.

In summary, a number of studies have reported that restitutive treatments, whether incorporating semantic or phonologic information, are effective in improving word retrieval for trained words. The best restitutive treatments appear to be those that combine semantic and phonologic information during the course of training to encourage word retrieval in a manner compatible with the normal lexical processes (Drew & Thompson, 1999). Little direct correlation is evident between the type of word-retrieval impairment (semantic or phonologic) and the most effective type of treatment, however (Hillis, 1993). Either semantic or phonologic treatment seems to improve word retrieval in individuals with either semantic or phonologic impairments, an observation that is compatible with the interactive nature of semantic and phonologic processing in the course of word retrieval during picture naming tasks (Raymer & Ellsworth, 2002).

Vicariative Naming Treatments

READING AND WRITING

Some patients with oral naming impairments, particularly those with dysfunction related to the phonologic output lexicon, may nonetheless have available some knowledge about a word's spelling. In turn, this spelling information may be used to vicariatively generate the spoken word through a phonemic self-cuing process. Patients have been taught to type letters corresponding to target words into a computer, which in turn generated the initial phoneme of the target word (Nickels, 1992). One patient was trained to write the first letters of target words and then to pronounce those sounds as a self-generated phonemic cue (Bastiaanse et al., 1996). Over time this written cuing technique led to improved naming for the trained words, even in the absence of the computer- or self-generated phonemic cues.

Hillis's (1998) remarkable patient spontaneously used retained print-to-sound conversion abilities when word retrieval failure occurred. The patient's naming errors were regularized pronunciations of intended words (e.g., "/sup/" for "cup"). Listeners familiar with this counterproductive strategy could often translate back to a plausible spelling to figure out the word the patient was attempting to say. To circumvent this awkward strategy, Hillis taught her patient to pronounce regularized spellings of common words with exceptional spellings (e.g., "kup" for "cup"). Improvements in oral reading also generalized to pronunciations in oral naming of the same words.

GESTURE

Individuals often spontaneously attempt to use pantomimes when naming failures occur, sometimes leading to correct production of the words. Luria (1970) was perhaps the first to suggest the use of "intersystemic gestural reorganization," using intact gesture abilities to activate the impaired language system. Cognitive models of praxis processing recognize the interactive nature of lexical and praxis systems (Rothi et al., 1997), suggesting that gesture may be a useful vicariative means to mediate word retrieval. In verbal plus gestural training for picture naming, the patient practices an appropriate gesture in isolation, the target word in isolation, and the gesture and word in combination. With repeated practice, the goal is for the gesture to facilitate retrieval of the target word. A number of studies have reported improved naming abilities in conjunction with gestural training (Pashek, 1998; Rose & Douglas, 2001). A positive outcome of verbal plus gestural training is that those who do not improve word retrieval often improve their use of gestures as a compensatory communication strategy. Even patients with severe limb apraxia, who may not be able to use pantomime as a viable communication mode before training, can improve their use of recognizable, communicative gestures following verbal plus gestural training (Raymer & Maher, 2001).

Crosson and his colleagues (Crosson, 2000; Richards et al., 2002) have used nonmeaningful limb movements rather than pantomimes during word-retrieval training. Patients are taught to perform a complex reaching and turning movement of the left arm in left space in an effort to engage prefrontal systems during the process of word retrieval. Participation in this "intentional" training has led to improved naming abilities in some individuals with nonfluent forms of aphasia. The advantage of nonsymbolic limb movements in training compared to pantomimes is that these movements can be implemented with any word, regardless of meaning. On the other hand, a benefit of pantomime training is that even when word-retrieval abilities do not improve, general communication abilities often are enhanced through the use of pantomimes.

Naming Training in Context

A number of treatment techniques have been shown to be effective in improving naming abilities in individuals with aphasia, as indicated by improvement observed in structured lexical tasks, usually picture naming. However, a problem with many of these techniques is that treatment effects may not generalize to improvements in word retrieval in natural conversational settings (Raymer & Rothi, 2001). Therefore, it is incumbent upon clinicians to incorporate training techniques to promote generalization of naming improvements to conversational discourse. For example, training with the Promoting Aphasics' Communicative Effectiveness (PACE) protocol can be a useful means to implement strategies and techniques in a natural communicative context

to improve naming (Li et al., 1988). Using a barrier activity, the patient must indicate to the clinician what concept is conveyed on a picture card. If the patient is unable to think of the exact word, strategies can be attempted to relate information verbally (e.g., description of the physical characteristics, function, category, or associated concepts), or using alternative modes of communication (e.g., gesture, writing, drawing).

Another method to enhance generalization of naming treatment effects is through role playing (Linebaugh, 1997). Conversational topics may be selected related to the concepts included in trained picture naming stimuli. Level of difficulty can be manipulated as conversational interchanges move from prepared monologues to structured dialogues between clinician and patient, to less structured conversations with familiar and unfamiliar listeners. Conversational interactions can be videotaped and analyzed for instances of naming breakdown, and the clinician and patient can discuss strategies that might have been attempted to alleviate the communication disruption (Boles, 1998). Caregivers can be advised of ways to gently aid the individual with aphasia as moments of word-retrieval difficulty arise.

Finally, participation in group aphasia treatment can be a valuable means of moving from individual didactic naming training to conversational use of specific training vocabulary and strategies. Multiple individuals with aphasia all can benefit in the group therapy environment. The effective use of a word retrieval strategy by one person with aphasia provides an excellent model for others who might need to attempt a similar strategy to improve their communication interactions. Individuals in the group can suggest to one another useful information or strategies to convey an intended message.

Pharmacologic Treatment

In addition to the variety of behavioral interventions for naming, recent years have seen a surge in interest in pharmacologic interventions for individuals with aphasia and word-retrieval impairments. Researchers have investigated a number of pharmacologic agents whose effects target distinct neurotransmitters and neural regions. Because cholinergic input seems to play a critical role in left hemisphere temporal and thalamic functioning, some investigators have explored effects of cholinergic drugs for word retrieval. Administration of cholinergic agents physostigmine (Jacobs et al., 1996) and bifemelane (Tanaka et al., 1997) has been associated with improved word-retrieval skills in some patients with fluent aphasia. In contrast, the left frontal lobe depends on dopaminergic input for proficient functioning. The dopaminergic agonist bromocriptine has been administered to a number of patients with nonfluent aphasia following left frontal lesions, and some (though not all) studies have documented improvements in word-retrieval accuracy and reduction of pausing in selected patients (Gold et al., 2000; Raymer et al., 2001).

Finally, the noradrenergic agonist dextroamphetamine, which has a general influence on neural plasticity, has been examined for its effects on recovery of aphasia. Walker-Batson and her colleagues (2001) have reported positive effects of amphetamine for aphasia recovery in general. However, McNeil and colleagues (1997), in a double-blind controlled study, examined effects of amphetamine for naming abilities specifically, and reported no differences between behavioral treatment administered with and without pharmacologic treatment. In general, the evidence for most pharmacologic interventions is lacking in well-designed studies contrasting behavioral and pharmacologic interventions. Although some findings are positive, until adequate studies are completed, clinicians should maintain caution in advocating pharmacologic interventions for word-retrieval impairments.

Conclusion

Naming impairments are a common manifestation of left hemisphere brain damage. The cognitive and neural bases of naming breakdown vary across individuals with aphasia, and characteristic patterns of impairment can be observed depending on whether semantic or phonologic stages of naming are disrupted. The purpose of naming assessment is to reveal the cognitive bases and the lexical characteristics of naming failure. This specified information allows the clinician to select rational treatment interventions and stimuli to most directly impact on the naming and communication abilities of the individual with aphasia. Patients should be reminded, however, that even following successful intervention, word-retrieval difficulties are likely to persist.

Acknowledgments

Preparation of this chapter was supported by a grant from the National Institutes of Health (P50 DC03888-01A1) to the University of Florida (subcontract to Old Dominion University), and a Department of Veterans Affairs Rehabilitation Research and Development grant to the Brain Rehabilitation Research Center, Gainesville, Florida.

References

Alexander, M.P., Hiltbrunner, B. & Fischer, R.S. (1989). Distributed Anatomy of Transcortical Sensory Aphasia. *Archives of Neurology, 46*, 885–892.

Bastiaanse, R., Bosje, J. & Franssen, M. (1996). Deficit-Oriented Treatment of Word-Finding Problems: Another Replication. *Aphasiology, 10*, 363–383.

Best, W. (2000). Category-Specific Semantic Deficits. In W. Best, K. Bryan, & J. Maxim (Eds.), *Semantic Processing: Theory and Practice* (pp. 80–107). London: Whurr.

Boles, L. (1998). Conversational Discourse Analysis as a Method for Evaluating Progress in Aphasia: A Case Report. *Journal of Communication, Disorders, 31*, 261–273.

Boyle, M. (2001). Semantic Feature Analysis: The Evidence for Treating Lexical Impairments in Aphasia. *ASHA Special Interest Division 2: Neurophysiology and Neurogenic Speech and Language Disorders, 11*, 23–28.

Caramazza, A. (2000). Aspects of Lexical Access: Evidence from Aphasia. In: Y. Grodzinsky, L. Shapiro & D. Swinney (Eds.), *Language and the Brain* (pp. 203–228). San Diego: Academic Press.

Caramazza, A. & Hillis, A.E. (1990). Where Do Semantic Errors Come From? *Cortex, 26*, 95–122.

Caramazza, A. & Hillis, A.E. (1991). Lexical Organization of Nouns and Verbs in the Brain. *Nature, 349*, 788–790.

Caramazza, A. & Shelton, J.R. (1998). Domain-Specific Knowledge Systems in the Brain: The Animate-Inanimate Distinction. *Journal of Cognitive Neuroscience, 10*, 1–34.

Collins, M.J. (1997). Global Aphasia. In: L.L. LaPointe (Ed.), *Aphasia and Related Neurogenic Language Disorders* (2nd ed., pp. 133–150). New York: Thieme.

Crosson B. (2000). Systems that Support Language Processes: Attention. In: S.E. Nadeau, L.J.G. Rothi & B. Crosson (Eds.), *Aphasia and Language: Theory to Practice* (pp. 372–397). New York: Guilford Press.

Damasio, H., Grabowski, T.J., Tranel, D., Ponto, L.L.B., Hichwa, R.D. & Damasio, A.R. (2001). Neural Correlates of Naming Actions and of Naming Spatial Relations. *NeuroImage, 13*, 1053–1064.

Damasio, A.R. & Tranel, D. (1993). Nouns and Verbs Are Retrieved with Differently Distributed Neural Systems. *Proceedings of the National Academy of Sciences, USA, 90*, 4957–4960.

Drew, R.L., & Thompson, C.K. (1999). Model-Based Semantic Treatment for Naming Deficits in Aphasia. *Journal of Speech, Language, & Hearing Research, 42*, 972–989.

Dronkers, N.F., & Ludy, C.A. (1998). Brain Lesion Analysis in Clinical Research. In: B. Stemmer & H.A. Whitaker (Eds.), *Handbook of Neurolinguistics* (pp. 173–187). San Diego: Academic Press.

Druks, J. & Masterson, J. (1999). *An Object and Action Naming Battery*. New York: Psychology Press.

Ennis, M.R. (1999). Semantic Versus Phonological Aphasia Treatments for Anomia: A Within Subject Experimental Design. Unpublished dissertation, University of Florida.

Ennis, M.R. (2001). Comprehension Approaches for Word Retrieval Training in Aphasia. *ASHA Special Interest Division 2: Neurophysiology and Neurogenic Speech and Language Disorders, 11*, 18–22.

Farah, M.J. (1990). *Visual Agnosia*. Cambridge, MA: MIT Press.

Foundas, A.L., Daniels, S.K. & Vasterling, J.J. (1998). Anomia: Case Studies with Lesion Localization. *Neurocase, 4*, 35–43.

Gold, M., VanDam, D. & Silliman, E.R. (2000). An Open-Label Trial of Bromocriptine in Nonfluent Aphasia: A Qualitative Analysis of Word Storage and Retrieval. *Brain and Language, 74*, 141–156.

Goodglass, H., & Wingfield, A. (1997). Word-Finding Deficits in Aphasia: Brain-Behavior Relations and Clinical Symptomatology. In: H. Goodglass & A. Wingfield (Eds.), *Anomia: Neuroanatomical and Cognitive Correlates* (pp. 3–27). San Diego: Academic Press.

Greenwald, M.L., Raymer, A.M., Richardson, M.E. & Rothi, L.J.G. (1995). Contrasting Treatments for Severe Impairments of Picture Naming. *Neuropsychological Rehabilitation, 5*, 17–49.

Hart, J. & Gordon, B. (1990). Delineation of Single-Word Semantic Comprehension Deficits in Aphasia, with Anatomical Correlation. *Annals of Neurology, 27*, 226–231.

Hillis, A.E. (1993). The Role of Models of Language Processing in Rehabilitation of Language Impairments. *Aphasiology, 7*, 5–26.

Hillis, A.E. (1998). Treatment of Naming Disorders: New Issues Regarding Old Therapies. *Journal of the International Neuropsychological Society, 4*, 648–660.

Hillis, A. (2001). The organization of the Lexical System. In: B. Rapp (Ed.), *The Handbook of Cognitive Neuropsychology* (pp. 185–210). Philadelphia: Psychology Press.

Hillis, A.E. & Caramazza, A. (1995a). Cognitive and Neural Mechanisms Underlying Visual and Semantic Processing: Implications from "Optic Aphasia." *Journal of Cognitive Neuroscience, 7*, 457–478.

Hillis, A.E. & Caramazza, A. (1995b). The Compositionality of Lexical Semantic Representations: Clues from Semantic Errors in Object Naming. *Memory, 3*, 333–358.

Hillis, A.E., Rapp, B., Romani, C. & Caramazza, A. (1990). Selective Impairment of Semantics in Lexical Processing. *Cognitive Neuropsychology, 7*, 191–243.

Hillis, A.E., Tuffiash, E., Wityk, R.J. & Barker, P.B. (2002). Regions of Neural Dysfunction Associated with Impaired Naming of Actions and Objects in Acute Stroke. *Cognitive Neuropsychology, 19*, 523–534.

Hinckley, J.J. & Craig, H.K. (1998). Influence of Rate of Treatment on the Naming Abilities of Adults with Chronic Aphasia. *Aphasiology, 12*, 989–1106.

Hirsh, K.W. & Ellis, A.W. (1994). Age of Acquisition and Lexical Processing in Aphasia: A Case Study. *Cognitive Neuropsychology, 11*, 435–458.

Howard, D. & Patterson, K. (1992). *Pyramids and Palm Trees*. Bury St. Edmunds: Thames Valley.

Howard, D., Patterson, K., Franklin, S., Orchard-Lisle, V. & Morton, J. (1985). Treatment of Word Retrieval Deficits in Aphasia. *Brain, 108*, 817–829.

Jacobs, D.H., Shuren, J., Gold, M., Adair, J.C., Bowers, D., Williamson, D.J.G. & Heilman, K.M. (1996). Physostigmine Pharmacotherapy for Anomia. *Neurocase, 2*, 83–91.

Kaplan, E., Goodglass, H. & Weintraub, S. (2000). *Boston Naming Test* (2nd ed.) Philadelphia: Lippincott Williams & Wilkins.

Kay, J., Lesser, R. & Coltheart, M. (1992). *PALPA: Psycholinguistic Assessments of Language Processing in Aphasia*. East Sussex, England: Lawrence Erlbaum.

Kemmerer, D. & Tranel, D. (2000). Verb Retrieval in Brain-Damaged Subjects: 1. Analysis of Stimulus, Lexical, and Conceptual Factors. *Brain and Language, 73*, 347–392.

Kertesz, A., Davidson, W. & McCabe, P. (1998). Primary Progressive Semantic Aphasia: A Case Study. *Journal of the International Neuropsychological Society, 4*, 388–398.

Kohn, S.E., Smith, K.L. & Alexander, M.P. (1996). Differential Recovery from Impairment to the Phonological Lexicon. *Brain and Language, 52*, 129–149.

Li, E.C., Kitselman, K., Dusatko, D. & Spinelli, C. (1988). The Efficacy of PACE in the Remediation of Naming Deficits. *Journal of Communication Disorders, 21*, 491–503.

Linebaugh, C.W. (1997). Lexical Retrieval Problems: Anomia. In: L.L. LaPointe (Ed.), *Aphasia and Related Neurogenic Language Disorders* (pp. 112–132). New York: Thieme.

Luria, A.R. (1970). *Traumatic Aphasia*. Hague: Mouton.

Marshall, J., Pound, C., White-Thomson, M. & Pring, T. (1990). The Use of Picture/Word Matching Tasks to Assist Word Retrieval in Aphasic Patients. *Aphasiology, 4*, 167–184.

McNeil, M.R., Doyle, P.J., Spencer, K.A., Goda, A.J., Flores, D. & Small, S.L. (1997). A Double-Blind, Placebo-Controlled Study of Pharmacological and Behavioural Treatment of Lexical-Semantic Deficits in Aphasia. *Aphasiology, 11*, 385–400.

Miceli, G., Amitrano, A., Capasso, R. & Caramazza, A. (1996). The Treatment of Anomia Resulting from Output Lexical Damage: Analysis of Two Cases. *Brain and Language, 52*, 150–174.

Miceli, G., Giustollisi, L. & Caramazza, A. (1991). The Interaction of Lexical and Non-Lexical Processing Mechanisms: Evidence from Anomia. *Cortex, 27*, 57–80.

Mitchum, C. & Berndt, R.S. (1994). Verb Retrieval and Sentence Construction: Effects of Targeted Intervention. In: M.J. Riddoch & G. Humphreys (Eds.), *Cognitive Neuropsychology and Cognitive Rehabilitation* (pp. 317–348). Hove, England: Erlbaum.

Mitchum, C.C., Ritgert, B.A., Sandson, J. & Berndt, R.S. (1990). The Use of Response Analysis in Confrontation Naming. *Aphasiology, 4*, 261–280.

Murray, L. (2000). The Effects of Varying Attentional Demands on the Word Retrieval Skills of Adults with Aphasia, Right Hemisphere Brain Damage, or No Brain Damage. *Brain and Language, 72*, 40–72.

Murtha, S., Chertkow, H., Beauregard, M. & Evans, A. (1999). The Neural Substrate of Picture Naming. *Journal of Cognitive Neuroscience, 11*, 399–423.

Nickels, L. (1992). The Autocue? Self-Generated Phonemic Cues in the Treatment of a Disorder of Reading and Naming. *Cognitive Neuropsychology, 9*, 155–182.

Nickels, L. (1997). *Spoken Word Production and Its Breakdown in Aphasia.* Hove, East Sussex, UK: Psychology Press.

Nickels, L. (2001). Spoken Word Production. In: B. Rapp (Ed.), *The Handbook of Cognitive Neuropsychology* (pp. 291–320). Philadelphia: Psychology Press.

Nickels, L. & Best, W. (1996). Therapy for Naming Disorders (Part II): Specifics, Surprises, and Suggestions. *Aphasiology, 10*, 109–136.

Nickels, L. & Howard, D. (1995). Aphasic Naming: What Matters? *Neuropsychologia, 33*, 1281–1303.

Ochipa, C., Maher, L.M. & Raymer, A.M. (1998). One Approach to the Treatment of Anomia. *ASHA Special Interest Division 2: Neurophysiology and Neurogenic Speech and Language Disorders, 15*, 18–23.

Pashek, G.V. (1998). Gestural Facilitation of Noun and Verb Retrieval in Aphasia: A Case Study. *Brain and Language, 65*, 177–180.

Patterson, J.P. (2001). The Effectiveness of Cueing Hierarchies as a Treatment for Word Retrieval Impairment. *ASHA Special Interest Division 2: Neurophysiology and Neurogenic Speech and Language Disorders, 11*, 11–18.

Raymer, A.M., Bandy, D., Schwartz, R.L., Adair, J.C., Williamson, D.J.G., Rothi, L.J.G. & Heilman, K.M. (2001). Effects of Bromocriptine in a Patient with Crossed Aphasia. *Archives of Physical Medicine and Rehabilitation, 82*, 139–144.

Raymer, A.M. & Berndt, R.S. (1996). Reading Lexically without Semantics: Evidence from Patients with Probable Alzheimer's Disease. *Journal of the International Neuropsychological Society, 2*, 340–349.

Raymer, A.M. & Ellsworth, T.A. (2002). Response to Contrasting Verb Retrieval Treatments: A Case Study. *Aphasiology, 16*, 1031–1045.

Raymer, A.M., Foundas, A.L., Maher, L.M., Greenwald, M.L., Morris, M., Rothi, L.J.G. & Heilman, K.M. (1997a). Cognitive Neuropsychological Analysis and Neuroanatomic Correlates in a Case of Acute Anomia. *Brain and Language, 58*, 137–156.

Raymer, A.M. & Maher, L.M. (2001). Effects of Verbal Plus Gestural Training on Limb Apraxia: A Case Study. *Journal of the International Neuropsychological Society, 7*, 248.

Raymer, A.M., Moberg, P., Crosson, B., Nadeau, S.E. & Rothi, L.J.G. (1997b). Lexical-Semantic Deficits in Two Patients with Dominant Thalamic Infarction. *Neuropsychologia, 35*, 211–219.

Raymer, A.M. & Rothi, L.J.G. (2001). Cognitive Approaches to Impairments of Word Comprehension and Production. In: R. Chapey (Ed.), *Language Intervention Strategies in Aphasia and Related Disorders* (4th ed., pp. 524–550). Philadelphia: Lippincott Williams & Wilkins.

Raymer, A.M., Thompson, C.K., Jacobs, B. & leGrand, H.R. (1993). Phonologic Treatment of Naming Deficits in Aphasia: Model-Based Generalization Analysis. *Aphasiology, 7*, 27–53.

Richards, K., Singletary, F., Koehler, S., Crosson, B. & Rothi, L.J.G. (2002). Treatment of Nonfluent Aphasia Through the Pairing of a Non-Symbolic Movement Sequence and Naming. *Journal of Rehabilitation Research & Development, 39*, 7–16.

Robson, J., Marshall, J., Pring, T. & Chiat, S. (1998). Phonologic Naming Therapy in Jargon Aphasia: Positive but Paradoxical Effects. *Journal of the International Neuropsychological Society, 4*, 675–686.

Rose, M. & Douglas, J. (2001). The Differential Facilitatory Effects of Gesture and Visualization Processes on Object Naming in Aphasia. *Aphasiology, 15*, 977–990.

Rothi, L.J.G. (1995). Behavioral Compensation in the Case of Treatment of Acquired Language Disorders Resulting from Brain Damage. In: R.A. Dixon & L. Mackman (Eds.), *Compensating for Psychological Deficits and Declines: Managing Losses and Promoting Gains* (pp. 219–230). Mahwah, NJ: Lawrence Erlbaum.

Rothi, L.J.G., Ochipa, C. & Heilman, K.M. (1997). A Cognitive Neuropsychological Model of Limb Praxis and Apraxia. In: L.J.G. Rothi & K.M. Heilman (Eds.), *Apraxia: The Neuropsychology of Action* (pp. 29–49). East Sussex, UK: Psychology Press.

Spencer, K.A., Doyle, P.J., McNeil, M.R., Wambaugh, J.L., Park, G. & Carroll, B. (2000). Examining the Facilitative Effects of Rhyme in a Patient with Output Lexicon Damage. *Aphasiology, 14*, 567–584.

Tanaka, Y., Miyazaki, M. & Albert, M.L. (1997). Effects of Increased Cholinergic Activity on Naming in Aphasia. *Lancet, 350*, 116–117.

Thompson, C.K., Lange, K.L., Schneider, S.L. & Shapiro, L.P. (1997). Agrammatic and Non-Brain-Damaged Subjects' Verb and Verb Argument Structure Production. *Aphasiology, 11*, 473–490.

Tranel, D., Damasio, H. & Damasio, A.R. (1997). On the neurology of naming. In: H. Goodglass & A. Wingfield (Eds.), *Anomia: Neuroanatomical and Cognitive Correlates* (pp. 65–90). San Diego: Academic Press.

Walker-Batson, D., Curtis, S., Natarajan, R., Ford, J., Dronkers, N., Salmeron, E., Lai, J., & Unwin, H. (2001). A Double Blind, Placebo-Controlled Study of the Use of Amphetamine in the Treatment of Aphasia. *Stroke, 32*, 2093–2098.

Wilshire, C.E. & Coslett, H.B. (2000). Disorders of Word Retrieval in Aphasia: Theories and Potential Applications. In: S.E. Nadeau, L.J.G. Rothi & B. Crosson (Eds.), *Aphasia and Language: Theory to Practice* (pp. 82–107). New York: Guilford Press.

Zingeser, L.B. & Berndt, R.S. (1988). Grammatical Class and Context Effects in a Case of Pure Anomia: Implications for Models of Language Production. *Cognitive Neuropsychology, 5,* 473–516.

Suggested Readings

Goodglass, H. & Wingfield, A. (Eds.) (1997). *Anomia: Neuroanatomical and Cognitive Correlates.* San Diego: Academic Press.

Hillis, A.E. (2001). Cognitive Neuropsychological Approaches to Rehabilitation of Language Disorders: Introduction. In: R. Chapey (Ed.), *Language Intervention Strategies in Aphasia and Related Disorders* (4th ed., pp. 513–523). Philadelphia: Lippincott Williams & Wilkins.

Nickels, L. (1997). *Spoken Word Production and Its Breakdown in Aphasia.* Hove, East Sussex, UK: Psychology Press.

Rapp, B.C. & Caramazza, A. (1998). Lexical Deficits. In: M.T. Sarno (Ed.), *Acquired Aphasia* (3rd ed., pp. 187–227). San Diego: Academic Press.

Wilshire, C.E. & Coslett, H.B. (2000). Disorders of Word Retrieval in Aphasia: Theories and Potential Applications. In: S.E. Nadeau, L.J.G. Rothi & B. Crosson (Eds.), *Aphasia and Language: Theory to Practice* (pp. 82–107). New York: Guilford Press.

6

Acquired Dyslexias: Reading Disorders Associated with Aphasia

Wanda G. Webb

In a highly technical society such as ours, most of us are inundated daily with written material. Signs are posted everywhere, many without ideographs. There are numerous forms to fill out and written directions to follow for almost every activity. If we desired, we could spend all of our leisure hours reading, with the monumental number of books, magazines, newspapers, and "on-line" or computer-generated reading material available. Thus, the person with an acquired dyslexia, or reading disorder, is at a serious disadvantage in this "age of literacy."

Retraining reading following the onset of acquired dyslexia clearly is the purview of the speech-language pathologist. To be most effective, this therapy must be highly individualized, requiring considerable ingenuity on the part of the clinician. The speech-language pathologist should have knowledge about the normal processes of reading. Evidence from research on teaching reading to normal readers and to persons with developmental dyslexia as well as acquired alexia should be taken into account. The ideas and information presented here are designed to provide background information and a core of treatment principles and suggestions to make the task a little less formidable.

Pathophysiology

Normal Reading Process

To understand what may go wrong in the process of reading, one should have a model of what occurs in normal reading. Marshall (1985) provides a flow diagram and explanation of an information-processing model of reading that breaks down the process into several different components. Recently, Beeson and Hillis (2001) have provided a model of reading that combines several of the components into larger processing stages and allows for a simpler, more "user-friendly" explanation of the complex process of reading single words aloud. It should be noted that most models of reading, even in contemporary literature, deal only with the comprehension and production of single words in reading. Comprehension at the level of connected text is not included. There is limited understanding of this critical step in reading at this point.

The model provided by Beeson and Hillis is modified and presented as a schematic in Fig. 6–1. Included in this schematic are the processes of early visual analysis (EVA) and letter representation (LR). These steps were included in the Marshall (1985) model. As

Written Stimulus

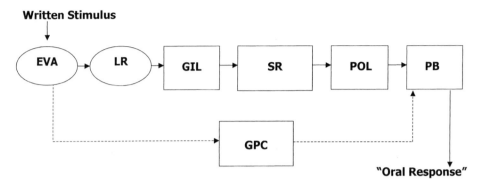

Figure 6–1. Model of processing of single words for oral reading. Visual features of the written stimulus are extracted through early visual analysis (EVA), and then letter representation (LR) processing assigns identities as graphemes to these features. The string of graphemes or letters is then fed to the graphemic input lexicon (GPC) and may be recognized as a familiar word and processed further in semantic representations (SR) where meaning is comprehended. For oral reading, the phonologic output lexicon (POL) is then accessed and graphemes are associated with phonemes. These patterns are held in the phonologic buffer (PB) until the word is pronounced. The dashed line indicates the sublexical route employed when the word is not familiar. The graphemes are processed through grapheme-phoneme conversion (GPC) and then held in the phonologic buffer until ready to be pronounced.

the initial step in reading a word, EVA extracts visual features from the stimulus array. This visual information is analyzed through the LR process and abstract letter identities are assigned. In other words, the visual stimulus is perceived as a grapheme, which is a letter or letter cluster that we associate with a single phoneme. For reading words, the perceived string of letters or graphemes is then fed into the graphemic input lexicon (GIL). It is in this lexicon that we mentally store strings of letters that we recognize as familiar words. In normal reading in which words are automatically processed, the graphemic input lexicon activates semantic representations (SR) in the semantic system and we comprehend the meaning of the word we are reading. If we are reading aloud, the phonologic output lexicon (POL) is accessed. It is believed that the POL is accessed at times even if a person is reading silently. Marshall (1985) conceives that during this process each grapheme is associated with the single phoneme that is its most frequent representation and an articulatory code is assigned. This pattern is held in the phonologic buffer (PB) until we

are ready to read the word aloud (or perhaps subvocally rehearse the word). Marshall labels this as reading through the *lexical route*. It is also known as the *lexical-semantic route*.

For normal readers an encounter with an unfamiliar word means there are no representations in the existing store of the graphemic input lexicon. Because we then cannot use the lexical (GIL to SR) route, we try to sound out the word by using a grapheme-to-phoneme conversion (GPC) (or letter-to-sound) approach. Beeson and Hillis note that this is considered a sublexical or nonlexical route by which reading can be accomplished. We can also use this process to pronounce pseudowords or nonwords (for example, "glaint" or "shanter"). Marshall labeled this form of reading as using the *phonologic route*.

Beyond the Routes

Schneider and Shiffrin (1977) have shown that most readers learn to use both automatic and controlled processing in reading. Automatic processing implies a learned association in long-term memory that occurs with consistent training. It operates in parallel with other simultaneous processes and does not require significant attention. In non–brain-injured persons, most of skilled reading, in terms of word identification and access to meaning, is probably through automatic processing. Controlled processing becomes necessary for new words or for comprehension of difficult text. Controlled processing requires more attention and active cognitive engagement.

Neurological Substrate of Reading

Earlier brain localization theories for reading depended primarily on studying patients with brain damage that impaired reading. The advent of functional magnetic resonance imaging (fMRI) has advanced the knowledge of brain activity during reading. Recent studies have helped shed light on the quest for information regarding neurologic substrates for normal reading.

Speech-language pathologists consider reading to be one of the five primary language modalities, along with listening, speaking, writing, and gesturing. As such, it is well agreed that reading is predominantly a left hemisphere function. All four lobes of the cortex appear to be involved in the process of reading. There is evidence for some participation of the right hemisphere and some subcortical structures also.

The occipital lobe is involved in early visual processing, and the area surrounding the striate cortex is the unimodal association area for visual information. The left fusiform gyrus has been implicated in holding prelexical representations of visual words (Dehaene et al., 2002). Older literature based on lesion data proposed that posterior cerebral infarction with damage to the geniculocalcarine pathways and the splenium of the corpus callosum effectively prevents visual information from an intact right hemisphere from reaching intact language areas in the left hemisphere, resulting in a classic syndrome known as "pure alexia" (or alexia without agraphia). Later studies have reported this syndrome with damage to the left occipital cortex without involvement of the splenium (Behrmann et al., 1990).

The left temporal lobe and the left inferior frontal gyrus have been found to be areas of primary activation during normal reading. Several recent studies support the temporal lobe's importance in reading (Nakada et al., 2001; Roder et al., 2002). The findings of one neuroimaging study (Pugh et al., 2001) seem to summate the findings of other studies, suggesting that skilled word identification in reading is dependent on the functional integrity of two posterior left hemisphere circuits, a dorsal (temporal-parietal) and a ventral (occipital-temporal) circuit.

The left inferior frontal gyrus (IFG) region appears to subserve both semantic and phonologic processing of words and sentences (Fiebach et al., 2002). Study of the functional link with posterior brain areas has supported the hypothesis that ventral/anterior left IFG is important for semantic processing and dorsal/posterior left IFG for phonologic processing (Bokde et al., 2001).

Thus, the current evidence seems to support the involvement in reading of cortical areas that we normally associate with language, the inferior frontal, temporoparietal, and temporo-occipital regions. As we unravel the mysteries of all forms of communication and attempt to provide simple models to explain processes, we should be constantly reminded that the models are quite simplified and often do not include the indirect associative pathways that are involved in most sensory processing. Keller et al. (2001) utilized fMRI to examine lexical and syntactic processes of reading comprehension and manipulated the cognitive demand on each of these processes. Their findings supported the involvement of the left perisylvian language areas, but further demonstrated that the factors studied also affected the activation in a network of left hemisphere areas. The findings imply that comprehension processes in reading may operate on different levels but draw on a shared infrastructure of cognitive resources. Many brain regions may contribute to more than one comprehension process. This study and others also show some engagement of the right hemisphere during difficult comprehension tasks

(Kircher et al., 2001). Thus, it must be acknowledged that problems with comprehension of written material can occur without specific damage to primary processing areas. Damage to cortical and subcortical association pathways, as may occur, for example, in traumatic brain injury, may result in difficulty with attention, reasoning, and/or memory. Any one of these difficulties could have devastating effects on functional reading, especially for the more complex comprehension tasks.

Nature and Differentiating Features of Acquired Dyslexias

As is typical with acquired language disorders, the symptomatology of acquired dyslexia is varied. Two approaches have been taken in attempts to classify these disorders and to differentiate among patterns of breakdown.

Traditional classifications have been emphasized by Benson (1979). In this classification system, reading disturbance is broken into two main categories: *alexia without agraphia* and *alexia with agraphia*. Alexia with agraphia can be further broken down into *aphasic alexia* and *agraphic alexia*.

Since 1973 when Marshall and Newcombe published an article on the psycholinguistic approach to studying acquired dyslexias, there has been great interest in looking for patterns of breakdown in reading. Primarily assessed through oral reading tasks, three major psycholinguistic classifications of reading disorders have been identified: deep dyslexia, surface dyslexia, and phonologic alexia. Disorders of both the traditional and the psycholinguistic classifications are described briefly in Table 6–1. See Kirshner (2002) and Greenwald (2000) for a more in-depth discussion of the symptomatology of these disorders.

Thus, there are various ways to look at the acquired dyslexias and to classify them. Classifications interrelate and individuals with acquired reading disorder may exhibit features of more than one category. More important than classifying the disorder is the correct identification of the deficits causing the difficulty with reading and the selection of appropriate treatment methods to address these deficits.

Evaluation

It is critical that the clinician realize that all of the acquired dyslexias affect the *comprehension* of written material in some way, and this is the primary question in evaluation and the primary target in treatment. Though assessment may be accompanied by the use of many oral reading tasks, the extent or severity of the alexia is measured by the effect on reading comprehension. In all of the acquired reading disorders, comprehension is impaired whether it be from inaccuracy of word identification, difficulty with comprehension of meaning carried by syntax, inability to remember and analyze what was read, or just because reading is so slow and laborious.

Always obtain a "literacy history" through interviewing the client or family regarding reading skills and the client's interest in reading. It is not feasible to teach the client skills that were not obtained premorbidly, and treatment will not be successful if the client has little interest in relearning reading.

A full language evaluation with assessment of all modalities usually is necessary. Strengths that are found in other modalities can be capitalized upon in treatment. We need to know if the lexical-semantic system is poorly organized across modalities or limited to written input only. For clients who seem to have difficulty reading single words, further assessment involving cross-modality matching (words to pictures or auditory stimuli) is needed using similar words as are used in evaluation of reading. Oral naming across different tasks (identifying words from pictures, associated sounds, oral spelling, description, etc.) should be assessed also. If the oral naming problem is limited only to the written word or is relatively poorer in comparison, the lexical and/or phonologic processing of written words is implicated.

When reading is targeted as a treatment modality, the clinician should gather more

Table 6–1. Disorders of the Traditional and the Psycholinguistic Classifications

Type of Disorder	Also Known as	Defining Characteristics	Possible Physiology
Alexia without agraphia	Pure alexia	Normal or nearly normal oral language and writing; letter-by-letter reading strategy; good comprehension of spelled words	Impaired access to graphemic input lexicon through normal route
Aphasic alexia (associated with Wernicke's aphasia		Usually parallels severity of auditory comprehension deficit, though there may be a modality bias	For both, likely impaired representations in graphemic input lexicon and/or impairment of semantic representations
Aphasic alexia (associated with Broca's aphasia)	"third alexia"; frontal alexia	"Whole word" reading strategy. Comprehension of contentives relatively good; obtaining meaning carried by syntax difficult Resembles deep dyslexia	
Agraphic alexia	Alexia with agraphia	Difficulty with letter and word identification as well as difficulty with all writing tasks	Impairment of access to and representations within the graphemic input lexicon and impairment of semantic representations
Deep dyslexia		Errors semantically related to target; unable to read pseudowords; little effect of length or spelling regularity; pronounced effect of frequency, part of speech and imageability	Disruption of semantic representations and impaired grapheme-to-phoneme conversion Phonemic output lexicon may be impaired also
Surface dyslexia	Surface alexia	Errors phonologically related to target Pronounced effect of spelling regularity	Impairment of access to graphemic input lexicon or of representations within
Phonologic alexia	Phonologic dyslexia	Unable to read pseudowords and difficulty with low-frequency words	Impairment of grapheme-to-phoneme conversion

in-depth information than an aphasia battery can yield. It is not enough to know that a person cannot read even single words or does not answer paragraph comprehension questions correctly after reading. The clinician must have a good idea of what is interfering with word recognition or comprehension of meaning. Beyond the language skills, there are factors that influence comprehension, such as knowledge base and cognitive resources of the reader. Questions must be answered regarding such things as attention and ability to access information not directly given in the text (i.e., inference). Testing of higher-level cognitive functions is recommended for the client who will be reading beyond a sentence level.

For all clients with acquired alexia, it is advisable to assess single-word reading with stimuli organized in word lists that vary features such as frequency, concreteness, spelling regularity, word length, etc. Sentences with homophones should be tested (for example: "She was dirty and there were tears in her clothing" vs. "She was sad and there were tears in her eyes"). Word/nonword lists for lexical decision tasks should also be included in the evaluation. The use of such tasks allows the clinician to establish a theory about the level at which processing begins to break down. A particular type of reading disorder, as laid out in Table 6–1, might be identified. Though the clinician could design word lists to include these features, there are also lists available that have been used for these tasks. The Psycholinguistic Assessments of Language Processing in Aphasia (PALPA) (Kay et al., 1972) contains word lists that are useful for this purpose. Rothi and Moss (1985), who designed and reported on a reading battery called the Battery of Adult Reading Function, use word lists divided into regular words (follow regular phoneme-grapheme conversion), rule-governed words (e.g., "marriage," "debt"), irregular words ("tomb," "shoes"), functor words, and nonsense words. This battery is unpublished. A previously unpublished list from the Johns Hopkins University (JHU) Dyslexia Battery has now been made available by Beeson and Hillis (2001).

Errors should be transcribed and categorized. Typical error types are: visual confusions ("bear" and "bean"), semantic confusions ("plane" and "jet"), derived errors ("wonder" and "wonderful"), regularization errors ("plaid" and "played"), and errors of grapheme-to-phoneme conversion ("Pete" and "pet"). No response and successful and unsuccessful corrections also should be noted. Timing should be noted for tasks of differentiating words from nonwords (lexical decision). Letter naming, grapheme-to-phoneme conversion, grapheme parsing (breaking words down into smaller units of sound), and sound blending may need to be tested, assessing processing at the nonlexical level. This route may be much stronger and could be used in treatment efforts. It is also vital to know if the client has significant impairment in the ability to use this type of processing.

The evaluation of the acquired dyslexias has not been given much emphasis in commercially available tests for brain-injured adults. The Reading Comprehension Battery for Aphasia (RCBA-2; LaPointe & Horner, 1998) is one of the few tests available with subtests that were carefully designed according to research findings concerning reading. It uses silent reading in all of the primary assessment tasks because it is designed for measuring comprehension. There are also supplementary oral reading tasks included to help analyze the nature of the reading impairment. Initial assessment at the sentence or short paragraph level can be done relatively well using the RCBA. The sentence-to-picture matching tasks are sufficiently complex to be assured that the client is able to process information at the simple and complex sentence level. The functional reading test of the RCBA is useful also. If the client can read the questions regarding the functional task, it is an indication that sentence comprehension is somewhat functional. If the client fails the functional task item itself, the clinician may want to read the question/directive aloud to make sure that the directive itself was not the problem. The client may be able to recognize how many minutes to cook a frozen vegetable when actually doing the task, but may not be able to comprehend the directive on the test that says to point to how many minutes to cook the vegetable.

The clinician evaluating reading should note that research on tests for reading in aphasia has shown that comprehension questions concerning short paragraphs were often answered correctly by both normal and aphasic subjects who had not even read the passages questioned (Nicholas et al., 1986; Rand et al., 1990). The RCBA was found to be the most passage-dependent of any of the tests or aphasia batteries evaluated in the Rand et al. study.

If the client can comprehend at a simple sentence/short paragraph level, the comprehension of longer text should be evaluated. This is usually done by answering multiple-choice questions concerning a written passage, by providing a word to fill in a blank placed within the text (the cloze procedure), or by retelling the narrative or performing a procedure written in the text. The Woodcock Reading Mastery Tests (Woodcock, 1998) contain useful measures at the paragraph and word level and are normed on adult readers. Tests from educational achievement testing may also be useful, although they can be difficult to access because they are usually group-administered tests. Informal reading inventories may be used to try to predict at what reading level (usually given in grade level) the person may fairly accurately comprehend connected text. The Slosson Oral Reading Test-Revised (Slosson & Nicholson, 1990) is a test of oral word reading that may assist in predicting reading level by using only word lists. The Burns-Roe Informal Reading Inventory (Roe & Burns, 1999) provides an inventory based on word recognition and paragraph comprehension. For more comprehensive testing, the Degrees of Reading Power-Revised (1995) is one of the better-designed tests for reading achievement. The most important information to be gained from any testing is where comprehension breaks down and what factors contribute to the breakdown. The design of these tests is such that the vocabulary and context gradually and systematically increases, and this design is helpful.

For those patients who can read at a paragraph level, the literature on the treatment of children and adults with developmental dyslexia is relatively convincing that the clinician should evaluate the patient's comprehension of longer text. To implement a more valid and helpful assessment, the clinician should have on hand many examples of reading passages at different grade levels. It is recommended that each one be ~500 words in length, as research has shown that the quality of the reading errors begins to change after the first 200 words, when the reader begins to develop meaning (Weaver, 1988). Therefore, it is preferable to ignore the errors that occur in the first 200 words of the text in this type of task. The passage should be complete in itself, that is, a story, a textbook chapter, an article, etc. A story should have a strong plot and an identifiable underlying theme. All material should use natural rather than stilted language. It is imperative that the reading material be something that the patient can understand and relate to, but it must be material that is novel to the reader. The most efficient way to gather such materials would probably be to enlist the aid of a curriculum librarian at an educational institution. The lengthier passages are harder to find for the lower grade levels. It is preferable to use adult literacy training materials such as those available through Laubach Literacy or Jamestown Education.

The client is asked to read the passage aloud, if possible. This is tape-recorded and then an error or "miscue" analysis is later done. This analysis documents omission, insertion, and reversal of words as well as repetition of a word or phrase when it is done apparently for reflection or for getting a "running start." The miscue should be analyzed by looking at whether it went with the preceding context or the following context, whether it preserved the essential meaning, and whether the error was corrected or meaning-preserving. Some errors result in no loss of meaning and no significant effect on comprehension.

Following the reading, the client should be asked to retell what was read, pretending the clinician has never read it. If this is not possible because of verbal limitations, a question-and-answer format with multiple-choice questions might be necessary. It is not a time to focus on insignificant details. Although the miscue or error analysis provides the clinician with information about how well the reader seems to comprehend during reading, the retelling gives an indication of how well the reader can remember and interpret what was read. The clinician may probe further and ask more verbal clients to use advanced reasoning by hypothesizing, explaining cause/effect relationships, or relating the story to themselves and situations they have experienced. Questioning or probing should assess inferential comprehension because subtle reading and cognitive deficits may be revealed by failure on inferential comprehension tasks.

Some clients will not comprehend well simply because they are reading aloud and are struggling too much with the verbalization or are accustomed only to silent reading. For these clients it will be necessary to do an oral reading for the miscue analysis and retelling as well as to select another comparable passage for silent reading and retelling. Memory and interpretation would then be assessed primarily from silent reading.

Treatment

There is a burgeoning literature of clinical descriptions of cases of acquired dyslexia and consequent hypotheses concerning the reading process and brain function. There is not, however, a vast literature on treatment of the acquired dyslexias. Most of the clinical research done in this area comes from single case studies, which indicates, perhaps, how variably the disorder manifests itself.

A special caution regarding visual deficits in these clients should be included here. Reading should be physically facilitated by making certain the print size is large enough, the material is placed in the visual field correctly, and there are no distractions. The person with acquired alexia may present as a severely impaired reader with visual perceptual or other visual deficits, such as neglect, and treatment of these problems may take precedence. The occupational therapist can often provide great assistance. There are also workbooks and computer software that may provide activities to target these areas. Heeringa (2002) has recently organized a manual addressing vision and near vision impairments that may result after traumatic brain injury (TBI) or stroke. The manual provides highly useful assessment tools, treatment strategies, and exercises for these types of deficits. It also provides excellent background information on visual processing and the breakdowns that may occur after trauma to the brain.

Treatment for acquired reading disorders is usually a long, arduous process and, as previously indicated, the client must be motivated strongly and committed to the objectives. To regain the ability to read, the client must read as much as possible; therefore, a commitment of time and effort is essential.

Specific Treatment Tasks

Treatment strategies for improving comprehension at the connected text level are emphasized in most discussions on treatment. However, clients cannot begin to read connected text without some ability to read at a single-word level. Much of what has been written concerning treatment of acquired alexia targets the recognition, comprehension, and oral naming of single words. It is crucial that analysis of single-word reading be done if there is any problem with oral word reading. It may be quite beneficial to design a treatment program targeting accurate reading of words. Some clients may be able to comprehend sentences, paragraphs, and longer text, once helped to access single words for reading.

Beeson and Hillis (2000) present an excellent discussion of treatment methods designed to target impairments in various reading process components (Fig. 6–1). Treatment suggestions are summarized here, but the reader is referred to Beeson and Hillis for more in-depth information on these techniques.

If it appears that the client's difficulty is at the level of failure to recognize a string of letters as a familiar word, yet the client can call the name of the individual letters, then the impairment is likely due to impaired access to the graphemic input lexicon. Such clients may be the ones with alexia without agraphia. Treatment methods that may improve access include brief exposure to whole words with the task being to make a decision about the word (example, "Is it a real word" or "Is it clothing?"). The success of this approach has been variable (Rothi et al., 1998). The clinician can also use brief exposure with a core vocabulary of semantically based words and continue to drill the client on recognition of these words, not allowing time for letter-by-letter reading. Over time, the person may become able to recognize many of the words by sight and expand the vocabulary. Beeson (1998) found a technique called multiple oral reading (Moyer, 1979) to be useful in improving whole word reading. This technique involves repeated readings of the same material, with the reading being done aloud.

It appears that the representations in the graphemic input lexicon are impaired or degraded in many of the clients with reading disorders. Depending on such features as familiarity, imageability, length, and frequency of occurrence, some words are recognized. However, others that were once easily recognized are now difficult. In normal reading when this difficulty is encountered, the sublexical route would be accessed for grapheme-to-phoneme conversion, that is, the reader would attempt to sound it out. For many clients this route is also impaired and letter-to-sound conversion must be targeted in treatment. Training may be done to help the client produce the appropriate phoneme for letters and digraphs that are common in English. Hillis (1993) trained letter-to-sound conversion by using nonsense words as training items and incorporated a technique that established an association between easily pronounced key words and specific graphemes (example: using the client's name *Sharon* to cue the [sh]). Improvement was found in trained and untrained words with both regular and irregular spellings.

Clients with milder impairment and retained ability for new learning may be able to learn a few phonic rules to assist in pronunciation of new words. May and Elliott (1973) conclude that only a few phonic rules are consistent enough or cover enough words to warrant spending valuable time when teaching children to read. These consistent rules are:

1. The "c rule." When *c* comes just before *a*, *o*, or *u*, it usually has the /k/ sound. Otherwise it usually has an /s/ sound.
2. The "g rule." When *g* comes at the end of words or just before *a*, *o*, or *u*, it sounds like /g/. Otherwise it has the /dz/ sound. *Get*, *give*, *begin*, and *girl* are important exceptions.
3. The VC pattern. In either a word or syllable, a single vowel letter followed by a letter, digraph, or blend usually represents a short vowel sound.
4. The VV pattern. In a word or syllable containing a vowel digraph, the first letter of the digraph usually represents a long vowel sound and the second is usually silent. This is fairly reliable for *ee, oa, ay, ea,* and *ai* but not as reliable for others.
5. The VCE pattern. In one-syllable words containing two vowels, one of which is a final *e*, the first vowel usually represents a long vowel and the final *e* is silent.
6. The CV pattern. When there is only one vowel letter in a word or syllable and it comes at the end, it usually represents a long vowel.
7. The "r rule." The letter *r* usually modifies the short or long sound of the preceding vowel.

If these are the only rules thought to be consistent enough to teach children, then it seems that we might limit our teaching to brain-injured patients also, at least initially. If the patient seems to be having success at learning rules such as these, a more traditional approach or a modified approach to teaching consonant sounds and then vowel sounds may be implemented.

Even clients with less severe impairment often have difficulty reading functor or other particular categories of words, such as verbs. Friedman et al. (2002) used paired associate learning in a rehabilitation program for two patients who could not access the phonologic route to learn now unfamiliar words. Employing a "reorganization approach," difficult words were paired with picturable homophones (example: "knows" with "nose") or near-homophone (example: "of" with "oven"). After training, their patients were able to achieve 90% accuracy on the targeted sets of words. Generalization to untrained words did not occur, however. Despite the lack of generalization the use of this approach may be helpful to train words that are critical to a reader's functional vocabulary.

In the reading of connected text, the reader should always use a strategy that allows for continued flow of reading. If a word cannot be pronounced but this failure does not reduce overall comprehension of the passage, the reader should just continue rather than struggle. This would be true, for example, if the word were a character's name or the name of a particular city or animal. If "what's-its-name" or "blank" could be inserted and the meaning unchanged, reading should continue. On the other hand, the reader does need a way to decode the word that carries more linguistic weight.

Targeting Comprehension

As stated previously, it is possible that reading of text may be reestablished by training oral reading of single words. Because of the damage to the language system as a whole, it is frequently necessary to go beyond this and directly target comprehension. The following sections give suggestions for working with clients with various degrees of reading impairment. Reading comprehension should be a generative process for understanding. There should be a cognitive interaction with the material. At all levels of training, opportunity for some type of additional interaction with what is being read is important.

The Severely Impaired Reader

For the person demonstrating very poor reading comprehension even at the single-word level, the basic goal is *survival reading skill*. If possible this patient should understand a reading vocabulary containing a functional vocabulary for signs, foods, financial transactions, TV, emergency procedures, etc. The most useful vocabulary list would be that designed with maximum input from the client and family members or friends, so that it is individualized to the reader's needs. The various methodologies for retraining oral reading of single words would be employed at this level to establish such a vocabulary. In selecting or designing the vocabulary or content, the properties or features of words that are known to have an effect on recognition and comprehension should be considered. These features are length, part of speech, frequency of occurrence, concreteness, imageability, and both linguistic and experiential familiarity. Every opportunity should be given for cognitive and functional interaction with this vocabulary. If real-life experiences can be designed to use the targeted words, it should be done. The vocabulary should continue to be increased as the client reaches 90% comprehension when a wide variety of choices are given.

If the more severely involved clients are able to develop a fairly extensive single-word functional reading vocabulary, they may be able to go further and begin to combine words for reading phrases and sentences. The clinician should make use of published materials written for adult literacy training. There are several that emphasize survival reading skills and functional activities of reading.

The Moderately Impaired Reader

The client who can read at the sentence level, even though poorly, is a better candidate for improving reading because there is obviously better underlying skill. This person should be reading contextual material in therapy. The initial assessment should provide information on the grade level at which the patient can read at an *instructional level*, that is, comprehension is at ~45 to 55% without help from someone. The readability of any text that is not graded can be determined individually by using the Fry Readability Scale (Fry, 1977). Microsoft Word gives a readability statistic for any document saved in its format. Knowing the readability is valuable because the client can choose the reading materials while the clinician determines the difficulty level and, perhaps, uses the information to sequence their presentation.

The client will need more work at the sentence level, increasing the complexity of the sentences to be comprehended. Some individuals may need therapy time concentrated on comprehension of meaning carried by different syntactical constructions and the accompanying semantic indicators. One useful treatment task for this involves giving the client sentences that contain syntactic and/or semantic errors. The task is to find the errors and, for some, to correct the errors. Syntactic errors have been shown to be more difficult for persons with aphasia to identify. The reader who can find the more subtle syntactic errors of subject-verb agreement or pluralization is probably reading closely and becoming able to comprehend meaning at a deeper level than surface semantics. There are also many workbooks available that provide materials at the sentence and simple paragraph level for patients with aphasia or TBI.

It is advisable to move the client into work on paragraph-level material as soon as possible. Passages should be more than 200 words in length and read both silently and aloud. Difficulty level for contextual reading can be advanced in two major ways: (1) increasing length, and (2) increasing vocabulary and syntactical complexity. The clinician should consider controlling one or the other as much as possible to be able to analyze reading comprehension failures.

Normal readers enhance comprehension of words and sentences by utilizing the preceding and following contexts, and research has shown this use of context also facilitates comprehension in brain-damaged patients (Germani and Pierce, 1992). In other words, readers use the context to make predictions about, or sometimes to guess, the meaning of words and sentences within the text. If readers do not seem to be using contextual information, they should be interrupted at errors that change meaning and they should be helped to analyze whether the error fits with the context. Then it should be read again correctly. If clients continue to make the same error when reading aloud, reading the sentence back to front may help them correct the reading. Comprehension assessment follows each reading, and the questions should require the patient to make use

of cognitive-linguistic processes such as association, deductive reasoning, sequencing, and analysis.

Another good approach for training monitoring and comprehension of context is to use material that involves following directions. The patient can select various items from home or work that include written directions (recipes, assembly manuals, equipment directions), or activities for auditory comprehension training can be adapted. Again, the self-monitoring of reading in terms of what makes sense and, in this case, the outcome is one of the primary objectives.

The Mildly Impaired Reader

The mildly impaired reader may be extremely frustrated with reading. Although these readers can read context at the appropriate grade level, reading may be slow and laborious. They may reread material continuously because they cannot synthesize or remember what has been read. They may read most words correctly, but read texts in an arduous, one-word-at-a-time fashion. If they are willing to devote the time and effort, reading can usually be improved. However, they may never regain the automaticity and ease with which they read premorbidly.

A clinical report (Webb, 1982) noted that techniques used in speed-reading training may assist these patients in increasing comprehension and speed. In this training much of the emphasis is on searching for the main idea, skimming unimportant details, and using comprehension strategies that promote easier interaction with the text. Treatment tasks to train rapid scanning may need to be used. Scanning the phone book for certain names or scanning context for particular facts are good training tasks. For readers who seem to use a word-by-word reading approach resulting in very decreased reading rate, speed-reading techniques suggest rapid fixation or perception exercises to force the reader to take in more information or more words at one visual fixation. Flash cards can be used, or a tachistoscopic program on a computer can be utilized. Many of these exercises can be found in speed-reading texts. There are software programs available that provide speed-reading training in which full pages of text are moved or scrolled at various rates. Both this method and tachistoscopic presentation should be assessed as to which seems more effective for a particular client. Intensive practice will be needed.

Reading comprehension is a process of using syntactic, semantic, and rhetorical information to reconstruct in the reader's mind a hypothesis or personal explanation that might account for the intended message of the writer (Smith, 1994). In this process readers use the knowledge of the world that they possess, plus appropriate cognitive and reasoning skill. If one accepts this definition of comprehension and the process it involves, it becomes clear that clients with brain damage must be constantly interacting with the text. It must be relevant to them, or they must find a way to make it relevant. Materials utilized in therapy should be as close as possible to what the individual would normally be using in reading for work or school or for leisure reading. As clients move into reading longer text, it is critical that they be trained in strategies that increase comprehension. These strategies involve planning and organization techniques that mandate interaction with the text. They are also useful for students relearning study skills. These strategies include such tactics as the following: (1) overview of the text prior to reading it, (2) setting up a purpose for reading or a lesson framework for the reader, (3) listing main ideas during reading, (4) outlining, (5) inserting questions for the reader in the text, (6) making timelines and charts, and (7) talking or writing about what was read. There are "fix-up" strategies that should be adopted for the times comprehension appears to be failing. Approaches such as changing the rate of reading, hypothesizing, ignoring small problems, and moving on and rereading or going to another source should be considered by every reader at those times.

Use of Computers and Other Equipment

Computers can be of great value in retraining reading. Computers may be used for training attention, vocabulary building drills, sentence comprehension, paragraph comprehension, and rapid scanning or perception exercises. Commercially there are more and more software programs available that target reading both for the normal and the impaired learner. These will be found most often through educational software companies, though there are programs that target aphasic populations. Other functions can be performed such as assessing readability or informally assessing reading grade level.

The clinician also may want to use a tape player at some point in training. The clinician may record a reading of contextual material and the client can follow along during practice before reading it independently.

Compensatory Strategies

Though we live in the "age of literacy," there are individuals who cannot read functionally but can carry on without that skill. For others, who need or want methods to compensate for reading, many books are now recorded on tape or CD and are available for loan at the public library or for sale in bookstores. Friends may also record books on tape for the patient. The student or working person may need the assistance of a "reading partner." This individual would be available to help with reading difficult material and would verify or correct comprehension. The use of a small portable speaking language master such as that available from Franklin Learning Resources can also be valuable for the impaired reader. The person types the word into the device and it pronounces the word. It can also give a definition, and some devices provide synonyms for further enhancing understanding. The utilization of this type of device allows the reader to move forward when reading a difficult passage instead of having to constantly struggle to decode troublesome words. This may increase reading speed and decrease the laboriousness for some clients.

Conclusion

Working with the acquired dyslexias is a stimulating challenge. There is much to be learned about better ways to facilitate reading both for the developmental and the acquired alexias. For the present, the speech-language pathologist can best prepare for treating clients with these disorders by learning how normal reading takes place, how reading is taught to non-brain-damaged learners, how brain injury affects the learning and reading process, and how others have treated the disorders. Armed with this information and plenty of creativity, the speech-language pathologist can, in most cases, target functional reading with optimism.

References

Beeson, P.M. (1998). Treatment for Letter-by-Letter Reading: A Case Study. In: N. Helm-Estabrooks & A.L. Holland (Eds.), *Approaches to the Treatment of Aphasia*. San Diego: Singular Publishing Group.

Beeson, P.M. and Hillis, A.E. (2001). Comprehension and Production of Written Words. In: R. Chapey (Ed.), *Language Intervention Strategies in Aphasia and Related Neurogenic Communication Disorders* (4th ed., pp. 572–604). Baltimore: Lippincott, Williams and Wilkins.

Behrmann, M., Black, S.E. & Bub, D. (1990). The Evolution of Pure Alexia: A Longitudinal Study of Recovery. *Brain and Language, 39(3)*, 405–427.

Benson, D.F. (1979). *Aphasia, Alexia and Agraphia*. New York: Churchill Livingstone.

Bokde, A.L., Tagamets, M.A., Friedman, R.B. & Horwitz, B. (2001). Functional Interaction of the Inferior Frontal Cortex During the Processing of Words and Word-Like Stimuli. *Neuron, 30*, 609–617.

Degrees of Reading Power-Revised. (1995). Brewster, NY: Touchstone Applied Science Associates.

Dehaene, S., Le Clec, H.G., Poline, J.B., Le Bihan, D. & Cohen, L. (2002). The Visual Word Form Area: A Prelexical Representation of Visual Words in the Fusiform Gyrus. *Neuroreport, 13*, 321–325.

Fiebach, C.J., Friederici, A.D., Muller, K. & von Cramon, D.Y. (2002). fMRI Evidence for Dual Routes to the Mental Lexicon in Visual Word Recognition. *Journal of Cognitive Neuroscience, 14*, 11–23.

Friedman, R.B., Sample, D.M. & Lott, S.N. (2002). The Role of Level of Representation in the Use of Paired Associate Learning for Rehabilitation of Alexia. *Neuropsychologica, 40*, 223–234.

Fry, E. (1977). Fry's Readability Graph: Clarification, Validity, and Extension to Level 17. *Journal of Reading, 21*, 242–251.

Germani, M.J. & Pierce, R.S. (1992). Contextual Influences in Reading Comprehension in Aphasia. *Brain and Language, 42*, 308–319.

Greenwald, M.L. (2000). The Acquired Dyslexias. In: S.E. Nadeau, L.J.G. Rothi & B. Crosson (Eds.), *Aphasia and Language* (pp. 159–183). New York: Guilford Press.

Heeringa, H.M. (2002). *A Manual for the Treatment of Acquired Reading and Writing Disorders*. Ann Arbor, MI: SLP Pathways.

Hillis, A.E. (1993). The Role of Models of Language Processing in the Rehabilitation of Language Impairments. *Aphasiology, 7*, 5–26.

Keller, R.A., Carpenter, P.A. & Just, M.A. (2001). The Neural Bases of Sentence Comprehension: A fMRI Examination of Syntactic and Lexical Processing. *Cerebral Cortex, 11*, 223–237.

Kircher, T.T., Brammer, M., Andreu, N.T., Williams, S.C. & McGuire, P.K. (2001). Engagement of Right Temporal Cortex During Processing of Linguistic Context. *Neuropsychologia, 39*, 798–809.

Kirshner, H.S. (2002). *Behavioral Neurology: Practical Science of Mind and Brain* (2nd ed.). Boston: Butterworth-Heinemann.

LaPointe, L.L. & Horner, J. (1998). *Reading Comprehension Battery for Aphasia*. Austin, TX: Pro-Ed.

Marshall, J.C. (1985). On Some Relationships Between Acquired and Developmental Dyslexias. In F.H. Duffy & N. Geschwind (Eds), *Dyslexia: A Neuroscientific Approach to Clinical Evaluation* (pp. 55–66). Boston: Little, Brown.

Marshall, J.C. & Newcombe, F. (1973). Patterns of Paralexia: A Psycholinguistic Approach. *Journal of Psycholinguistic Research, 2*, 175–186.

May, F.B. & Elliott, S. (1973). *To Help Children Read: Mastery Performance Modules for Teachers in Training*. Columbus, OH: Charles C. Merrill.

Moyer, S. (1979). Rehabilitation of Alexia: A Case Study. *Cortex, 15*, 139–144.

Nakada, T., Fujii, Y., Yoneoka, Y. & Kwee, I.L. (2001). Planum Temporale: Where Spoken and Written Language Meet. *European Neurology, 46*, 121–125.

Nicholas, L.E., MacLennon D.L. & Brookshire R.H. (1986). Validity of Multiple-Sentence Reading Comprehension Tests for Aphasic Adults. *Journal of Speech and Hearing Disorders, 51*, 82–87.

Pugh, K.R., Mencl, W.E., Jenner, A.R., Katz, L., Frost, S.J., Lee, J.R., Shaywitz, S.E. & Shaywitz, B.A. (2001). Neurobiological Studies of Reading and Reading Disability. *Journal of Communication Disorders, 34*, 479–492.

Rand, M.B., Trudeau, M.D. & Nelson, L.K. (1990). Reading Assessment Post Head Injury: How Valid Is It? *Brain Injury, 4*, 155–160.

Roder, B., Stock, O., Neville, H., Bien, S. and Rosler, F. (2002). Brain Activation Modulated by the Comprehension of Normal and Pseudo-Word Sentences of Different Processing Demands: A Functional Magnetic Resonance Imaging Study. *Neuroimage, 15*, 1003–1014.

Roe, B.D. & Burns, P.C. (1999). *Burns-Roe Informal Reading Inventory*. Boston: Houghton Mifflin.

Rothi, L.G., Greenwald, M., Maher, L.M. & Ochipa, C. (1998). Alexia Without Agraphia: Lessons from a Treatment Failure. In: N. Helm-Estabrooks & A.L. Holland (Eds.), *Approaches to the Treatment of Aphasia* (pp. 179–201). San Diego: Singular Publishing Group.

Rothi, L.G. & Moss, S.E. (1985). Alexia/Agraphia in Brain-Damaged Adults. Paper presented at the convention of the American Speech-Language-Hearing Association, Washington, DC.

Schneider, W. & Shiffrin, R.M. (1977). Automatic and Controlled Information Processing in Vision. In: D. LaBerge & S.J. Samuels (Eds.), *Basic Processes in Reading: Perception and Comprehension* (pp. 127–154). Hillsdale, NJ: Lawrence Erlbaum.

Slosson, R.L. & Nicholson, C.L. (1990). *Slosson Oral Reading Test-Revised*. Aurora, NY: Slosson Educational Publications, Inc.

Smith, F. (1994). *Understanding Reading*. Hillsdale, NJ: Lawrence Erlbaum.

Weaver, C. (1988). *Reading Process and Practice: From Sociopsycholinguistics to Whole Language*. Portsmouth, NH: Heinemann Educational Books.

Webb, W.G. (1982). Intervention Strategies in Mild Reading Disorders Associated with Aphasia. Paper presented at the annual convention of the American Speech-Language-Hearing Association, Toronto.

Woodcock, R.W. (1998). *Woodcock Reading Mastery Tests-Revised/Normative Update*. Circle Pines, MN: American Guidance Service.

7

Acquired Neurogenic Agraphias: Writing Problems

MALCOLM R. MCNEIL AND CHIN-HSING TSENG

Writing is one major expressive communication channel that is parallel, rather than subordinate, to speaking. Acquired disorders of writing occur for many reasons. These include those that are related to anatomic changes of the writing apparatus (e.g., visual impairment, blindness, limb or hand injury), psychiatric disorders (e.g., depression), psychological or physiologic adaptation (e.g., avoidance or compensation due to pain from arthritis; neural reorganization), or to a host of neurocognitive conditions including executive dysfunctions, linguistic impairments, and a range of sensorimotor disorders affecting the corticospinal system. Except on rare occasions, these disorders reflect the neurologic dysfunctions of a complex and interactive cognitive system. We define acquired neurogenic agraphias as the family of writing disorders resulting from central or peripheral neurologic damage. Implied in this very general definition is the exclusion of anatomic disorders affecting writing, as well as psychiatric and affective disorders, such as schizophrenia or depression, from those conditions more clearly attributable to peripheral and central nervous system (PNS/CNS) insult or disease. This chapter discusses acquired agraphias that occur in adulthood, and summarizes the current paradigm reported in theoretical and clinical literature on acquired agraphias.

Among the various communication disorders that result from PNS and CNS lesions, acquired agraphia has received the least attention from researchers and clinicians, for several reasons. First, speech is often better appreciated as the major functional communication means, and thus spoken language disorders are the primary target of assessment and intervention. Second, writing is considered as secondary to speech in neural organization and order of acquisition (Marcie & Hecaen, 1979), which leads to a common attitude that the linguistic problems (e.g., grammatical and word retrieval errors) evidenced in writing are only the mirror images of those in speech (Goodglass, 1981; Goodglass & Hunter, 1970). Finally, investigations of normal writing have received little scientific attention until recent decades (Ellis, 1989; Frith, 1980; Hansen & McNeil, 1986; Hansen et al., 1987; Kao et al., 1986). Without tests of pathologic writing on normal subjects and without normal reference data, the evaluation of writing disorders remains subjective and continues to lead to uninterpretable experimental results and imprecise or inaccurate clinical decisions.

As a highly sophisticated skill, effective writing can be performed only with a large ensemble of intact subskills: limb and hand sensorimotor control (calligraphy), orthography, visual-perceptual orientation, and a cascade of linguistic capacities (Benson, 1979; Taylor, 1985). Education plays a significant role in the shaping of these skills (Hansen et al., 1987; Keenan & Brassell, 1974; Roeltgen, 1993).

Undoubtedly, agraphias can have various clinical manifestations cross-linguistically, as orthographies are notoriously diverse. The alphabetical system in which letters are linearly mapped onto the sounds of spoken language is not universal. For instance, the orthographic system originated in China but later adopted by other East Asian nations does not have the phoneme-to-grapheme rules found in English and many other languages. As such, agraphias arising from the nonalphabetic systems may have different manifestations than those arising from alphabetical ones. In the past decade, a surge of interest has been observed in agraphias of Asian languages, most notably Japanese (Hashimoto et al., 1998; Kim & Na, 2000; Kokubo et al., 2001; Maeshima et al., 2002; Otsuki et al. 1999; Sakurai et al., 1994, 1997; Seki et al., 1998). Research has concentrated on the selective impairment of one writing system (e.g., kana or phonogram) compared with another well-preserved system (e.g., kanji or ideogram) in the same patient. Finally, even within the alphabetical systems, orthographies differ in the degree to which letters correspond to phonemes in a regular manner, and thus whether spelling regularity and graphemic consistency are crucial factors in understanding agraphia has also been addressed. Luzzati et al. (1998) concluded that "current psycholinguistic models of written language also apply to languages [e.g., Italian, Spanish] with shallow orthography [i.e., with more regular spellings]" (p. 1731). However, they also pointed out that spelling retrieval routes (see below) should be differentially weighted among languages (see also Iribarren et al., 2001).

With so many sources of variability even in healthy adults, it can be imagined that the underlying mechanisms of agraphic performance are not always easy to determine. Although several neuropsychological models have been proposed to account for the various forms of agraphia, little is agreed upon as to the neuroanatomic substrates subserving the various processes of writing. To date, the pathophysiologic mechanisms

of writing disorders can be described only in tentative terms.

Pathophysiology

Localization: A Cortical Center for Writing?

Since the late 19th century, academic battle has been waged among the opponents and proponents of a single brain center for writing. In 1881, Exner postulated that the writing function resided at the foot of the left second frontal convolution (Leischner, 1969). This idea, however, was not accepted without challenge by Exner's contemporaries such as Wernicke and Dejerine. Their challenge was waged on the basis of several assumptions: first, written language is a later-acquired skill on phylogenic and ontogenic scales; second, writing movements are nothing more than the visual copying of the oral language; and third, writing can be achieved only through a combination of many skills, all of which appear to be localized in disparate locations of the brain.

Hecaen and Angelergues (1964) conducted a clinicoanatomic study in which the severity of functional disturbances in seven communication domains was correlated with the locus of the lesion. A five-point equal-appearing interval scale, with a score of 0 representing intact writing, was used to quantify the deficits. They concluded that no single lobe could be totally responsible for writing disturbances. They stated, "Writing disturbances due to impairment of one lobe manifest themselves clearly among temporal (1.35) and parietal (1.13) lesions. When the lesion affects two lobes, agraphia is most noticeable when the parietal lobe is involved (parietotemporal lesion, 2; parieto-occipital lesion, 2; and fronto-parietal, 1.18); but the degree of agraphia is always more marked among massive lesions and predominates in posterior impairment (3.66 compared with 2.83)" (p. 241). The numbers in parentheses are the average scale values for severity of the writing deficits. Furthermore, they claimed, "The degree of writing disturbances is coupled in a preferential fashion with the parietal factor . . . but the temporal factor remains important . . . , and the occipital . . . and rolandic factors are not negligible; the frontal factor is non-existent . . ." (p. 243).

The numerous case studies reported in the neurologic literature seemed to confirm Hecaen and Angelergues's (1964) notion against a single neural substrate for writing. Most neurogenic dysgraphias can most profitably be considered as a composite of writing deficits arising from widely distributed neural substrates, and the failure to identify a circumscribed brain area for writing is taken as a rule, more than an exception. The strict localizationist view has been gradually (though not universally) replaced by a neural-network notion that assumes that basic mental operations are localized in different brain areas and that writing is performed by a network of widely distributed neural systems (Posner & Raichle, 1994). Thus far, the left/right, the anterior/posterior, and the cortical/subcortical distinctions have been suggested to reflect specialized features of agraphias and perhaps the specialized neurologic and psycholinguistic processes that support writing functions. In addition, agraphias are also often associated with a few distinct neurologic disorders such as Gerstmann's syndrome, Alzheimer's disease, Parkinson's disease, and confusional states, as well as a necessary component of aphasia (McNeil & Pratt, 2001).

Left Versus Right Hemisphere

A well-accepted principle in neurology is that a dominant portion of language-specific representation and processing functions are lateralized to the left hemisphere in most humans (Benson & Geschwind, 1985; Bradshaw & Nettleton, 1983). In addition, for as yet unknown reasons, most people are left hemisphere dominant for the planning and programming of limb (Bradshaw & Nettleton, 1983) and speech (McNeil et al., 2000) movements. Writing, a limb motor act involving linguistic formulation, is thus thought to be mediated, if not controlled, primarily by the left hemisphere. The essential elements of the

writing disturbance known as paragraphia, neologism, and agrammatism are frequently observed in the writing of left hemisphere-damaged patients. Other defects, such as the inability to form letters and the difficulty in using either cursive or print, but not both, have also been identified in the writing of some persons with left hemisphere lesions.

During the past two decades, the role of the right hemisphere in language processing has gained support (Myers, 1999; Tompkins, 1995; Zaidel, 1978, 1985). The agraphia literature has also documented several cases of writing disturbances resulting from right hemisphere damage (e.g., Hashimoto et al., 1998; Hecaen & Marcie, 1974; Klatka et al., 1998; Kokubo et al., 2001; Rothi et al., 1987; Seki, et al., 1998; Silveri, 1996; Silveri et al., 1997). These case reports, however, appeared to verify the ancillary role of right hemisphere in linguistic stages of writing. Such "peripheral" processes as visuospatial, proprioceptive (Hecaen & Marcie, 1974; Silveri, 1996), and subconscious (or automatic) operations (Simerniskaya, 1974) and some high-level inferencing operations that are required for a successful writing act are said to be subserved by the right hemisphere. Therefore, right hemisphere–damaged individuals present alignment (writing form) problems, such as unusual left or top margins and line slopes, awkward grapheme configurations (often with extra strokes), left agnosia or neglect, and other deviant spatial features. In addition, it has been proposed that the right hemisphere may be involved substantively in one mode of lexical writing, namely, the direct access of word spelling from the word engram without a phoneme-to-grapheme transformation procedure (Rothi et al., 1987). Damage to the right hemisphere may result in a particular type of agraphia called, by some, *lexical agraphia* (see below).

Anterior Versus Posterior

Benson and Geschwind (1985) divided agraphias associated with aphasia into anterior or posterior types according to the lesion location. This anatomically based classification parallels a common typology based on spoken language performance in aphasia. Misspellings, agrammatism, and some abnormal mechanical anomalies (due to the nonpreferred hand's lack of experience and practice in writing movements) are said to be the predominant characteristics of the writing produced by anterior-lesioned persons. By contrast, well-formed letter configurations are seen more often in individuals with posterior lesions who show frequent spelling errors, word order abnormalities (verbal paragraphias), and word omissions. Kaplan and Goodglass (1981) proposed that persons with Broca's aphasia (anterior) more commonly used block printing, whereas cursive writing was more frequently used in persons with Wernicke's aphasia (posterior). These authors also suggested that patients with parietal lesions typically demonstrated pathologic writing and reading under the agraphia with alexia syndrome label. Summaries of the literature (e.g., Rapcsak & Beeson, 2000) have not taken the anterior-posterior dichotomy into serious consideration, and have essentially abandoned the distinction.

Cortical Versus Subcortical

In contrast with cortical lesions, to which most attention has been paid, subcortical lesions (particularly of the thalamus) have become more seriously linked with speech and language (including writing) deficits (Crosson, 1992; Nadeau & Crosson, 1997; Nadeau & Gonzalez-Rothi, 2001). Lesions in the thalamus (in the left hemisphere) are often associated with a transient grammatical aphasia, anomia with perseveration, verbal memory deficits, and contralateral motor neglect (Mateer & Ojemann, 1983). According to Nadeau and Crosson (1997), the major psycholinguistic deficits seen in thalamic aphasia stem from lexical-semantic impairments.

Little systematic effort has been made to analyze subcortical agraphia as opposed to cortical agraphia. This distinction is so imprecise as to be uninformative because variation in signs produced with lesions within both the cortical and subcortical regions is as great as the variation of signs produced between the regions. Margolin and Wing (1983) compared agraphia in subcortical patients (with Parkinson's disease) and in a patient with cortical lesions. The cortical agraphia, supposedly *apraxic agraphic* (see below), was characterized by frequent but inconsistent letter malformations, better performance on copying than other writing tasks, and superior block printing to cursive writing. In contrast, the subcortical patients (with presumed basal ganglia involvement) showed *micrographia*, or abnormally small writing. An analysis of the spatiotemporal characteristic of the handwriting produced by these subcortical patients revealed a significant increase in movement time and decrease in letter height. Margolin and Wing (1983) hypothesized that the increase in movement time appeared to be an attempt to compensate for an underlying diminution in force. In other words, the Parkinsonian patients with micrographia "were able to access an intact graphic motor pattern but could not generate the proper neuromuscular activity to produce a letter of adequate size" (p. 282). Writing disturbances in other subcortical structures, including thalamus (Ohno et al., 2000), caudate nucleus and internal capsule (Laine & Marttila, 1981), putamen (Tanridag & Kirshner, 1985), and corticocerebellar pathways (Rosenbek et al., 1981; Silveri et al., 1997), have also been reported with vastly different language, motoric, and other cognitive mechanisms involved in these patients' disparate dysgraphic behaviors.

Gerstmann's Syndrome

Gerstmann's syndrome is characterized by four behavioral signs that are necessary and sufficient for its diagnosis: finger agnosia, right-left disorientation, acalculia, and agraphia. In addition to the debate over the syndrome's existence, equally controversial is the issue of whether there is a single unifying mechanism for those seemingly disparate signs (Benton, 1992). Some proponents of the syndrome have considered a lesion in the left parietal lobe as the pathogenesis for a disorder of spatiotemporal sequencing, which in turn creates the four clinical signs. However, a study by Wingard et al. (2002) found that these signs did not statistically cluster together, as revealed by the data from Alzheimer's patients, and thus questioned the validity of a monolithic mechanism. Often associated with the syndrome is apraxic agraphia, as suggested by Benson and Geschwind (1985). However, by Roeltgen's (1985) account, all subtypes of agraphia may co-occur with it.

Alzheimer's Disease

Agraphia is common in dementia of the Alzheimer type as revealed by an increasingly large body of literature (Henderson et al., 1992; LaBerge et al., 1992; Lambert et al., 1996; Neils et al., 1995; Neils-Strunjas et al., 1998; Penniello et al., 1995). Both linguistic and motor deficits in writing are associated with this population. LaBerge et al. (1992) compared writing errors made by persons with Alzheimer's disease and by normal controls. Although significantly more errors were found with the persons with Alzheimer's disease, a discriminant function analysis could not reliably distinguish the persons with Alzheimer's disease from the normally aging participants. It should be noted, however, that dysgraphic errors such as capitalization and punctuation errors, paraphasias, uncrossed *t*'s, and undotted *i*'s increased with the severity of dementia. Similar findings were also reported by Horner et al. (1988), who found that dementia severity and visuoperceptual impairment were the most important predictors of writing deficits in this population. One interesting suggestion made by these investigators was that agraphia is an early important sign of Alzheimer's disease, with the *lexical* subtype preceding the *phonologic* subtype (see below) as the disease evolves.

Confusional States

Patients with various confusional states have been reported to demonstrate attentional disturbances as their primary clinical feature. The etiology for these confusional states varies from head injury to metabolic-toxic encephalopathy, especially of rapid onset (Mesulam, 1985). Interestingly, writing by the confused patients has been reported to be more defective than speech (Chedru & Geschwind, 1972). Further, in a study designed to compare communication functions among four patient groups (aphasia, general intellectual impairment, apraxia of speech, and confusion), Halpern et al. (1973) found that writing to dictation ranked third among several speech and language functions in impairment in the confused patient group, but was less impaired in the other groups. Chedru and Geschwind (1972), in an attempt to dismiss the idea of *pure agraphia* (agraphia unassociated with any other neurologic signs), documented the writing disturbances in 33 of 34 acutely confused patients. According to these authors, agraphia in these patients involved motor, spatial, syntactic, and, most remarkably, spelling aspects of writing. They suspected that previous researchers might have misidentified (at least in some cases) agraphia associated with confusional states as *pure* agraphia.

Nature and Differentiating Features

Clinical Symptomatology

In this section we summarize the salient features associated with various subtypes of agraphias. Although numerous classification systems have been developed, such as the central (spelling-related) and peripheral (letter production) distinction discussed by Rapcsak and Beeson (2000), we restrict our discussion to those generated from the neuropsychological/psycholinguistic models of agraphia.

Lexical (Surface) Agraphia

Lexical agraphia arises from a difficulty in spelling words that do not follow the ordinary sound-to-letter conversion rules (irregular words) with writing to dictation errors approximating the phonologic shape of the target words (Hatfield & Patterson, 1985).

For example, "kom" might be written for "comb" or "telafon" for "telephone." Beauvois and Derousene (1981) described a patient who could write nonwords to dictation (invoking the sound-to-letter rules of the language) with 99% accuracy but wrote irregular real words with only 38% accuracy. Similarly, Iribarren et al. (2001) reported a Spanish patient who made 39% (31 of 80), mostly phonologically plausible errors, on irregularly spelled words, but only 15% (3 of 20) nonword errors on a dictation task. It was speculated that brain damage had compromised the *lexical* route(s) (or variably termed *graphemic output lexicon, orthographic knowledge,* etc.) of the normal writing procedures such that accurate spelling could be accomplished only by means of the *nonlexical* (*sublexical,* or *phoneme-to-grapheme*) route. In other words, it is said that a patient with lexical agraphia does not recall the "engram" of the whole word but has to analyze the sound on the spot and convert it into a pronounceable spelling.

Phonologic Agraphia

If one can write from dictation a word that is regular or irregular in spelling but has difficulty in writing a nonword, phonologic agraphia is said to exist (Baxter & Warrington, 1985; Ellis, 1982; Shallice, 1981). Iribarren et al. (2001) also reported the performance of one individual who made only two errors out of 160 on real regular and irregular words (<1%), but produced 100% errors on a 20-item nonword dictation task. According to contemporary model builders, a "functional lesion" of the *phoneme-to-grapheme* conversion rules was presumably responsible for this performance, so that an appropriate letter sequence could not be mapped onto an unfamiliar vocalization. On the other hand, this individual was able to correctly spell irregular words through the recall of the whole word engram. Bub and Kertesz (1982a) reported that the spelling performance of persons with phonologic dysgraphia is often influenced by linguistic attributes of a word such as

imageability and by form class. This suggests that these individuals might recall the orthographic shape of the word with the help of the word's meaning(s) and its syntactic functions.

Deep Agraphia

Deep agraphia can be conceived as a variant of phonologic agraphia. The profiles of the two look similar, except that deep agraphia is associated with more frequent semantic paragraphias (Bub & Kertesz, 1982b). Bub and Kertesz (1982b) presented an individual who had good comprehension of written and spoken words, showed telegraphic speech, and performed well on automatic writing and copying tasks. In writing words to dictation, she made many semantic errors (e.g., "happy" written as "funny"), and her performance on nouns and concrete words, respectively, was better than on function words and abstract words. In addition, she had great difficulty generating nonwords. Consistent with neuropsychological dysgraphia models, the semantic errors in deep agraphia can only have resulted from multiple deficits; that is, the spoken word cannot activate the orthographic memory of the whole word directly (through the lexical route), indirectly (through the lexical-semantic route), or phonologically (with the help of phoneme-to-grapheme conversion). Hillis et al. (1999) reported an individual with deep agraphia whose semantic errors were abundant in writing to dictation but were almost absent in oral naming. The authors explained this individual's clinical profile by the damaged lexical and phonologic routes, with a spared semantic system.

Graphemic Buffer Impairment

This dysgraphia subtype has gained little attention until recent decades (Caramazza et al., 1987; Hillis & Caramazza, 1989; Katz, 1991; McCloskey et al., 1994; Miceli et al., 1985; Posteraro et al., 1988). According to Jonsdottir et al. (1996), only eight patients had been reported to have the impairment of graphemic buffer before 1996. The graphemic buffer is assumed to be a working memory storage for orthographic representations of words or nonwords before they are fed into the subsequent motor processes for handwriting or oral spelling. As the graphemic buffer stands at the juncture between the spelling routes and the motor output, an impairment of the buffer would imply errors (letter additions, deletions, substitutions, or transpositions) across many tasks (copying, written naming, spontaneous writing, oral spelling, or writing to dictation). In "pure graphemic buffer impairments" the productions are expected to be free of lexical, semantic errors because the computations preceding the selection and serial ordering of the abstract graphemes are presumably completed without error. Errors for nonwords should be similar to those for words because both the lexical and the nonlexical routes converge into the same graphemic buffer. Finally, errors tend to cluster in the middle of the words and are likely to increase with the length of the word, as might be expected from the characteristics of the working memory system. Discussion of this subtype in the literature has focused on the theoretical issues such as the nature of the graphemic buffer, whose elucidation is beyond the scope of this chapter (Annoni et al., 1998; Jonsdottir et al., 1996; Tainturier & Caramazza, 1996).

Peripheral Agraphias

Agraphias that are not attributed to psycholinguistic deficits are classified in the literature as peripheral agraphias. These include allographic impairment, apraxic agraphia, and spatial agraphia (Rapcsak & Beeson, 2000; Roeltgen, 1993). Bifurcated downstream from the graphemic buffer are an allographic conversion system (for writing) and a grapheme-letter name conversion system (for oral spelling), as postulated in most models. The abstract graphemes are converted into upper- or lower-case, script or print, via the allographic system; thus, the

damage to the system may yield substitution errors in writing but not necessarily in oral spelling. The patient may write worse in one case than another or even intersperse graphemes in both forms (De Bastini & Barry, 1989; Goodman & Caramazza, 1986). It is worth noting that there is converging validation for this model of writing errors, with the model invoked differentially accounting for and explaining the array of sound-level speech production errors. For example, those of phonemic paraphasia are attributed to impairments of phonologic assembly/encoding (Dell, 1984, 1988; McNeil et al., 2004), which is analogous to graphemic buffer dysgraphia; some aspects of apraxia of speech are attributed to a disorder of motor planning (McNeil et al., 2004; Van der Merwe, 1997), which is analogous to allographic or apraxic dysgraphia; and other aspects of apraxia of speech and some of the dysarthrias (McNeil et al., 2004; Van der Merwe, 1997) are analogous to afferent or spatial dysgraphia. A person with apraxic agraphia may be able to spell orally or with anagram letters but have difficulty producing letter shapes in handwriting, and their letter malformations are not attributable to sensorimotor deficits or limb apraxia (Crary & Heilman, 1988; Roeltgen & Heilman, 1983). According to Alexander et al. (1992), apraxic agraphia has been variously explained as a loss of graphic motor pattern, a loss of letter-form knowledge, a disconnection of visuokinesthetic engrams from motor executors, and as a visuospatial impairment. However, the peripheral agraphias attributable to the last two factors are sometimes classified as afferent or spatial agraphia. Thus some confusion of terminology exists about the sensorimotor end of the agraphias (Destreie et al., 2000; Hodges, 1991; Miozzo & De Bastiani, 2002; Zesiger et al., 1994).

The so-called afferent or spatial agraphia refers to the peripheral writing disorder due to visual or proprioceptive feedback disruptions. Afferent agraphia is characterized by omission and duplication of strokes and letters, alignment and spacing problems, and the tendency to write on the right-hand side of the page (Ellis et al., 1987; Lebrun, 1976; Seki et al., 1998; Silveri, 1996; Silveri et al., 1997). This subtype of agraphia is often associated with the right hemisphere lesions or cerebellar pathologies. Although the attribution and classification of the motoric characteristics of dysgraphia are considerably less developed than their analogous motor speech counterparts, the similarities are obvious and the study of the dysgraphias could benefit from closer academic and clinical cross-fertilization with those derived from and utilized in motor speech disorders.

A Caveat

As outlined in this section, agraphias are described and explained with the language of "functional architecture" postulated by contemporary researchers. Different patterns of impairment are described and attributed to the malfunction of a particular component (e.g., sound-to-letter conversion) of the "machine" that would otherwise make the cognitive act of writing successful. Because new patterns of deficits are frequently reported, these functional architectures continue to evolve. The major benefit of this approach is to improve understanding of the cognitive disorders in a logical-analytic manner, with some scientific method. However, readers are cautioned against overinterpretation of a functional deficit as having the neuroanatomic reality to which the models frequently adhere. Additionally, a selective impairment in many studies represents no more than a differential performance level among tasks. A functional deficit so defined can be incomplete, allowing for explanations other than the identification of an isolable mental module that is represented by a true dissociation (Odell et al., 1995). Suffice it to say that the functional architecture approach is convenient for simplifying clinical and theoretical complexities, yet is still an analogic tool that requires a substantive measure of caution in its application.

Evaluation

Reasons for Assessing Acquired Dysgraphia

As with the evaluation of any memorial, attentional, motor, linguistic, or communicative function, the procedures used in the evaluation reflect the philosophy of the test's authors relative to the nature of the hypothesized deficits as well as the purpose(s) for which the test was constructed. Likewise, the test will reflect the clinician's or researcher's philosophy and beliefs about the nature of the deficit under investigation. The philosophical decisions involve those discussed above (see Nature and Differentiating Features).

The purposes of developing (and eventually administering) a test of handwriting parallel those purposes for the assessment of the other features of neurogenic speech, language, memory, attention, and sensorimotor disorders (McNeil, 1984). As such, assessment often goes beyond localizing a deficit in the model. Although the specific writing tasks (e.g., copying versus writing to dictation), the stimuli used to elicit the response (e.g., copying letters versus copying sentences; writing orthographically regular versus irregular words), and the analysis procedures (e.g., counting misspelled words versus measuring intergraphemic distance) used to assess writing may differ among the different purposes, a single task can often serve more than one purpose. Multiple test purposes have been designed into some of the standardized and published aphasia tests. The purposes of assessing handwriting are summarized in Table 7–1, along with two commonly used tools and one unpublished experimental protocol judged to address each purpose.

Published and Experimental Dysgraphia Tests

Unlike tests for auditory or reading processing and comprehension, there are no standardized and published tests solely for the evaluation of writing associated with neurogenic

Table 7–1. Purposes of Assessment Achieved (Marked with an X) by Various Standardized Writing Assessment Protocols Relative to Neuropsychologic Classification System (Superscript Numbers Indicate Relevant Supporting Literature)

Assessment Purpose	PICA[1]	WAB[1]	NDB[1]
Detection of dysgraphia	X[7]		X[17,18]
Lesion localization	X[19]		
Differential diagnosis among neurogenic disorders	X[4,5,6,8,15,16]	X[2,3]	X[17,18]
Prediction of recovery	X[9,10,11,12,13]		
Classification via neuropsychologic subtype			X[17,18]
Scaling of severity	X[13]		
Treatment focus via subtype	X[14]		X[17,18]
Measure of change	X[13]		
Treatment termination criteria			

PICA, Porch Index of Communicative Ability; WAB, Western Aphasia Battery; NDB, Neurogenic Dysgraphia Battery.
[1]Tseng & McNeil (1997), [2]Horner et al. (1987), [3]Kertesz (1979), [4]Duffy and Keith (1980), [5]Watson & Records (1978), [6]Metzler & Jelinek (1977), [7]Porch et al. (1976), [8]Selinger et al. (1987), [9]Aten & Lyon (1978), [10]Porch & Callaghan (1981), [11]Wertz et al. (1980), [12]Deal et al. (1979), [13]Porch (1971), [14]Porch (1986), [15]Brauer et al. (1989), [16]Brauer (1989), [17]Hansen & McNeil (1986), [18] Hansen et al. (1987), [19]Porch (1978).

disorders, although some researchers have attempted to develop such a specific-purpose tool (Goodman & Caramazza, 1985; Hansen and McNeil, 1986), and only the Psycholinguistic Assessments of Language Processing in Aphasia (PALPA) (Kay et al., 1992) can be said to generally conform to the neuropsychological model of dysgraphia presented above. However, because the PALPA, like the Boston Diagnostic Aphasia Examination (BDAE) (Goodglass et al., 2001), lacks basic psychometric development/documentation, they are not reviewed in Table 7–1. Writing and dysgraphia are usually assessed as part of a larger battery of tests, and as such, most standardized tests of aphasia and related disorders possess several writing subtests. Most test authors, however, have not been explicit in either theory or purpose of the writing subtests. Additionally, although some classification of impairments among the various types of dysgraphia discussed above can be accomplished from the aphasia batteries reviewed [Porch Index of Communicative Ability (PICA) and Western Aphaisa Battery (WAB)], none of the batteries have systematically manipulated stimuli or tasks so as to conform to the models discussed above.

It is essential that future research describe the performance of various neurologically impaired samples on the same protocol, with the same analysis procedures to provide data useful in differentiating normal variations in writing from writing disorders that have neuropathologically predictable substrates. This call for appropriate reference data has gone unattended to the present. Indeed, although writing performance has received the least attention of any modality in the assessment of language and communication among the neurogenic populations, it has been shown to be a critical modality for many of the purposes of assessment. No area of neurogenic language and communication research is in greater need of valid, reliable, and standardized assessment procedures than the area of dysgraphia. The ad hoc adoption of tasks and scoring procedures from the experimental literature on dysgraphia does not substitute for a well-standardized and psychometrically sound assessment battery. Using informal, unstructured, observational, or custom-designed assessment techniques that have not stood the rigor of psychometric design, standardization, and evaluation will not provide the assurance of replicability, predictability, or comparability among populations or individuals that are needed for accurate detection, classification, lesion localization, and the various treatment-related issues. Continued research with the standardized and published tests currently available, along with continued research on experimental protocols such as the one previously reported (Tseng & McNeil, 1997), may eventually provide the tools needed in this most neglected area of neurogenic language and communication production assessment.

Treatment

Although the literature on the nature and assessment of dysgraphia is relatively lean, the literature on the treatment of dysgraphia is skeletal. In spite of the paucity of treatment data, several theoretical approaches to the clinical management of neurogenic dysgraphia can be culled from an amalgamation of the theoretical and the treatment literature (Martin, 1981). One approach is a rather utilitarian one in which the behaviors observed are evaluated against some internal standard of the clinician, and a direct assault is made on the behavior believed to account for the discrepancy between the observed and the expected. Typically the clinician hypothesizes about the origin of the identified behavior. Following the traditional model of neurogenic dysgraphias, the hypotheses involve the attribution of the deficit to a specific visual-spatial, motoric, linguistic, or other cognitive (e.g., memorial or attentional) origin. If a more current information-processing model is imputed, then the hypotheses might involve the attribution of the deficit to a specific subcomponent of the phonologic route or to a subcomponent of the lexical-semantic route (Mitchum & Berndt, 1991; Seron & de Partz, 1993).

Particularly important for this discussion is the fact that models of normal writing can serve as legitimate heuristics for many neurogenic dysgraphias. In other words, what is known about the processes of writing from the study of normal subjects under idealized or degraded conditions (e.g., without kines-

thetic or visual feedback or under conditions of divided attention) may have relevance for the understanding and treatment of disordered writing. In addition, what is known about all aspects of all of the neurogenic dysgraphias influences their management. As Hatfield (1983) described, there is a clear correspondence between reading and writing, and because more work has been done on reading, familiarity with the relevant constructs is essential to understanding dysgraphia. It takes little expansion of logic to realize that a full account of spelling, semantics, phonology, lexical storage and access, phoneme-to-grapheme conversion, graphemic buffers, limb motor control, attention, memory, and a myriad other legitimate areas of inquiry are necessary for the development of a theory of handwriting and its disorders and for the application of this theory to clinical management. Therefore, a parochial view of writing impedes the development of a theory of dysgraphia and delays a full accounting of the relevant variables and procedures needed for its most efficacious treatment. Even if such a theory were developed and available, it would be beyond the scope of this chapter to even review its outline. It suffices to be aware that the cognitive (including linguistic) and motor processes involved in handwriting never operate in isolation. Although much of the dysgraphia literature has developed around the search for dissociations among finite processes or computations, writing errors are rarely, if ever, attributable to a simple or single mechanism.

Following the observation of the deficit and the application of the theoretical model, one of three treatment strategies is usually adopted. The disordered behavior is (1) retrained directly or indirectly, (2) compensated for by strengthening a system capable of assuming the same function, or (3) conveyed and practiced through an alternative system or modality. The clinician needs to make three decisions before instituting one of these treatment strategies: (1) target a behavior or a process for remediation, including the context in which this treatment is to be administered (see discussion of context in

Tseng & McNeil, 1997); (2) decide on the technique(s) to be used to manipulate or influence the behavior in some direct or indirect way so as to effect change in the specific observable writing behavior; and (3) specify the criteria and the exact measurement techniques to be used to decide whether to change or terminate treatment. This final process involves specifying the single subject design that will allow the differentiation of any change in the specified behaviors to be measured that are attributable to the treatment versus those that are due to the myriad other factors that could cause the change. If the efficacy of a particular technique can be applied with a reasonable degree of confidence based on its previously documented efficacy, then step number three can be simplified or perhaps even eliminated (McNeil & Kennedy, 1984; Yoder & Kent, 1988).

Dysgraphia Treatment Literature

A cursory review of the aphasia treatment efficacy literature (Basso et al., 1979; Butfield & Zangwill, 1946; Hagen, 1973; Vignolo, 1961; Wertz et al., 1981) provides ample evidence that dysgraphia associated with aphasia can be improved with therapy. However, of necessity, these general efficacy studies do not provide sufficient detail to the rationale or structure of this treatment to be of much value to the clinician. Although a thorough review of the rationale and methods of these studies is beyond the scope of this chapter, consultation with the original sources provides some insight into the successful and unsuccessful treatment of writing associated with aphasia. Summarized in Table 7–2 are studies directed specifically toward the remediation of dysgraphia. These phase 1 or phase 2 evidence studies, mostly reported as case studies or as single-subject experimental studies, provide evidence that treating dysgraphia can be effective, especially if careful analyses of the mechanisms causing the specific deficits are addressed. They also serve to illustrate that not all treatments are effective with all subjects. Although the quantity of evidence supporting a particular

treatment's efficacy for a specific hypothesized deficit is extremely sparse, these preliminary studies provide important heuristics for clinicians and motivation for continued study.

In addition to the treatment studies summarized in Table 7–2, a variety of prosthetic devices (Brown & Chobor, 1989; Brown et al., 1983; Friedland, 1990; Leischner, 1983; Lorch, 1995a,b; Lorch & Whurr, 1991; Whurr & Lorch, 1991) have been proposed as rehabilitation tools, with a variety of neurologic explanations for the assumed effects. Although the results, and their neuropsychological explanations, are intriguing, they are uniformly without adequate experimental design to conclude either that the effects are attributable to the prosthetic device or that the person with dysgraphia had learned in the sense that writing was improved in the absence of the prosthetic device (however, see Lorch, 1995a). Research in this area has been slow to appear. Likewise, both magnetic field stimulation (Sandyk, 1996; Sandyk & Iacono, 1994) and pharmacologic agents (Gerken et al., 1991) have been shown to effect positive changes in neurogenic dysgraphias, primarily in neurodegenerative diseases such as Parkinson's disease or in pharmacologically induced dyskinesia. However, because of space limitations, these modalities of treatment are not reviewed here.

Specific Treatment Procedures

In the absence of minimally adequate experimental evidence on which to base treatment for dysgraphia, the phase 1 and phase 2 clinical evidence summarized in Table 7–2, along with expert opinion and sound theoretical/clinical logic, will guide the treatment of persons with dysgraphia. Several treatment protocols and suggested hierarchies have been proposed that can assist as models or heuristics in this enterprise. For example, Amster and Amster (1995) proposed a treatment for dysgraphia that is grounded in the premise that the "most effective procedures for retraining writing may be those that initiate instruction through a 'top-down' or

Table 7–2. Summary of Dysgraphia Treatment Studies with Both Positive and Negative Outcomes

Positive Treatment Studies

Citation	Subject N and Design	Treatment Focus (Goals)	Treatment Tasks (Stimuli)	Treatment Technique	Treatment Context	Results
Pizzamiglio & Roberts (1967)	10 each in 2 treated groups	Evaluate treatment dosage (daily versus every other day)		Spelling feedback	Teletype machine practice	Daily treatment yielded greater acquisition but equal maintenance
Mills & Kaufman (1978)	1, Single subject/case study	Improve writing letters to dictation and generalize to longer units	Writing letter names to dictation	Weigl's auditory-to-visual transcoding (finger spelling)	One-to one patient/clinician drill	Improved PICA graphic scores
Hatfield (1983)	1 "surface" dysgraphia/case study	Spontaneously writing functor words by form class	Homophone writing in isolation and in sentences	Didactic teaching of spelling rules/cuing vowels and diphthongs	One-to one patient/clinician drill	20-30% improvement on both tasks
Hatfield (1983)	3 "deep" dysgraphia/case studies	Spontaneously write functor words by form class	Homophone writing in isolation and in sentences	Dictation with feedback	One-to one patient/clinician drill isolation and in sentences	Clinician's subjectively judged improvement
Hillis & Caramazza (1987)	1 "graphemic buffer" subject/single subject multiple-baseline	Improve written spelling	Identifying correctly spelled words from sentences	Dictation with feedback	One-to-one patient/clinician drill by teaching (1) rules, and (2) a "searching" self-correction strategy	Both techniques yielded acquisition but only the self-correction strategy generalized
Behrmann (1987)	1 "surface dysgraphic" subject/pre-test-post test design (with baselines)	Improve written spelling	Paired written homophones with pictures	Clinician supplied feedback	One-to-one patient/clinician drill by linking orthography with word meaning	Significant acquisition but little generalization of homophones and good generalization to untreated irregular words

Study	Design/Subjects	Goal	Task	Feedback	Format	Outcome
de Partz, Seron & Van der Linden (1992)	1 "surface dysgraphic" subject / pretest-posttest design with trained and untrained lists	Improve written spelling	Writing words, sentences, to dictation and text completion	Error correction with explanation and copying	One-to-one patient/clinician drill by teaching (1) rules, and (2) visual imagery	"Rule"-based treatment yielded significant regular word improvement while irregular and ambiguous words did not; imagery yielded significant trained > untrained lists and good maintenance.
Aliminosa, McCloskey, Goodman-Schulman & Sokol (1993)	1 "mixed" dysgraphic / equivalently disordered treated and untreated lists without baselines; subsequent treatment of untreated list	Improve written spelling to trained and untrained word lists	Delayed copying of words and writing to dictation	Clinician supplied feedback with correction until accurate	One-to-one patient/clinician drill	Acquisition from 40% to 100% with delayed copying and no significant generalization to untrained words; following training of untrained list, acquisition reached 100%
Mitchum, Haendiges & Berndt (1993)	1 person with agrammatic aphasia / pretest-posttest without reported baselines	Writing main verbs and morphological links to verbs in sentences	Write: (1) main verb and inflections depicted in pictures and sentences, (2) construction of grammatical frames	Semantic and graphemic cueing	One-to-one patient/clinician drill	Improved main verb but not inflection retrieval with cued pictured words but not sentences. Grammatical frame generation improved and generalized
Beeson (1999)	1 person with "Wernicke's aphasia" / 4 separate multiple-baseline designs	Improve single-word noun and verb writing and single word writing as a pragmatic support for conversation	Anagram spelling and copying and writing from memory	Clinician supplied feedback with copying	One-to-one patient/clinician drill and independent homework	Improvement on drill and homework on treated nouns and verbs without generalization within or between word classes

(Continued)

Table 7–2. Summary of Dysgraphia Treatment Studies with Both Positive and Negative Outcomes (Continued)

Positive Treatment Studies

Citation	Subject N and Design	Treatment Focus (Goals)	Treatment Tasks (Stimuli)	Treatment Technique	Treatment Context	Results
Beeson, Hirsh, & Rewega (2002)	2 person with "global," 1 with "Broca," and 1 "anomic" aphasia/ each a single subject multiple-baseline design	Improve single word writing	Anagram spelling + copying (ACT) and writing from memory or ACT or homework copying	Clinician supplied feedback with anagram and copying or homework review	One-to-one patient/clinician drill and independent homework	ACT + Homework = 100% acquisition in 2 to 7 sessions with no generalization; homework alone = 100% acquisition in 2 sessions without generalization all subjects maintained

Negative Treatment Studies

Citation	Subject N and Design	Treatment Focus (Goals)	Treatment Tasks (Stimuli)	Treatment Technique	Treatment Context	Results
Schwartz, Nemeroff & Reiss (1973)	Two groups of 8 and 6 persons with aphasia	Generally improve writing performance	Group 1 multiple tasks and stimuli; group 2 multiple language (non writing) tasks	Group 1 writing alphabet, pictured nouns, words to dictation; group 2 general language stim.	One-to-one pt./ clinician drill	Post-test PICA graphic subtests improved sig. for writing group but not for general language stim. group
McNeil, Prescott & Lemme (1976)	4 persons with aphasia/pretest-posttest	Reduce general muscle tension during error productions	Various writing tasks	EMG biofeedback during difficulty graded writing tasks	One-to-one pt./ clinician drill	No significant change on PICA subtests
Mills & Kaufman (1978)	1 subject/case study		Writing letter names to dictation	60 weeks - multimodality stimulation	One-to-one pt./ clinician drill	No change on PICA graphic subtests

macroprocessing approach that exploits re-tained cognitive strengths" (p. 459). The au-thors site the work of Armus et al. (1989), who demonstrated that script knowledge was available to a large degree in individuals with aphasia, though not necessarily in writing tasks. The assumption behind this approach is that writing treatments that subordinate motor aspects, various linguistic levels, and such cognitive processes as phoneme-to-grapheme conversion rules to communicative intent processes are not only most consistent with writing instruction for children and language-learning disordered youths, but are appropriate for persons with aphasia as well. Amster and Amster (1995) outline a framework for treating dysgraphia that incor-porates both "bottom-up" and "top-down" mental operations. A similar approach stress-ing the use of premorbid traits in treatment has been espoused by Parr (1995), using "functional therapy" involving activities, strategies, and patient adjustment.

Haskins' (1976) treatment paradigm illus-trates a hierarchy of tasks frequently used in the treatment of dysgraphia. In addition to these suggestions, the availability of several treatment workbooks (Brubaker, 1978; Keith, 1980; Stryker, 1975) provides a variety of tasks that appear to be well developed both con-ceptually and technically.

None of these authors, however, provides direct evidence that his or her approach is either more efficient than any other approach or is efficacious in its own right. Without exception, these treatment tasks are as yet unaccompanied by sufficient data on their efficacy or effectiveness to allow them to be recommended for use without careful vigi-lance to their effectiveness for each patient for whom they are employed. Although these frameworks and hierarchies might be help-ful for the structure of a treatment regimen and a reasonable place to start for the begin-ning clinician, their ordering and adapta-tion to individual patient's strengths and weaknesses is necessary. As LaPointe (1985) stated, "Failure to underscore the importance of hand-tailoring the goals and techniques of therapy to the individual would be folly.

On the other hand, the attitude that specific suggestions or examples of therapy tasks cannot, or must not, be given has left begin-ning clinicians with the queasy and dually frustrating feeling of being both impotent and empty handed" (p. 206).

Although the theoretical frameworks and the tasks used in the treatment efficacy stud-ies summarized above are certainly reason-able for some individuals with some specific dysgraphic deficits, the diagnostically or the-oretically unmotivated application of any hierarchy to any individual with neurogenic dysgraphia would be folly.

Conclusion

Attempts to categorize writing disorders and relate them to the location of lesions or to the disease process thought to have caused them have been documented and summarized in this chapter. A brief review of the assessment and treatment literature on dysgraphia was also provided. From this summary it is evi-dent that acquired neurogenic dysgraphia has held a diminished status as a particu-larly essential or enlightening window into the mystery of language processing and lan-guage breakdown. This conclusion is reflected in the neglect of dysgraphia in the major aphasic taxonomies, the lack of standard-ized psychometric tests and instrumental procedures evaluating dysgraphia, and the paucity of treatment research on the topic. Although recent interest in spelling pro-cesses involved in both reading and writing may signify the coming of a new era of dys-graphia research, caution must be exercised to avoid too narrow a focus on spelling pro-cesses and the biases that may accompany the reposing on a single explanation or theory. To manage the total communication of the neurogenic patient, a complete account of language production, including that of writ-ing and the performance factors that influence it, needs to be presented.

We have attempted to summarize the current relevant state of knowledge on writ-ing and its disorders. Although this state of knowledge leaves us wanting in many domains, we hope that it has some factual and theoretic information that serves to guide the search for an understanding of acquired neurogenic dysgraphia along with its most efficacious management strategies.

References

Alexander, M.P., Fischer, R.S. & Friedman, R. (1992). Lesion Localization in Apractic Agraphia. *Archives of Neurology, 49,* 246–251.

Aliminosa, D., McCloskey, M., Goodman-Schulman, R. & Sokol, M. (1993). Remediation of Acquired Dysgraphia as a Technique for Testing Interpretations of Deficits. *Aphasiology, 7,* 55–69.

Amster, W.W. & Amster, J.B. (1995). Treatment of Writing Disorders in Aphasia. In: R. Chapey (Ed.), *Language Intervention Strategies in Adult Aphasia* (pp. 458–466). Baltimore: Williams & Wilkins.

Annoni, J.-M., Lemay, M A., Pimenta, M.A.D.M. & Lecours, A.R. (1998). The Contribution of Attentional Mechanisms to an Irregularity Effect at the Graphemic Buffer Level. *Brain and Language, 63,* 64–78.

Armus, S.R., Brookshire, R.H. & Nicholas, L.E. (1989). Aphasic and Non-Brain-Damaged Adults' Knowledge of Script for Common Situations. *Brain and Language, 36,* 518–528.

Aten, J.L. & Lyon, J.G. (1978). Measures of PICA Subtest Variance: A Preliminary Assessment of Their Value as Predictors of Language Recovery in Aphasic Patients. *Clinical Aphasiology, 8,* 106–116.

Basso, A., Capitani, E. & Vignolo, L.A. (1979). Influence of Rehabilitation of Language Skills in Aphasic Patients: A Controlled Study. *Archives of Neurology, 36,* 190–196.

Baxter, D.M. & Warrington, E.K. (1985). Category Specific Dysgraphia. *Neuropsychologia, 23,* 653–666.

Beauvois, M.-F. & Derousene, J. (1981). Lexical or orthographic agraphia. *Brain, 104,* 21–49.

Beeson, P.M. (1999). Treating Acquired Writing Impairment: Strengthening Graphemic Representations. *Aphasiology, 13,* 767–785.

Beeson, P.M., Hirsch, F.M. & Rewega, M.A. (2002). Successful Single-Word Writing Treatment: Experimental Analyses of Four Cases. *Aphasiology, 16,* 473–491.

Behrmann, M. (1987). The Rites of Righting Writing: Homophone Remediation in Acquired Dysgraphia. *Cognitive Neuropsychology, 4,* 365–384.

Benson, D.F. (1979). *Aphasia, Alexia, and Agraphia.* New York: Churchill Livingstone.

Benson, D.F. & Geschwind, N. (1985). Aphasia and Related Disorders: A Clinical Approach. In: M.-M. Mesulam (Ed.), *Principles of Behavioral Neurology* (pp. 193–238). Philadelphia: FA Davis.

Benton, A.L. (1992). Gerstmann's Syndrome. *Archives of Neurology, 49,* 445–447.

Bradshaw, J.L. & Nettleton, N.C. (1983). *Human Cerebral Asymmetry.* Englewood Cliffs, NJ: Prentice-Hall.

Brauer, D. (1989). Differentiation of Learning Disabled, Aphasic and Normal Adults' Language Performance on Selected Aphasia Batteries. Unpublished master's thesis, University of Wisconsin.

Brauer, D., McNeil, M.R., Duffy, J.R., Keith, R.L. & Collins, M.J. (1989). The Differentiation of Normal from Aphasic Performance Using PICA Discriminant Function Scores. *Clinical Aphasiology, 18,* 117–129.

Brown, J. & Chobor, K. (1989). Therapy with Prosthesis for Writing in Aphasia. *Aphasiology, 3,* 709–715.

Brown, J., Leader, B. & Blum, S. (1983). Hemiplegic Writing in Severe Aphasia. *Brain and Language, 19,* 204–215.

Brubaker, S.H. (1978). *Workbook for Aphasia.* Detroit: Wayne State University Press.

Bub, D. & Kertesz, A. (1982a). Evidence for Lexicographic Processing in a Patient with Preserved Writing Over Oral Single Word Naming. *Brain, 105,* 697–717.

Bub, D. & Kertesz, A. (1982b). Deep Agraphia. *Brain and Language, 17,* 146–165.

Butfield, E. & Zangwill, O. (1946). Re-Education in Aphasia: A Review of 70 Cases. *Journal of Neurology, Neurosurgery and Psychiatry, 9,* 75–79.

Caramazza, A., Miceli, G., Villa, G. & Romani, C. (1987). The Role of the Graphemic Buffer in Spelling: Evidence from a Case of Acquired Dysgraphia. *Cognition, 26,* 59–85.

Chedru, F. & Geschwind, N. (1972). Writing Disturbances in Acute Confusional States. *Neuropsychologia, 10,* 343–353.

Crary, M.A. & Heilman, K.M. (1988). Letter Imagery Deficits in a Case of Pure Apraxic Agraphia. *Brain and Language, 34,* 147–156.

Crosson, B. (1992). *Subcortical Functions in Language and Memory.* New York: Guilford Press.

Deal, J.L., Deal, L.A., Wertz, R.T., Kitselman, K. & Dwyer, D. (1979). Right Hemisphere PICA Percentiles: Some Speculations about Aphasia. *Clinical Aphasiology, 9,* 30–37.

De Bastini, P. & Barry, C. (1989). A Cognitive Analysis of an Acquired Dysgraphic Patient with an "Allographic" Writing Disorder. *Cognitive Neuropsychology, 6,* 25–41.

Dell, G.S. (1984). Representation of Serial Order in Speech: Evidence from the Repeated Phoneme Effect in Speech Errors. *Journal of Experimental Psychology: Learning, Memory, and Cognition, 10,* 222–233.

Dell, G.S. (1988). The Retrieval of Phonological Forms in Production: Tests of Predictions from a Connectionist Model. *Journal of Memory and Language, 27,* 124–142.

De Partz, M-P., Seron, S. & Van der Linden, M. (1992). Re-education of a Surface Dysgraphia with a Visual Imagery Strategy. *Cognitive Neuropsychology, 9,* 369–401.

Destreie, N.D.G., Farina, E., Alberoni, M., Pomati, S., Nichelli, P. & Mariani, C. (2000). Selective Uppercase Dysgraphia with Loss of Visual Imagery of Letter Forms: A Window on the Organization of Graphomotor Pattern. *Brain and Language, 71,* 353–372.

Duffy, J.R. & Keith, R.C. (1980). Performance of Non-Brain Injured Adults on the PICA: Descriptive Data and a Comparison in Patients with Aphasia. *Aphasia-Apraxia-Agnosia, 1,* 1–29.

Ellis, A.W. (1982). Spelling and Writing (and Reading and Speaking). In A.W. Ellis (Ed.), *Normality and Pathology in Cognitive Functions* (pp. 113–146). London: Academic Press.

Ellis, A.W. (1989). *Reading, Writing and Dyslexia.* Hove, UK: LEA Publishers.

Ellis, A.W., Young, A.W. & Flude, B.M. (1987). "Afferent Dysgraphia" in a Patient and in Normal Subjects. *Cognitive Neuropsychology, 4*, 465–486.

Friedland, J. (1990). Accessing Language in Agraphia: An Examination of Hemiplegic Writing. *Aphasiology, 4*, 241–257.

Frith, U. (1980). *Cognitive Processes in Spelling*. London: Academic Press.

Gerken, A., Wetzel, H. & Benkert, O. (1991). Extrapyramidal Symptoms and Their Relationship to Clinical Efficacy Under Perphenazine Treatment: A Controlled Prospective Handwriting-Test Study in 22 Acutely Ill Schizophrenic Patients. *Pharmacopsychiatry, 24*, 132–137.

Goodglass, H. (1981). The Syndromes of Aphasia: Similarities and Differences in Neurolinguistic Features. *Topics in Language Disorders, 1*, 1–14.

Goodglass, H. & Hunter, M.A. (1970). Linguistic Comparisons of Speech and Writing in Two Types of Aphasia. *Journal of Communication Disorders, 3*, 28–35.

Goodglass, H., Kaplan, E. & Barresi, B. (2001). *The Assessment of Aphasia and Related Disorders* (3rd ed.). Philadelphia: Lea and Febiger.

Goodman, R.A. & Caramazza, A. (1985). *The Johns Hopkins Dysgraphia Battery*. Baltimore: Johns Hopkins University.

Goodman, R.A. & Caramazza, A. (1986). Dissociation of Spelling Errors in Written and Oral Spelling: The Role of Allographic Conversion in Writing. *Cognitive Neuropsychology, 3*, 179–206.

Hagen, C. (1973). Communication Abilities in Hemiplegia: Effect of Speech Therapy. *Archives of Physical Medical Rehabilitation, 54*, 454–463.

Halpern, H., Darley, F.L. & Brown, J.R. (1973). Differential Language and Neurological Characteristics in Cerebral Involvement. *Journal of Speech and Hearing Disorders, 38*, 162–173.

Hansen, A.M. & McNeil, M R. (1986). Differences Between Writing with Dominant and Nondominant Hand by Normal Geriatric Subjects on a Spontaneous Writing Task. *Clinical Aphasiology, 16*, 166–122.

Hansen, A.M., McNeil, M.R. & Vetter, D.K. (1987). More Differences Between Writing with Dominant and Nondominant Hand by Normal Geriatric Subjects: Eight Perceptual and Eight Computerized Measures on a Sentence Dictation Task. *Clinical Aphasiology, 17*, 152–157.

Hashimoto, R., Tanaka, Y. & Yoshida, M. (1998). Selective Kana Jargonagraphia Following Right Hemisphere Infarction. *Brain and Language, 63*, 50–63.

Haskins, S. (1976). A Treatment Procedure for Writing Disorders. *Clinical Aphasiology, 6*, 192–199.

Hatfield, F.M. (1983). Aspects of Acquired Dysgraphia and Implications for Re-education. In: C. Code & D.J. Muller (Eds.), *Aphasia Therapy* (pp. 157–169). London: Edward Arnold.

Hatfield, F.M. & Patterson, K.E. (1985). Phonological Spelling. *Quarterly Journal of Experimental Psychology, 35A*, 451–468.

Hecaen, H. & Angelergues, R. (1964). Localizations of Symptoms in Aphasia. In: A. DeReuck & M. O'Connor (Eds.), *Disorders of Language* (pp. 223–260). London: Ciba Foundation.

Hecaen, H. & Marcie, P. (1974). Disorders of Written Language Following Right Hemisphere Lesions: Spatial Dysgraphia. In: S.J. Dimond & J. Beaumont (Eds.), *Hemisphere Function in the Human Brain* (pp. 345–366). London: Elek Science.

Henderson, V.W., Buckwalter, J.G., Sobel, E., et al. (1992). The Agraphia of Alzheimer's Disease. *Neurology, 42*, 776–784.

Hillis, A.E. & Caramazza, A. (1987). Model-Driven Remediation of Dysgraphia. *Clinical Aphasiology, 17*, 84–105.

Hillis, A.E. & Caramazza, A. (1989). The Graphemic Buffer and Attentional Mechanisms. *Brain and Language, 36*, 208–235.

Hillis, A.E., Rapp, B.C. & Caramazza, A. (1999). When a Rose Is a Rose in Speech but a Tulip in Writing. *Cortex, 35*, 337–356.

Hodges, J.R. (1991). Pure Apraxic Agraphia with Recovery After Drainage of a Left Frontal Cyst. *Cortex, 27*, 469–473.

Horner, J., Heyman, A., Dawson, D. & Rogers, H. (1988). The Relationship of Agraphia to the Severity of Dementia in Alzheimer's Disease. *Archives of Neurology, 45*, 760–763.

Horner, J., Lathrop, D.L., Fish, A.M. & Dawson, D. (1987). Agraphia in Left and Right Hemisphere Stroke and Alzheimer Dementia Patients. *Clinical Aphasiology, 17*, 73–83.

Iribarren, I.C., Jarema, G. & Lecours, A.R. (2001). Two Different Dysgraphic Syndromes in a Regular Orthography, Spanish. *Brain and Language, 77*, 166–175.

Jonsdottir, M.K., Shallice, T. & Wise, R. (1996). Phonological Mediation and the Graphemic Buffer Disorder in Spelling: Cross-Language Differences? *Cognition, 59*, 169–197.

Kao, H.S.R., van Galen, G.P. & Hoosain, R. (1986). Graphonomics. Amsterdam: Elsevier.

Kaplan, E. & Goodglass, H. (1981). Aphasia-Related Disorders. In: M.T. Sarno (Ed.), *Acquired Aphasia* (pp. 303–325). New York: Academic.

Katz, R.B. (1991). Limited Retention of Information in the Graphemic Buffer. *Cortex, 27*, 111–119.

Kay, J., Lesser, R. & Coltheart, M. (1992). *Psycholinguistic Assessments of Language Processing in Aphasia (PALPA)*. Hillsdale, NJ: Erlbaum.

Keenan, I.S. & Brassell, E.G. (1974). Factors Influencing Linguistic Recovery in Aphasic Adults. *Journal of Speech and Hearing Disorders, 39*, 1–12.

Keith, R.L. (1980). *Speech and Language Rehabilitation: A Workbook for the Neurologically Impaired*. Danville: Interstate Printers and Publishers.

Kertesz, A. (1979). *Aphasia and Associated Disorders: Taxonomy, Location and Recovery*. New York: Grune and Stratton.

Kim, H. & Na, D.L. (2000). Dissociation of Pure Korean Words and Chinese-Derivative Words in Phonological Dysgraphia. *Brain and Language, 74*, 134–137.

Klatka, L.A., Depper, M. H. & Marini, A. (1998). Infarction in the Territory of the Anterior Cerebral Artery. *Neurology, 51*, 620–622.

Kokubo, K., Suzuki, K., Yamadori, A. & Satou, K. (2001). Pure Kana Agraphia as a Manifestation of Graphemic Buffer Impairment. *Cortex, 37*, 187–195.

LaBerge, E., Smith, D.S., Dick, L. & Storandt, M. (1992). Agraphia in Dementia of the Alzheimer's Type. *Archives of Neurology, 49*, 1151–1156.

Laine, T. & Marttila, R.J. (1981). Pure Agraphia: A Case Study. *Neuropsychologia, 19*, 311–316.

Lambert, J., Eustache, F., Viader, F., Dary, M., Rioux, P. & Lechevalier, B. (1996). Agraphia in Alzheimer's Disease: An Independent Lexical Impairment. *Brain and Language, 53,* 222–233.

LaPointe, L.L. (1985). Aphasia Therapy: Some Principles and Strategies for Treatment. In: D.F. Johns (Ed.), *Clinical Management of Neurogenic Communicative Disorders* (pp. 179–241). Boston/Toronto: Little, Brown.

Lebrun, Y. (1976). Neurolinguistic Models of Language and Speech. In: H. Whitaker & H.A. Whitaker (Eds.), *Studies in Neurolinguistics* (vol. 1, pp. 1–30). New York: Academic Press.

Leischner, A. (1969). The agraphias. In: P.J. Vinken & C.W. Bruyn (Eds.), *Handbook of Clinical Neurology* (vol. 4, pp. 141–180). Amsterdam: North-Holland Publishing.

Leischner, A. (1983). Side Differences in Writing to Dictation of Aphasics with Agraphia: A Graphic Disconnection Syndrome. *Brain and Language, 18,* 1–19.

Lorch, M.P. (1995a). Language and Praxis in Written Production: A Rehabilitation Paradigm. *Aphasiology, 9,* 280–282.

Lorch, M.P. (1995b). Laterality and Rehabilitation: Differences in Left and Right Hand Productions in Aphasic Agraphic Hemiplegics. *Aphasiology, 9,* 257–271.

Lorch, M.P. & Whurr, M. (1991). Hemiplegic Writing with the Use of a Prosthesis in an Aphasic Agraphic Patient. *Grazer Linguistische Studien: Neuro-und Patholinguistik, 35,* 214–227.

Luzzatti, C., Laiacona, M., Allamano, N., De Tanti, A. & Inzaghi, M.G. (1998). Writing Disorders in Italian Aphasic Patients: A Multiple Single-Case Study of Dysgraphia in a Language with Shallow Orthography. *Brain, 121,* 1721–1734.

Maeshima, S., Ueyoshi, A., Matsumoto, T., Okita, R., Yamaga, H., Ozaki, F., et al. (2002). Agraphia in Kanji After a Contusional Haemorrhage in the Left Temporo-Occipital Lobe. *Journal of Neurology, Neurosurgery, and Psychiatry, 72,* 126–127.

Marcie, P. & Hecaen, H. (1979). Agraphia: Writing Disorders Associated with Unilateral Lesions. In: K.M. Heilman & E. Valenstein (Eds.), *Clinical Neuropsychology* (pp. 92–127). New York: Oxford University Press.

Margolin, D.E. & Wing, A.M. (1983). Agraphia and Micrographia: Clinical Manifestations of Motor Programming and Performance Disorders. *Acta Psychologica, 54,* 263–283.

Martin, A.D. (1981). The Role of Theory in Therapy: A Rationale. *Topics in Language Disorders, 1,* 63–72.

Mateer, C.A. & Ojemann, G.A. (1983). Thalamic Mechanisms in Language and Memory. In: S.J. Segalowitz (Ed.), *Language Function and Brain Organization* (pp. 171–191). New York: Academic.

McCloskey, M., Badecker, W., Goodman-Schulman, R.A. & Aliminosa, D. (1994). The Structure of Graphemic Representations in Spelling: Evidence from a Case of Acquired Dysgraphia. *Cognitive Neuropsychology, 11,* 341–392.

McNeil, M.R. (1984). Current Concepts in Adult Aphasia. *International Rehabilitation Medicine, 6,* 128–134.

McNeil, M.R., Doyle, P.J. & Wambaugh, J. (2000). Apraxia of Speech: A Treatable Disorder of Motor Planning and Programming. In: S.E. Nadeau,

L.J. Gonzalez Rothi & B. Crosson (Eds.), *Aphasia and Language: Theory to Practice* (pp. 221–266). New York: Guilford Press.

McNeil, M.R. & Kennedy, J.G. (1984). Measuring the Effects of Treatment for Dysarthria: Knowing When to Change or Terminate. *Seminars in Speech and Language: Dysarthria: Nature and Assessment, 5,* 337–358.

McNeil, M.R. & Pratt, S.R. (2001). Defining Aphasia: Some Theoretical and Clinical Implications of Operating from a Formal Definition. *Aphasiology, 15,* 901–912.

McNeil, M.R., Pratt, S.R. & Fossett, T.R.D. (2004). Differential Diagnosis of Apraxia of Speech. In: B. Maassen, R.D. Kent, H.F.M. Peters, P.H.M.M. Van Lieshout & W. Hulstijn (Eds.), *Speech Motor Control in Normal and Disordered Speech* (pp. 389–413). Oxford, UK: Oxford Medical Publications.

McNeil, M.R., Prescott, T.E. & Lemme, M.L. (1976). An Application of Electromyographic Biofeedback to Aphasia/Apraxia Treatment. *Clinical Aphasiology, 6,* 151–171.

Mesulam, M.-M. (1985). Attention, Confusional States, and Neglect. In: M.-M. Mesulam (Ed.), *Principles of Behavioral Neurology* (pp. 125–168). Philadelphia: FA Davis.

Metzler, N.G. & Jelinek, I.E.M. (1977). Writing Disturbances in Patients with Right Cerebral Hemisphere Lesions. *Clinical Aphasiology, 7,* 214–225.

Miceli, G., Silveri, M.C. & Caramazza, A. (1985). Cognitive Analysis of a Case of Pure Agraphia. *Brain and Language, 25,* 187–212.

Mills, R.H. & Kaufman, E. (1978). Gestural Signing: Treatment for a Letter Writing to Dictation Impairment. *Clinical Aphasiology, 8,* 188–200.

Miozzo, M. & De Bastiani, P. (2002). The Organization of Letter-Forma Representations in Written Spelling: Evidence from Acquired Dysgraphia. *Brain and Language, 80,* 366–392.

Mitchum, C.C. & Berndt, R.S. (1991). Diagnosis and Treatment of "Phonological Assembly" in Acquired Dyslexia: An Illustration of the Cognitive Neuropsychological Approach. *Journal of Neurolinguistics, 6,* 103–137.

Mitchum, C.C., Heandiges, A.N. & Berndt, R.S. (1993). Model-Guided Treatment to Improve Written Sentence Production: A Case Study. *Aphasiology, 7,* 71–109.

Myers, P.S. (1999). *Right Hemisphere Damage.* San Diego: Singular.

Nadeau, S.E. & Crosson, B. (1997). Subcortical Aphasia. *Brain and Language, 58,* 355–402.

Nadeau, S.E. & Gonzalez-Rothi, L.J. (2001). Rehabilitation of Subcortical Aphasia. In R. Chapey (Ed.), *Language Intervention in Aphasia and Related Neurogenic Communication Disorders* (pp. 457–471). Philadelphia: Lippincott Williams & Wilkins.

Neils, J., Roeltgen, D.P. & Greer, A. (1995). Spelling and Attention in Early Alzheimer's Disease: Evidence for Impairment of the Graphemic Buffer. *Brain and Language, 49,* 241–262.

Neils-Sturnjas, J., Shuren, J., Roeltgen, D. & Brown, C. (1998). Perseverative Writing Errors in a Patient with Alzheimer's Disease. *Brain and Language, 63,* 303–320.

Odell, K.H., Hashi, M., Miller, S.B. & McNeil, M.R. (1995). A Critical Look at the Notion of Selective Impairment. *Clinical Aphasiology, 23,* 1–8.

Ohno, T., Bando, M., Nagura, H., Ishii, K. & Yamanouchi, H. (2000). Apraxic Agraphia Due to Thalamic Infarction. *Neurology, 54*, 2336–2339.

Otsuki, M., Soma, Y., Arai, T., Otsuka, A. & Tsuji, S. (1999). Pure Apraxic Agraphia with Abnormal Writing Stroke Sequences: Report of a Japanese Patient with a Left Superior Parietal Haemorrhage. *Journal of Neurology, Neurosurgery, and Psychiatry, 66*, 223–237.

Parr, S. (1995). Everyday Reading and Writing in Aphasia: Role Change and the Influence of Pre-morbid Literacy Practice. *Aphasiology, 9*, 223–238.

Penniello, M.-J., Lambert, J., Eustache, F., Petit-Taboue, M.C., Barre, L., Viader, F., et al. (1995). A PET Study of the Functional Neuroanatomy of Writing Impairment in Alzheimer's Disease: The Role of the Left Supramarginal and Left Angular Gyri. *Brain, 118*, 697–706.

Pizzamiglio, L. & Roberts, M. (1967). Writing in Aphasia: A Learning Study. *Cortex, 3*, 250–257.

Porch, B.E. (1971). *Porch Index of Communicative Ability* (vol. 2). Administration and Scoring. Palo Alto, CA: Consulting Psychologist Press.

Porch, B.E. (1978). Profiles of Aphasia: Test Interpretation Regarding the Localization of Lesions. *Clinical Aphasiology, 8*, 78–92.

Porch, B.E. (1986). Therapy Subsequent to the Porch Index of Communicative Ability. In: Chapey R (Ed.), *Language Intervention Strategies in Adult Aphasia* (pp. 295–303). Baltimore: Williams & Wilkins.

Porch, B.E. & Callaghan, S. (1981). Making Predictions About Recovery: Is There HOAP? *Clinical Aphasiology, 11*, 187–200.

Porch, B.E., Friden, T. & Porec, J. (1976). Objective Differentiation of Aphasic Versus Non-Organic Patients. Paper presented at the meeting of the International Neuropsychology Association, Santa Fe, New Mexico.

Posner, M. & Raichle, M.E. (1994). *Images of Brain.* New York: Scientific American Library.

Posteraro, L., Zinelli, P. & Mazzucchi, A. (1988). Selective Impairment of the Graphemic Buffer in Acquired Dysgraphia: A Case Study. *Brain and Language, 35*, 274–286.

Rapcsak, S.Z. & Beeson, P.M. (2000). Agraphia. In: S.E. Nadeau, L.J. Gonzalez-Rothi & B. Crosson (Eds.), *Aphasia and Language: Theory to Practice* (pp. 184–220). New York: Guilford Press.

Roeltgen, D.P. (1985). Agraphia. In: K.M. Heilman & E. Valenstein (Eds.), *Clinical Neuropsychology* (pp. 75–96). New York: Oxford University Press.

Roeltgen, D.P. (1993). Agraphia. In: K.M. Heilman & E. Valenstein (Eds.), *Clinical Neuropsychology* (pp. 63–89). New York: Oxford University Press.

Roeltgen, D.P. & Heilman, K.M. (1983). Apraxic Agraphia in a Patient with Normal Praxis. *Brain and Language, 18*, 35–46.

Rosenbek, J.C., McNeil, M.R. & Teetson, M. (1981). Syndrome of Neuromotor Speech Deficit and Dysgraphia? *Clinical Aphasiology, 9*, 309–315.

Rothi, L.J.G., Roeltgen, D.P. & Kooistra, C.A. (1987). Isolated Lexical Agraphia in a Right-Handed Patient with a Posterior Lesion of the Right Cerebral Hemisphere. *Brain and Language, 30*, 181–190.

Sakurai, Y., Matsumura, K., Iwatsubo, T. & Momose, T. (1997). Frontal Pure Agraphia for Kanji or Kana:

Dissociation Between Morphology and Phonology. *Neurology, 49*, 946–952.

Sakurai, Y., Sakai, K., Sakuta, M. & Iwata, M. (1994). Naming Difficulties in Alexia for Kanji After a Left Posterior Inferior Temporal Lesion. *Journal of Neurology, Neurosurgery, and Psychiatry, 57*, 609–613.

Sandyk, R. (1996). Brief Communication: Electromagnetic Fields Improve Visuospatial Performance and Reverse Agraphia in a Parkinsonian Patient. *International Journal of Neuroscience, 87*, 209–217.

Sandyk, R. & Iacono, R.P. (1994). Reversal of Micrographia in Parkinson's Disease by Application of Picotesla Range Magnetic Fields. *International Journal of Neuroscience, 77*, 77–84.

Schwartz, L., Nemeroff, S. & Reiss, M. (1973). An Investigation of Writing Therapy for the Adult Aphasic: The Word [sic] Level. *Cortex, 9*, 278–283.

Seki, S., Ishiai, S., Koyama, Y., Sato, S., Hirabayashi, H., Inaki, K. & Nakayama, T. (1998). Effects of Unilateral Neglect on Spatial Agraphia of Kana and Kanji Letters. *Brain and Language, 63*, 256–275.

Selinger, M., Prescott, T.E. & Katz, R. (1987). Handwritten Vs Computer Responses on Porch Index of Communicative Ability Graphic Subtests. *Clinical Aphasiology, 17*, 136–142.

Seron, X. & de Partz, M.P. (1993). The Re-education of Aphasia: Between Theory and Practice. In: A.L. Holland & M.M. Forbes (Eds.), *Aphasia Treatment: World Perspectives* (pp. 131–144). San Diego: Singular.

Shallice, T. (1981). Phonological Agraphia and the Lexical Route in Writing. *Brain, 104*, 413–429.

Silveri, M.C. (1996). Peripheral Aspects of Writing Can be Differentially Affected by Sensorial and Attentional Defect: Evidence from a Patient with Afferent Agraphia and Case Dissociation. *Cortex, 32*, 155–172.

Silveri, M.C., Misciagna, S., Leggio, M.G. & Molinari, M. (1997). Spatial Dysgraphia and Cerebellar Lesion: A Case Report. *Neurology, 48*, 1529–1532.

Simerniskaya, E.G. (1974). On Two Forms of Writing Defect Following Local Brain Lesions. In: S.J. Diamond & J. Beaumont (Eds.), *Hemisphere Function in the Human Brain.* London: Elek Science.

Stryker, S. (1975). *Speech After Stroke: A Manual for the Speech Pathologist and the Family Member.* Springfield, IL: Charles C Thomas.

Tainturier, M.J. & Caramazza, A. (1996). The Status of Double Letters in Graphemic Representations. *Journal of Memory and Language, 35*, 53–73.

Tanridag, O. & Kirshner, H S. (1985). Aphasia and Agraphia in Lesions of the Posterior Internal Capsule and Putamen. *Neurology, 35*, 1797–1801.

Taylor, I. (1985). The Sequence and Structure of Handwriting Competence: Where Are the Breakdown Points in the Mastery of Handwriting? *Occupational Therapy, 40*, 205–207.

Tompkins, C.A. (1995). *Right Hemisphere Communication Disorders: Theory and management.* San Diego: Singular Publishing Group.

Tseng, C-H. & McNeil, M.R. (1997). Nature and Management of Acquired Neurogenic Dysgraphias. In: L.L. LaPointe (Ed.), *Aphasia and Related Neurogenic Language Disorders* (2nd ed., pp. 172–200). New York: Thieme.

Van der Merwe, A. (1997). A Theoretical Framework for the Characterization of Pathological Speech Sensorimotor Control, In: M.R. McNeil (Ed.), *Clinical Management of Sensorimotor Speech Disorders* (pp. 1–26). New York: Thieme.

Vignolo, L.A. (1961). Evolution of Aphasia and Language Rehabilitation: A Retrospective Exploratory Study. *Cortex, 1,* 344–367.

Watson, J.M. & Records, L.E. (1978). The Effectiveness of the Porch Index of Communicative Ability as a Diagnostic Tool in Assessing Specific Behaviors of Senile Dementia. *Clinical Aphasiology, 8,* 93–105.

Wertz, R.T., Collins, M.J., Weiss, D., Kurtzke, J.F., Frieden, T., Brookshire, R.H., et al. (1981). Veterans Administration Cooperative Study on Aphasia: A Comparison of Individual and Group Treatment. *Journal of Speech and Hearing Research, 24,* 580–594.

Wertz, R.T., Deal, L.A. & Deal J.L. (1980). Prognosis in Aphasia: Investigation of the High-Overall (HOAP) and the Short-Direct (HOAP Slope) Method to Predict Change in PICA Performance. *Clinical Aphasiology, 10,* 164–173.

Whurr, M. & Lorch, M. (1991). The Use of a Prosthesis to Facilitate Writing in Aphasia and Right Hemiplegia. *Aphasiology, 5,* 411–418.

Wingard, E.M., Barrett, A.M., Crucian, G.P., Doty, L. & Heilman, K.M. (2002). The Gerstmann Syndrome in Alzheimer's Disease. *Journal of Neurology, Neurosurgery and Psychiatry, 72,* 403–405.

Yoder, D.E. & Kent, R.D. (Eds.) (1988). *Decision Making in Speech and Language Pathology.* Toronto: BC Decker.

Zaidel, E. (1978). Lexical Organization in the Right Hemisphere. *INSERM Symposium, 6,* 177–197.

Zaidel, E. (1985). Language in the Right Hemisphere. In: D.F. Benson & E. Zaidel (Eds.), *The Dual Brain* (pp. 205–231). New York: Guilford Press.

Zesiger, P., Pegna, A. & Rilliet, B. (1994). Unilateral Dysgraphia of the Dominant Hand in a Left-Hander: A Disruption of Graphic Motor Pattern Selection. *Cortex, 30,* 673–683.

8

Broca's Aphasia

KEVIN P. KEARNS

Although a variety of language disorders had been recognized prior to the mid-19th century (Benton, 1998) the study of aphasia can be directly traced to the work of a 37-year-old surgeon and anthropologist, Pierre Paul Broca (1861). Ironically, the first patient described by Broca did not appear to have the syndrome that bears his name (A. Damasio, 1998). Broca was primarily interested in localizing the faculty of articulated speech (i.e., motor aspects of speech production), and not the "general faculty of language" (Head, 1963).

Broca's aphasia is perhaps the most frequently occurring and widely recognized aphasia syndrome (Kertesz, 1982). The core features of Broca's aphasia include a nonfluent, halting verbal output that is characterized by incomplete and syntactically simplified sentences, reduced phrase length, a prosodic disturbance, and awkward articulation. The verbal output problems of individuals with Broca's aphasia often reflect a concomitant apraxia of speech, and agrammatism is a common, although not invariant, feature. Those having Broca's aphasia often omit function words (i.e., articles, conjunctions, pronouns, auxiliary verbs, and prepositions) and grammatical morphemes from their speech while retaining a relatively greater proportion of content words (i.e., nouns, verbs, and adverbs). Some individuals produce a relative paucity of verbs in their speech.

Auditory comprehension, although impaired, is relatively spared and often functional for everyday conversation. Repetition of spoken words and phrases and confrontation naming ability are also impaired in this syndrome. Writing is also impaired, and written errors may qualitatively resemble verbal production errors. Similarly, reading comprehension is deficient to a degree that generally parallels auditory comprehension.

There was an ongoing debate about localization of cerebral functions during the meetings of the French Anthropology Society in 1861 (Head, 1963). Unfortunately, the debate consisted mostly of logical arguments and rigid opinions rather than data-based presentations. While immersed in this professional atmosphere, Broca had the opportunity to examine a patient who presented with loss of speech and other clinical signs of frontal lobe damage. He viewed this patient as a possible test case of the theory of localization of the faculty of speech to the frontal lobes. The patient, Leborgne, had been an epileptic throughout his life, but he had functioned quite well prior to being hospitalized after he had lost the use of his speech. He had been in the hospital for more than 20 years prior to his referral to Broca. Head (1963) notes that Broca could not determine if the patient's speechlessness had occurred suddenly or gradually. However, the patient appeared to have normal hearing, and he could understand almost all that was said to him. He could not speak or write. Fortunately for science, but unfortunately for Leborgne, he died several days after Broca's clinical examination.

Broca was reportedly a superb anatomist, and he had the foresight to perform an autopsy on his patient. He presented his observations to the Anthropology Society the day after the postmortem examination. Broca concluded that his case supported the claim that the frontal lobes were indeed responsible for the "faculty of articulate language." Despite the fact that Broca provided the first objective findings to support the localizationist position, the response to his conclusions were underwhelming. As Head (1963) reports, "It is customary to speak of Broca's discovery as if it came like a clap of thunder from a clear sky; this was by no means the case" (p. 17).

In August 1861, Broca subsequently presented a precise anatomic description of his autopsy findings on Leborgne to the French Anatomical Society, and Broca labeled the loss of the "special faculty for articulated language" as "aphemia." (The term *aphasia* was coined by Trousseau in 1864 and was adopted in place of "aphemia" despite Broca's objections.) Later that year Broca had the good fortune to examine a second patient who, years earlier had collapsed and "lost the power of speech." Similar to Leborgne, this patient appeared to be intelligent and could understand most or all of what was said to him. His verbal output was restricted to a limited vocabulary of poorly articulated words.

This second patient also died while under Broca's care and was subsequently autopsied. Despite rather extensive and diffuse damage, Broca relied on neuroanatomical concepts of his day to conclude that "the aphemia was the result of a profound, but accurately circumscribed lesion of the posterior third of second and third frontal convolutions" (Head, 1963). Postmortem examination of his two patients led to Broca's now famous conclusion that the faculty for articulate speech could be localized to the third frontal convolution. The posterior-

inferior frontal gyrus of the left cerebral hemisphere continues to be referred to as "Broca's area."

Broca's contributions to aphasiology were not confined to the discovery that speech production capabilities were localizable to the posterior portion of the frontal lobes. He rejected the popular phrenologic approach to cerebral localization, and he observed that the left cerebral hemisphere appeared to be specialized for expressive language functions. [Although Dax discussed hemispheric specialization 30 years prior to Broca, Dax's observations were unpublished and relatively unknown (Critchley, 1964).] Broca (1865) is also credited with linking left hemisphere dominance for language with handedness, in commenting on embryologic differences between the hemispheres, and for noting that the right hemisphere has receptive language capabilities. From a clinical perspective, it is remarkable that Broca concluded that the right hemisphere could subsume left hemisphere functions and that language rehabilitation could benefit aphasic patients. It seems impossible to overestimate Broca's influence on aphasiology. Broca was largely responsible for elevating the study of aphasia from a minor curiosity to its current position as a disorder with diagnostic implications for identifying focal brain damage and cerebral localization (Benton, 1998; Roth & Heilman, 2000).

Pathophysiology

Early clinical-anatomic correlations of the localizationists and holists alike provided limited insight and resolution into the controversy surrounding the localization of language abilities because the interval between ictus and examination was often not documented in early autopsy studies, and there was a lack of specificity with regard to the nature of the aphasic deficits (Kertesz, 1979; Mohr et al., 1978). Despite renewed interest in aphasia and localization following the Second World War, significant advances in our views regarding the localization of language abilities in specific cortical areas, such as Broca's area, remained relatively stagnant until modern advances in brain imaging techniques permitted in vivo studies of cerebral changes following brain injury. Following is a brief summary of lesion localization information relating to Broca's aphasia. This topic is covered extensively in recent reviews of neuroimaging techniques and their contributions to aphasia (Demmonet & Thierry, 2001; Hillis, 2002).

The advent of computerized axial tomography (CT) has led to new insights into brain-behavior relationships in aphasia, and it has led to a refinement of our view of the role of Broca's area in language processing and aphasia (A. Damasio, 1998). Naeser and Hayward (1978) examined the relationship between CT findings and language profiles in 19 stable aphasic subjects who had suffered a single left hemisphere stroke. Their results support the classical schema for localization of Wernicke's, Broca's, conduction, and global aphasia. Subsequent studies have replicated the general finding that there is a significant correlation between lesion localization and type of aphasia. However, Mohr et al.'s (1978) extensive review of the literature in conjunction with his examination of autopsy data and neuroradiodiagnostic findings has modified our view of the role of Broca's area in language production and aphasia. Mohr et al. concluded that small lesions confined to Broca's area "[do] not cause what traditionally and currently considered to be Broca's aphasia. . . . The principal deficit in this syndrome is best described as dyspraxia of speaking aloud" (p. 321).

Naeser et al.'s (1986) findings support and extend Mohr's conclusion that extensive lesions are typically found in Broca's patients. However, Naeser et al. report that some patients with significant Broca's area lesions and sparing of other neuroanatomic areas recover speech fluency to a remarkable degree. They suggest that the extent of lesion in the subcallosal fasciculus and periventricular white matter and the middle one-third of periventricular white matter may play a critical role in the recovery of spontaneous speech.

Although the results of CT studies demonstrate a significant correlation between lesion sites and aphasia classification, there are many exceptions to predictions based on classical localization of the aphasias. For example, cases have been reported of patients diagnosed with Broca's aphasia who did not have Broca's area infarction (Naeser et al., 1986). Moreover, patients having lesions in Broca's area have exhibited transcortical motor aphasia rather than a Broca's aphasia as traditionally expected (Naeser and Hayward, 1978). One can speculate that individual differences in cerebral localization in part may account for the unusual localization findings in these cases.

Recent technical advances that have permitted examination of the metabolic status of patients with brain lesions have made significant contributions to our understanding of the pathoanatomy of the aphasias. Positron emission tomography (PET), for example, has been used to measure the rate of glucose metabolism in the brain, thereby providing a better understanding of how structural lesions affect cerebral metabolism. For example, Metter et al.'s (1987) study of 11 Broca's patients compared CT and PET findings. They reported that "lesions seen on computerized tomography demonstrated consistent damage to the anterior internal capsule and the lenticular nuclei with variable cortical changes, whereas glucose metabolism was found to be decreased throughout the hemisphere" (p. 134). These and subsequent findings (Metter et al., 1992) provide convincing evidence that changes in the brain's metabolic activity in regions outside of Broca's area contribute to the pattern of language impairment in Broca's aphasia.

Modern neuroradiographic techniques have been used to obtain data that call in question the commonly held notion that Broca's aphasia results from a lesion to Broca's area. Taken together, data support the position that a lesion to Broca's area is neither necessary nor sufficient to produce Broca's aphasia. H. Damasio (1998) summarizes the pathophysiology of Broca's aphasia: "In general, it is fair to say that lesions in

Broca's area not only encompass the frontal operculum ([Brodmann's] area 44 and 45), but also premotor and motor regions immediately behind and above, in addition to extending to underlying white matter and basal ganglia as well as the insula. As might be expected, the extension of damage into these many different regions correlate(s) with diverse accompanying deficits and with the extent of recovery" (p. 54).

The cumulative results of recent localization studies of Broca's aphasia reinforce Kertesz's (1979) caution that, "only lesions causing impairment are localizable, not the impairment itself" (p. 142). Classical pathoanatomic descriptions of the aphasias, including Broca's aphasia, are gradually yielding to more sophisticated models of brain and language relationships. Although far from complete, these models have attempted to account for findings regarding the influence of distant and especially subcortical regions on language ability and patterns of aphasic impairments (Crosson, 1985; Metter et al., 1988; Naeser et al., 1986). Recent research using functional imaging techniques, such as PET, functional magnetic resonance imaging (fMRI), and single photon emission computed tomography (SPECT), have significantly contributed to our understanding of aphasia (Mlcoch & Metter, 2001). Recent dynamic imaging research has increasingly focused on refining our understanding of specific aspects linguistic processing involving Broca's area (Warburton et al., 1996). At the same time, it is becoming increasingly clear that broad areas of cortical structures and activation are involved in language processing. Newer imaging techniques, such as magnetic resonance perfusion imaging (Hillis et al., 2001) and magnetencephalographic (MEG) imaging (Dale & Halgren, 2001), will further elucidate our understanding of the pathophysiology of Broca's aphasia, particularly when neuroimaging procedures are combined to provide spatial and temporal mapping of language and cognitive activity through the integration of multiple imaging techniques.

The Features of Broca's Aphasia

Although the classical taxonomies of aphasia are less than adequate in terms of models of language processing (Badecker and Caramazza, 1985), a cogent theory of normal or pathologic language that accounts for the rich variety of aphasic impairments does not currently exist. It is unlikely that a universally agreed upon alternative to the classical taxonomies of aphasia into fluent and nonfluent subtypes is forthcoming, and the classical system continues to provide a valuable heuristic for clinicians faced with the day-to-day care of aphasic patients. The classical descriptions of aphasic syndromes enhance cross-disciplinary dialogue by providing a common vocabulary for communication and interaction, thereby encouraging multidisciplinary research and patient care efforts. In addition, the reemergence of the classical taxonomies has coincided with an increased effort by clinical researchers to develop and investigate specific language treatment approaches for subtypes of aphasic patients. The classical taxonomies will continue to serve an important role in the clinical arena. In the remainder of this section, we will examine the nature and underlying features of Broca's aphasia.

The Nature of Broca's Aphasia

For ease of discussion, hypotheses relating to the nature of Broca's aphasia are described below as nonlinguistic and linguistic explanations. This dichotomy is somewhat arbitrary because nonlinguistic explanations of agrammatism are not totally void of linguistic or psycholinguistic descriptions or explanations. The nonlinguistic theories discussed herein are not, however, based on models of linguistic processing per se, and their emphasis is on nonlanguage factors that contribute to the pattern of deficits in Broca's aphasia. Only representative examples of the range of linguistic and nonlinguistic explanations of Broca's aphasia are presented below. More comprehensive reviews of the nature of agrammatism and

Broca's aphasia are available elsewhere (Berndt, 1998; Kean, 1985).

NONLINGUISTIC HYPOTHESES

Explanations of the nature of Broca's aphasia have stressed the importance of nonlinguistic factors, such as impaired processing and memory capacity, the effect of stimulus variables on verbal output, and aphasic individuals' compensatory strategies on language production. In attempting to understand the nature of Broca's aphasia, aphasiologists have often scrutinized various aspects of agrammatism. As noted earlier, agrammatism is a frequent sequela of Broca's aphasia that is characterized by the omission of low information lexical items and grammatical morphemes from speech. The verbal output of agrammatic individuals may sound "telegraphic" because of the paucity of articles, conjunctions, auxiliary verbs, and word endings. Similar to a telegraph, the verbal output of agrammatic speech is often the production of short strings of content words (e.g., nouns and verbs) that convey a fractured but successful message. Agrammatic Broca's patients have particular difficulty retrieving verbs, and they often produce an overabundance of nouns when speaking. It is generally felt that a better understanding of agrammatism will lead to a greater appreciation of the underlying nature of Broca's aphasia.

Pick (1931) provided one of the earliest nonlinguistic explanations of agrammatism when he postulated that the deletion of low information lexical items from agrammatic speech resulted from patients' attempts to conserve effort during speech production (Brown, 1973). This proposition has intuitive appeal because the nonfluent speech output of Broca's patients is halting, hesitant, and apraxic, and an economy-of-effort explanation suggests that agrammatism is a compensatory strategy to circumvent these expressive problems.

Several contemporary aphasiologists have also proposed explanations that attribute agrammatism to compensatory strategies. Heeschen (1985), for example, proposes an avoidance hypothesis that purports that persons having Broca's aphasia learn to speak agrammatically by monitoring their aphasic utterances and then adapting to the language problem by only producing constructions that present relatively little difficulty for them. Heeschen's position is similar to the "economy-of-effort" theory. He writes, "Agrammatism is something that must be learned by the patient. . . . The advantage to the patient is obvious; his speech gains a certain systematicity for the listener and the patient spares himself enormous efforts by simply omitting all these 'terrible small words,' the production of which is really vexing for the patient" (p. 241). The avoidance hypothesis is in part based on evidence that shows that agrammatic speakers who are experimentally deprived of the opportunity to avoid difficult words and syntactic constructions show marked reductions in the number of omissions of grammatical items.

Kolk et al. (1985) proposed an "adaptation" theory of agrammatism. This theory claims that agrammatic speech is a reflection of a decrease in computational resources necessary for sentence production rather than an underlying impairment to syntactic competence. Agrammatism reflects the way in which aphasic individuals adapt to their reduced capacity for the temporal computation of language. Delayed processes that underlie agrammatism may include a slowing down of the application of syntactic rules, or there may be a general slowing of lexical retrieval. The adaptation theory contends that, by opting to speak agrammatically, aphasic individuals minimize the effect of delayed processing. Kolk et al. (1985) contend that patients may not be fully conscious of their decision to speak agrammatically. Research has also shown that some elicitation conditions significantly reduce agrammatic features and result in production of more complete sentences for individuals with Broca's aphasia (Kolk and Heeschen, 1990, 1992).

The view that at least some of the characteristics of agrammatic speech are a consequence of adapting to or compensating for underlying processing impairments are evident clinically.

Goodglass (1993), for example, terms the compensations and adaptations of agrammatic patients as "positive symptoms." Among the stylistic features that Goodglass identifies are the stringing together of words or short phrases with the use of "and" as the only conjunctions, acting out events with the assistance of onomatopoeic sounds, exclamations, and direct quotes, and spared expressions, such as those expressing time.

Goodglass and his colleagues have argued against economy-of-effort explanations, noting that agrammatism rarely improves to any significant degree with prompting. Even repeated attempts at self-correction by individuals with Broca's aphasia are largely unsuccessful. Goodglass and Menn (1985) describe a partial explanation of agrammatism called the stress-salience hypothesis: "A basic feature of Broca's aphasia is the increased threshold for mobilizing the speech output system, . . . and the response threshold . . . requires an emphatic or salient element in the message to overcome the elevated threshold and begin the flow of speech" (p. 252). Goodglass et al. define salience as the result of informational load, affective tone, and increased amplitude and intentional stress.

They note that, nonfluent Broca's subjects who suffer from impaired prosody and fluency do not have the facilitory effects of fluency available to help overcome their tendency to omit functors and grammatical morphemes. This proposal suggests that patients' fluency interacts with and in part determines the extent of agrammatism.

Thus far, we have sampled several nonlinguistic explanations of the nature of agrammatism and Broca's aphasia. It is clear that no single account can satisfactorily explain the variety and complexity of symptoms that occur in Broca's aphasia and agrammatism. In the following section, we briefly examine selected linguistic theories that attempt to account for the same phenomenon.

Linguistic Hypotheses

Jakobson (1952) provided the earliest linguistic description of aphasic disorders.

Agrammatism was viewed as a contiguity disorder in which there was a deficit in the sequential combining of words into grammatical sentences. Formal linguistic theory has played an increasingly important role in aphasia research, and studies of aphasic individuals have been used with increasing frequency to examine theoretical linguistic constructs. This is particularly true in the study of Broca's aphasia, where detailed studies of aphasic patients have been used to formulate and explore linguistic and psycholinguistic explanations of syntactic deficits. Of particular relevance to the current discussion, researchers have extensively examined the hypothesis that agrammatism in Broca's aphasia is the result of a syntactically based, central linguistic deficit. (Grodzinsky, 1990; Shapiro & Thompson, 1994).

Although there are actually several versions of the central syntactic deficit theory, the primary assumption underlying each is that agrammatism is a manifestation of a central disruption of the syntactic parsing component of the language system (Berndt and Caramazza, 1980). If the syntactic impairments of Broca's patients result from a single central deficit, then one would predict that parallel deficits would be found across language modalities.

The central syntactic deficit hypothesis has been challenged by data from reports of patients who were expressively but not receptively agrammatic (Kolk and Heeschen, 1992). Studies provided evidence that countered the assumption of the existence of parallel agrammatic deficits across modalities that was key to the central syntactic deficit hypothesis. A dissociation of impairments across modalities is problematic for theories ascribing agrammatism to a central linguistic deficit that presumably causes similar impairments in expressive and receptive modalities. Despite evidence that has ultimately led to the demise of the central syntactic deficit hypothesis (Menn & Obler, 1990; Schwartz et al., 1985), this theory stimulated a tremendous amount of linguistically based research into the nature of Broca's aphasia.

Alternative linguistic explanations of the nature of agrammatism and Broca's aphasia have examined phonologic factors (Kean, 1985), retrieval difficulties for closed class morphology (i.e., functors, etc.) (Petocz and Oliphant, 1988), difficulty mapping semantic roles onto sentence constituents (Saffran et al., 1980; Schwartz et al., 1985), and violations of phrase structure rules (Grodzinsky, 1990). Of particular relevance to this discussion are two accounts of agrammatism that have led to experimental treatments for Broca's aphasic individuals: the mapping hypothesis (Marshall, 1995), and linguistic approaches that have been based on Chomsky's (1986) theory of government and binding.

The mapping hypothesis attributes the symptoms of agrammatism to a deficit in the ability to map semantic roles onto sentence constituents (Saffran et al., 1980; Schwartz et al., 1985). Saffran et al. (1980) challenged the central syntactic deficit theory when they demonstrated that the comprehension difficulties of Broca's subjects could not have resulted from syntactic complexity. These researchers also demonstrated that Broca's subjects were able to identify grammatical violations present in spoken sentences, and this finding was also inconsistent with a syntactic parsing account of agrammatism. Based on analysis of production as well as comprehension data, Schwartz and her colleagues (1985) concluded that Broca's subjects have difficulty abstracting thematic meaning from verb roles (e.g., agent-action-object) of sentence constituents. That is, rather than resulting from a syntactic deficit per se, individuals with Broca's aphasia are seen as being unable to map sentence structure (i.e., syntax) to meaning (Marshall, 1995). This account of agrammatism has given rise to a method of treatment, referred to as mapping therapy, in which the goal of intervention is to overcome the problem of mapping the thematic roles of sentence constituents onto syntax (Mitchum & Berndt, 2001; Mitchum et al., 2000; Schwartz et al., 1994).

Another linguistic theory that has led to experimental treatments for aphasia is the government and binding theory of Chomsky

(1986). Grodzinsky (1990) has applied this theory to aphasia and provided a theoretical explanation of agrammatism. In Chomsky's theory, sentences that vary from the basic (canonical) word order leave a trace (t) in the position where the original noun or pronoun was moved from when an agent-action-object (i.e., S-V-O) sentence is transformed from an active to a passive voice. For example, in the sentence "The boy was licked by the dog," there would be a trace (t) of the object boy following the verb "licked" to help mark the correct object in the sentence. Grodzinsky indicates that agrammatic patients are unable to determine whether the object of such sentences is the "boy" or the "dog" because they are insensitive to the residual trace (I) that marks the true object. This type of theoretical framework has been used to develop experimental treatment protocols for investigating treatment and generalization issues with Broca's aphasic subjects (Ballard & Shapiro, 1998; Shapiro & Thompson, 1994; Thompson, 2001; Thompson and Shapiro, 1994).

SUMMARY OF NONLINGUISTIC AND LINGUISTIC HYPOTHESES

Aphasiologists have examined wide-range linguistic and nonlinguistic hypotheses regarding the nature of agrammatism in Broca's aphasia. Nonlinguistic hypotheses that have been proposed to account for agrammatism have included an economy of effort theory (Pick, 1931), the adaptation theory (Kolk and Heeschen, 1990, 1992; Kolk et al., 1985), and the stress, salience, and fluency hypothesis (Goodglass, 1993; Goodglass & Menn, 1985). Linguistic explanations of agrammatism have also proliferated since Jakobson's (1952) seminal work in neurolinguistics. In particular, considerable research effort has been expended on testing various forms of the central syntactic deficit theory of agrammatism (Zurif et al., 1972), mapping theory (Saffran et al., 1980; Schwartz et al., 1985), and theoretical positions based on Chomsky's (1986) government and binding theory (Grodzinsky, 1990; Shapiro and Thompson, 1994).

At the present time, no single theory can fully account for the variety of research findings and clinical observations regarding agrammatism and Broca's aphasia. The current status of research in this area, as aptly summarized by Goodglass and Menn's (1985), remains relevant today: "One thing is certain: No single explanation of agrammatism, whether based on syntax, phonology, or economy of speaking effort, can yield the observed intricate patterns of within-modality and cross-modality dissociation. Parsimony as a metatheoretical principle in neurolinguistics is dead" (p. 19).

Although caution is necessary as we attempt to apply neurolinguistic theory to the clinical arena (Davis, 2000; Holland, 1994), evaluation and treatment procedures that have evolved from a theoretical perspective have demonstrated the potential clinical contributions that may come from this research in the future. Clinicians can obtain valuable clinical information from the research in this area despite the lack of theoretical parsimony. Our discussion of clinical issues begins with a consideration of the distinguishing characteristics of Broca's aphasia.

Differentiating Features

As noted earlier, the hallmark of Broca's aphasia is nonfluent, effortful, and slow speech output with reduced phrase length and syntactic complexity, and awkward articulation. Verbal output may include an overabundance of content words, especially nouns, and relatively few functors and grammatical word endings. Despite a tendency toward "telegraphic" speech, the verbal output of individuals with Broca's aphasia usually contains sufficient informational content to communicate reasonably well in daily, contextually rich situations. Repetition and confrontation naming are often moderately to severely impaired in Broca's patients. Auditory comprehension ability is relatively preserved and often functional for everyday conversation. Reading and writing ability are also variable but may parallel auditory

comprehension and verbal output, respectively (A. Damasio, 1998; Goodglass, 1993; Goodglass et al., 2000; Kertesz, 1982).

Broca's aphasia can be differentiated from other types of aphasia by examining patients' relative performance on spontaneous verbal output (i.e., speech fluency), auditory comprehension, confrontation naming, and repetition tasks. It should be apparent that a relative comparison across language modalities such as these results in rather broad and inclusive patient categories. The constellation of symptoms in Broca's aphasia varies considerably in terms of verbal ability, for example, depending on the presence and severity of agrammatism. Some of those patients classified as having Broca's aphasia may be restricted to one- or two-word responses, whereas others may display a relatively mild interruption of speech fluency. In addition to the degree of individual variability within each type of aphasia, many individuals seen clinically do not fit unequivocally into one of the classical types of aphasia because many aphasic patients have large lesions that result in mixed symptoms (Goodglass, 2000). Finally, the fact that there are no invariant features common to all patients within a given aphasia subtype further complicates attempts to classify. These cautionary remarks should be kept in mind during the following discussion of features that differentiate Broca's from other types of aphasia.

A relative comparison of aphasic patients on speech fluency, auditory comprehension, repetition, and confrontation naming results in the following classification schema (Goodglass, 1993; Goodglass et al., 2000; Kertesz, 1982).

Examination of Table 8–1 reveals the basic dichotomy between fluent and nonfluent aphasia. Speech fluency is one of the most reliable features for differentiating the aphasias, and it has become an important clinical criterion for classification (Goodglass, 2000; Kertesz, 1982). Nonfluent aphasic speech is characterized by decreased speech rate, increased effort, reduced phrase length,

Table 8–1. Basic Classification of Aphasic Syndromes

	Fluency	Auditory Comprehension	Repetition	Naming
Nonfluent				
Broca's	−	+	=	=
Global	−	−	−	−
Transcortical motor	−	+	+	=
Fluent				
Wernicke's	+	−	−	=
Transcortical sensory	+	−	+	=
Conduction	+	+	−	=
Anomic	+	+	+	−

Key: (+) Relatively unimpaired; (−) Impaired; (=) Variable impairment across patients.

and dysprosody. In addition, nonfluent aphasic individuals have difficulty initiating speech production, and their overall quantity of speech also tends to be reduced. As shown in the table, Broca's, global, and transcortical motor aphasia are classified as nonfluent aphasias.

In contrast to nonfluent aphasic speech, the speech rate of fluent aphasic patients is essentially normal or even somewhat increased. The speech of fluent aphasic patients is effortless, melodic, and flowing. Fluent aphasic patients substitute inappropriate words (verbal paraphasias), nonwords (jargon), and phonemes (literal paraphasias) while speaking, yet they do so smoothly and effortlessly without interruption of the flow or melody of speech. Thus, despite near-normal prosody and speech rate, there is often a considerable decrease in the amount of information conveyed by fluent aphasic speakers. Hesitations and pauses occur in the speech of fluent aphasic patients, but they often precede and follow uninterrupted fluent, sometimes meaningless speech. The fluent aphasias include Wernicke's, transcortical sensory, conduction, and anomic aphasia (Table 8–1).

The nonfluent speech of Broca's patients can be briefly contrasted with the fluent speech of patients with Wernicke's aphasia to demonstrate qualitative differences between fluent and nonfluent types of aphasia.

In response to the request, "Tell me what you do with a cigarette," a person with chronic Broca's aphasia replied, "Uh . . . uh . . . cigarette [pause] smoke it." This response was halting and agrammatic, but it clearly conveyed an accurate response to the request. In response to the same request, a patient with chronic Wernicke's replied, "This is a segment of a pegment. Soap a cigarette." This fluent individual's response is strikingly different from that of the person with Broca's aphasia in several respects. First, despite a lack of informational content, there appears to a basic syntactic integrity to the response. That is, basic word order constraints were not apparently violated, and the small connective words were also retained, despite the fact that the response was replete with jargon. By contrast, the Broca's speaker simply juxtaposed a correct noun, verb, and pronoun. Finally, despite a halting, disconnected style of speaking, the person with Broca's aphasia communicated successfully. On the other hand, the fluent speech sample was melodic and uninterrupted, but it was essentially devoid of any meaning.

The overall pattern of impairments determines patient classification rather than performance on a single variable per se, and standardized tests are available to assist with the challenging task of differential diagnosis (Goodglass et al., 2000; Helm-Estabrooks, 1992; Kertesz, 1982). Thus, in addition to the fluency distinction, the person with Broca's aphasia in the previous example had a mild auditory comprehension deficit on standardized testing, whereas the person with Wernicke's aphasia had severely impaired auditory comprehension ability. Individuals with Broca's aphasia frequently demonstrate a high level of awareness of their language problems, and they also tend to demonstrate varying degrees of frustration when they make errors. This is in marked contrast to those with Wernicke's aphasia, who often show little frustration or error awareness.

Within the general category of nonfluent aphasias, those with Broca's can be readily differentiated from individuals classified as having global and transcortical motor aphasia. As the comparison in Table 8–1 demonstrates, individuals classified as global are severely impaired across all language modalities. Their verbal output is limited to a few nonfunctional, automatic phrases or stereotypic responses, and they have severely impaired auditory comprehension skills. By contrast, Broca's patients often communicate effectively through the use of one- and two-word responses, and their comprehension is adequate for following simple commands and understanding basic conversations.

The clinical profile of Broca's aphasia most closely resembles the clinical profile of transcortical motor aphasia (Table 8–1). Similar to Broca's, a transcortical motor profile reveals an overall reduction in verbal output, and signs of agrammatism may be present. Another similarity is that Broca's and transcortical motor patients have relatively good auditory comprehension skills. One important qualitative difference between these two syndromes in that individuals with transcortical aphasia demonstrate a paucity of spontaneous speech and marked initiation difficulties (Goodglass et al., 2000; Kertesz, 1979, 1982). Although Broca's patients' spontaneous speech is effortful and halting, they often spontaneously initiate communicative interactions. Another subtle difference between these nonfluent aphasias is that the transcortical group exhibits a

greater degree of stumbling, repetitive, even stuttering spontaneous output, in conjunction with motor prompts, such as foot stomping. Echolalia may also present in transcortical motor aphasia, but it is rarely evident in Broca's patients.

In addition to these rather subtle differences, one major factor, repetition ability, distinguishes these two syndromes. Whereas the ability to repeat aurally presented information is moderately to severely impaired in Broca's aphasia, repetition ability is relatively preserved in transcortical motor aphasia. A striking preservation of repetition skills in combination with impoverished spontaneous speech and good auditory comprehension ability are characteristic of transcortical motor aphasia.

The preceding examples demonstrate how fluency, auditory comprehension, repetition, and confrontation naming can be used to distinguish Broca's aphasia from the other classical types of aphasia. In the next section we explore associated signs and symptoms that co-occur with Broca's aphasia. Knowledge of these associated characteristics can contribute to the differential diagnosis of aphasia and related disorders.

ASSOCIATED SIGNS AND SYMPTOMS

Aphasia-causing lesions are often rather large; therefore, it is not surprising that aphasia frequently co-occurs with other communication, motor, and sensory problems that result from brain damage. Because lesions that cause Broca's aphasia also interrupt adjacent cortical motor fibers and deep fiber tracts, it is predictable that patients with Broca's aphasia frequently exhibit contralateral hemiparesis. Similarly, because Broca's area lesions may disrupt one's ability to plan and implement coordinated motor activity, apraxia of speech is a common and predictable concomitant impairment. Another common sequela of large Broca's area lesions is a mild dysarthria. Although severe dysarthria and dysphagia most often occur following bilateral involvement, Broca's patients may have difficulty with intraoral transit of food, and the possibility of increased risk for aspiration should not be overlooked.

Prior to formal speech and language testing, astute clinicians will observe their patients and note any associated motor or behavioral conditions that will contribute to a differential diagnosis of the disorder. The constellation of impairments associated with Broca's patients may lead clinicians to explore some diagnostic possibilities and eliminate others. Thus, a person with acute Broca's aphasia may be confined to a wheelchair as a result of right-sided hemiplegia (i.e., paralysis); his right arm may be in a protective sling, his right shoulder may droop, and he may show a flattening of the nasolabial folds and other signs of weakness of the muscles on the right side of the face. In time, people with acute Broca's aphasia may recover the ability to ambulate, often with the assistance of a leg brace, cane, or walker. The amount of recovery achieved with the right arm and hand is usually less than the amount of improvement apparent in the leg and foot. The amount of facial weakness, drooling, and other signs of muscular involvement also tend to subside over time until there may be only minimal residual deficit. In contrast to the pattern of involvement seen in Broca's aphasia, in fluent Wernicke's aphasia signs of physical impairment may be subtle or nonexistent.

As noted above, Broca's patients often have a mild dysarthria that can impact on speech intelligibility. The dysarthric involvement of Broca's patients tends not to be severely debilitating because speech musculature is bilaterally innervated and the aphasia-causing lesion affects only one side of the speech apparatus. However, the dysarthric component of speech may interact with apraxia of speech to a degree that is greater than a simple additive effect of the two impairments. That is, the cumulative effect of even mild dysarthria and apraxia of speech can significantly impair intelligibility and complicate clinical management.

Wertz et al. (1984b) define apraxia of speech as "neurogenic phonologic disorder resulting from sensorimotor impairment to the capacity to select, program, and/or execute in coordinated and normally timed sequences, the positioning of speech musculature for the volitional production of speech sounds. . . . Prosodic alteration, that is, changes in speech stress, intonation, and/or rhythm, may be associated with the articulatory disruption either as a primary part of the condition or in compensation for it" (p. 4). Unlike dysarthria, apraxia is not a result of muscular weakness, slowness, or incoordination and, although linguistic factors interact with apraxia, the disorder is most often viewed as being distinct from aphasic language impairments. Consequently, apraxia of speech requires an approach to clinical management that is quite distinct from language intervention strategies for aphasia (Duffy, 1995).

Although exact figures are not available, it is clear that apraxia of speech frequently coexists with Broca's aphasia. Duffy (1995) reports that motor speech disorders represented ~50% of the primary diagnoses of acquired neurogenic communication disorders at the Mayo Clinic over a 3-year period. It is obviously prudent to assume that the incidence of co-occurrence of apraxia of speech with Broca's aphasia is sufficiently high to merit routine screening in clinical settings.

As is the case with all differential diagnostic endeavors, clinicians interested in distinguishing Broca's aphasia with apraxia of speech from other clinical populations should examine the overall pattern of involvement before affixing a diagnostic label. The presence of any single differentiating feature alone is insufficient for diagnosing apraxia of speech and distinguishing Broca's apraxic individuals from other categories of aphasia. With this in mind, Wertz et al. (1984b) have summarized the clinical characteristics of apraxia of speech as follows:

1. "Effortful, trial and error, groping articulatory movements and attempts at self-correction.
2. Dysprosody unrelieved by extended periods of normal rhythm, stress, and intonation.

3. Articulatory inconsistency on repeated attempts of the same utterance.
4. Obvious difficulty initiating utterances" (p. 81).

This cluster of behaviors provides a cursory clinical guideline for diagnosing apraxia of speech in Broca's patients, and it should also prove useful for differentiating apraxia of speech from the speech characteristics of fluent aphasic patients. Duffy (1995) provides a detailed and insightful review of these topics. Additional evaluation procedures for diagnosing Broca's aphasia and developing appropriate intervention strategies are considered below.

Evaluation

The clinical evaluation of aphasia is undertaken to aid differential diagnosis, treatment planning, establishing a prognosis, monitoring change, and evaluating the maintenance of treatment gains. More often than not, evaluations serve these and other purposes simultaneously. Given the multifaceted nature of the evaluation process, it is not surprising that formal assessment measures are often supplemented with informal procedures including nonstandardized tests, behavioral observations, and clinical probes. The variety and complexity of assessment procedures underscores the need to view the evaluation process within the framework of a generalization planning approach to patient management (Kearns, 1989).

Traditional approaches to the clinical process often consider evaluation, treatment, generalization, and maintenance as discrete, relatively independent and sequential phases of patient management. This view is at variance with a generalization planning approach in which each phase of the clinical process is integrally related and overlapping with all other phases. Unlike the traditional approach, a generalization planning approach views the generalization of treatment effects as the primary goal of intervention. Consequently, formal test results are supplemented with probes of patient performance in the clinic, in natural environments, and in simulated natural environments and conditions as well. The evaluation phase of a generalization plan is ongoing, and it involves periodic administration of formal tests and probes so that on-line adjustments can be made in therapy as soon as they are needed.

The remainder of this section focuses on a description of procedures commonly used for diagnosing Broca's aphasia and planning clinical intervention. Ideally, the assessment suggestions discussed here will be administered in conjunction with clinical probes and in vivo observations of patients and significant others so that a successful generalization plan can be developed and implemented.

Aphasia Batteries and Patient Classification

For the purposes of our discussion the Boston Diagnostic Aphasia Examination (BDAE) (Goodglass et al., 2000) will be used to demonstrate aphasia testing and patient classification. Although there are important differences between the BDAE and other standardized batteries that lead to patient classification, including the Western Aphasia Examination (WAB; Kertesz, 1982) and the Aphasia Diagnostic Profiles (ADP; Helm-Estabrooks, 1992), these tests adhere to essentially the same classification system and approach exemplified in this discussion. Comprehensive reviews of standardized batteries for aphasia are available elsewhere (Brookshire, 2003; Davis, 2000).

The BDAE is a comprehensive test battery that can be used to examine fluency of verbal output, conversational and expository speech, auditory comprehension, articulation, recitation, music, repetition, naming, paraphasias, reading and writing auditory comprehension, oral expression, understanding written language, and writing. The BDAE is comprehensive, and administration of the entire battery can take several hours. The newest edition of the test provides a standardized short form that can be given in approximately 1 hour. Although the scoring procedure used for each subtest varies, the BDAE provides percentile rankings that permit across-task comparisons of the relative severity of performance.

The BDAE provides a well-described procedure for categorizing patients into one of the classical types of aphasia, and it is sufficiently comprehensive to provide valuable information for making treatment decisions. The authors freely admit that many patients seen in the clinic may not be unambiguously categorized with their test, and hold that the classic syndromes serve "as anchor points in our thinking about aphasia" (Goodglass et al., 2000). The authors provide sample profiles of the range of speech and language characteristics of Broca's, global, transcortical motor, Wernicke's, conduction, anomic, transcortical sensory aphasia, and mixed nonfluent aphasias. The authors also recognize and discuss so-called pure aphasia. These rare cases of aphasia affect a single language modality while leaving all others intact. These syndromes include aphemia, pure alexia, optic aphasia, pure word deafness, and pure agraphia.

Classification of the aphasias into fluent and nonfluent subtypes is largely based on ratings of parameters of conversational and expository speech, which are captured on the Rating Scale Profile of Speech Characteristics. The clinician evaluates the dimensions: articulatory agility, phrase length, grammatical form, melodic line (prosody), paraphasias in running speech, and word-finding difficulty relative to fluency. Scores for objective subtests for repetition and auditory comprehension are also noted. The ratings of each of these dimensions is placed on the seven-point rating scale profile and the overall pattern of speech characteristics is subsequently compared with expected ranges of performance for each for the various types of aphasia to determine patient classification.

An expected range of performance for Broca's aphasia on the Rating Scale Profile of Speech Characteristics is provided in the test book. These patients lie below the scale midpoint (4) for articulatory agility, phrase

length, grammatical form, and melodic line. They may produce occasional literal or verbal paraphasias but not for multiword utterances. At the more severe end of the rating scale, those with Broca's aphasia may have essentially no intonational contour (i.e., melodic line), produce only single-word "phrases," and have minimal articulatory agility and essentially no variety of grammatical constructions. Those less severely involved individuals have appropriate intonational contour only for short phrases and stereotypes; their longest occasional uninterrupted phrase length is approximately four words; their articulatory agility facility is normal only in familiar words and phrases; and the variety of grammatical form is limited to simple declaratives and stereotypes. Ratings of word-finding may also vary. Whereas the spontaneous speech of more severe individuals with Broca's aphasia may be restricted to production of content words, the speech of less severe individuals may be rated as having informational content that is proportional to their fluency.

In addition to the Rating Scale Profile of Speech Characteristics, performance on BDAE subtests is summarized on the Summary Profile of Standardized subtests. The profile summarizes a severity rating, fluency ratings, conversational and expository speech, and the remaining subtests for auditory comprehension, repetition, naming, reading and writing, etc. As noted above, the scores for the various subtests are easily converted to percentile scores for each of the standardized tests of the BDAE. Goodglass et al. (2000) note that individuals with Broca's aphasia are usually rated as severe (i.e., rating 1 or 2) on the five-point severity rating scale because of effortful, nonfluent nature of their verbal output. Patients rated above 4 on the overall severity rating scale are generally not classified as having Broca's aphasia.

The aphasia subtest summary profile typically shows that fluency and severity scales are lower than auditory comprehension and naming scores. The cumulative auditory comprehension percentile for those with

Broca's aphasia is above the 50th percentile of aphasic patients in the standardization sample. On repetition subtests, individuals with Broca's aphasia range from not being able to repeat a single high-probability phrase, such as "You know how," to being able to produce four of eight progressively longer phrases.

The comprehensive nature of the BDAE and its usefulness as a means of classifying patients make the test a valuable tool in the clinical armamentarium. Of particular clinical utility is the qualitative analysis of spontaneous speech and fluency that is incorporated into the BDAE. However, syndrome classification on the BDAE is based largely on subjective clinical ratings, and classification relies to some extent on the knowledge base and experience of the examiner.

Supplemental Evaluation Procedures

The information obtained from standardized test batteries, such as the BDAE, is often supplemented with modality-specific and nonstandardized test results. Supplemental evaluation procedures are used to obtain additional information about known deficit areas, to probe communicative abilities that are not sufficiently covered in standardized test batteries, and to rule out or help explain clinical observations that do not fit expected patterns. Supplemental testing often includes examination of functional communication abilities with instruments such as the communicative Abilities of Daily Living (CADL; Holland, 1980) or the American Speech and Hearing Association (ASHA) Functional Assessment of Communicative Skills for Adults (ASHA FACS; Frattali, Thompson, Holland et al, 1995). In addition, a wide range of modality-specific tests and nonstandardized assessments are also available and used in clinical practice. A comprehensive summary of aphasia testing is beyond the scope of this chapter. Recent reviews of this information are available elsewhere (Brookshire, 2003; Davis, 2000; Holland & Thompson, 1998). The following overview introduces selected assessment tools that are

commonly used in clinical practice and have been found useful for evaluating individuals with Broca's aphasia.

The Psycholinguistic Assessments of Language Processing in Aphasia (PALPA; Kay et al., 1997) is a nonstandardized battery that adopts a neurolinguistic approach to aphasia assessment. It provides valuable information for identifying impairments at the spoken and written language (form and content) at the word level. Other research tools, including the Northwestern University Sentence Comprehension Test and the Verb Production Battery (Thompson, 2001), may prove useful as supplemental tests for patients with Broca's aphasia.

The verbal impairments in Broca's aphasia are often the most obvious and debilitating communication deficit, and many individuals place a high premium on obtaining as much recovery of premorbid verbal abilities as possible. Consequently, a thorough examination of the verbal skills is essential to the development of a comprehensive intervention strategy. Helm-Estabrooks and colleagues (1981, 1986) developed an aphasia syntax training program using a story completion format to probe specific syntactic constructions of speakers with Broca's aphasia that may not be produced in spontaneous speech samples. This program also can be used to treat syntactic deficits in aphasic individuals.

In addition to probing ability to produce specific constructions, clinicians may also be interested in examining spontaneous use of grammatical constructions, compensatory strategies used to avoid difficult constructions, ability to initiate and maintain conversational topics, and aspects of discourse. The type of speech sample, elicitation procedure, stimuli, length, and conditions of sampling (e.g., monologue versus dialogue) vary according to the specific goals of the evaluation. For example, a clinician may choose a picture description format to examine the content and efficiency of a language sample and also examine dyadic communication in context. Regardless of the sampling context, spontaneous speech samples can be reliably collected and analyzed, and they provide valuable clinical information that cannot be obtained from standardized tests (Brookshire, 2003; Doyle, 1994; Nicholas and Brookshire, 1993). Carefully analyzed spontaneous speech samples provide a rich source of phonologic, grammatical, and semantic and quantitative aspects of spontaneous speech for planning treatment for aphasic individuals.

Although verbal impairments are usually the most obvious deficits in Broca's aphasia, other modalities may also require additional testing beyond that provided by standardized test batteries. In particular, it is important that clinicians closely examine auditory comprehension skills because mild comprehension deficits are relatively easy to overlook in this population. The various forms of the Token Test are particularly useful for identifying subtle auditory comprehension impairments (DeRenzi and Vignolo, 1962; McNeil and Prescott, 1978). In addition, the shortened version of the Token Test is relatively quick and easy to administer (~20 minutes), and severity cutoff scores and preliminary normative data are available (DeRenzi & Faglioni, 1978).

Other clinically useful tests of auditory comprehension ability include the Auditory Comprehension Test for Sentences (ACTS; Shewan, 1979) and the Functional Auditory Comprehension Test (FACT; LaPointe and Horner, 1978). The ACTS examines comprehension of sentences that systematically vary in terms of length, vocabulary level, and syntactic difficulty. The test was standardized on Broca's and other classical types of aphasia so that clinicians can compare the performance of individual patients to group normative data. The FACT was designed to overcome what the authors perceived as shortcomings of the Token Test. It consists of three levels of auditory commands that systematically increase in length and apparent complexity.

The Discourse Comprehension Test (DCT; Brookshire and Nicholas, 1993) is the first well-controlled assessment of discourse level comprehension specifically designed for aphasia. It is a useful supplement to any comprehensive test battery, particularly when subtle comprehension deficits are suspected. According to Brookshire and Nicholas, "The Discourse Comprehension Test was designed to assess comprehension and retention of spoken narrative discourse by adults with aphasia, right-brain damage, or traumatic brain injury. The test contains ten stories and sets of yes/no questions for each story. The questions systematically assess a listener's comprehension and retention of directly stated and implied main ideas and details from a homogeneous set of stories" (p. 3). The test is intended to examine auditory comprehension ability and provide information about how clients would perform in more natural communication interactions. Listening comprehension and silent reading versions of the test are included in the manual. The DCT is useful for assessment, treatment planning, and patient and family counseling.

Standardized test results and initial clinical impressions provide clues to the direction of supplemental testing. The clinician's task is to interpret initial test data and follow the lead in a direction that will provide valuable differential diagnostic or treatment information. In some instances additional testing may be required for a modality that has already been carefully examined. Still other leads may take the clinician in new directions that have not previously been explored. For example, the clinician may desire additional information about a client's reading (LaPointe and Horner, 1998) or gestural ability (Duffy and Duffy, 1984). Whatever form and direction supplemental testing takes, however, it is imperative that the clinician does not lose sight of the need to step back from testing and observe his or her patient's communicative abilities under more naturalistic conditions. Holland (1980) reminds us to ask spouses about their partners' communication skills, observe aphasic individuals with at least one other individual besides ourselves, and observe our clients in at least one naturalistic environment. These types of observations can be enlightening with regard to realistic goal setting. More importantly, naturalistic probes also provide information needed to develop a comprehensive generalization plan that attempts to facilitate improvement of communicative abilities to people, settings, and situations where they are needed most (Kearns, 1989).

Treatment

There has been a proliferation of treatment research involving Broca's patients, and the vast majority of studies in this area were designed to enhance verbal abilities (Thompson, 1989). Given the preponderance of studies designed to improve verbal skills, it is not surprising that reviews of treatment procedures for individuals with Broca's aphasia emphasize treatment procedures for expressive impairments. The present overview is no exception to this trend.

This section examines representative treatment approaches for the communication impairments apparent in Broca's aphasia. The emphasis is on the verbal treatment options that have been outlined in the literature. A variety of intervention and other programs are also appropriate for individuals with Broca's aphasia, and clinicians may wish to examine and try these options (Katz and Wertz, 1997; Lyon, 1992, 1995; Simmons et al., 1987). Our review begins with a discussion of treatment philosophy and proceeds to a brief consideration of treatment approaches.

A Treatment Philosophy

Language therapy for aphasia is an inexact science that is influenced by clinicians' training and their philosophy about the nature of aphasia. In addition, patient-specific considerations, such as the severity of language involvement, the presence of associated impairments, time postonset of aphasia, and patients' communication environments, also influence treatment decisions. For example, a clinician who is treating an acute Broca's client with a moderately severe apraxia of speech may elect to intensely treat the apraxia prior to treating the patient's syntactic prob-

lems. Guidelines are available to assist the clinician in making difficult treatment decisions, ranging from the selection of clinical goals and choice of stimuli used in treatment, to the ordering of tasks within each treatment session (Brookshire, 2003; Davis, 2000).

Another area of clinical decision making for which clinical aphasiologists must be prepared is the development and evaluation of procedures that facilitate generalization. (Kearns, 1989; Thompson, 1989) Although aphasiologists have historically assumed that generalization is a natural and expected outcome of intervention (e.g., Schuell et al., 1964), this has turned out to be an erroneous assumption (Thompson, 1989). Importantly, wholesale acceptance of this assumption may have inadvertently discouraged serious investigation of generalization issues in aphasia. Because we now know that generalization is not an automatic by-product of language intervention for aphasia, it is imperative that clinicians actively plan intervention in a manner that will increase the probability of obtaining generalization. Thompson (1989) has outlined the following steps for accomplishing this goal:

1. "Select functional targets and plan to program response generalization, if necessary, across structurally or functionally different responses.
2. . . . Design probes carefully for measuring generalization across response and stimulus conditions and to administer them periodically throughout treatment.
3. . . . Establish criteria for generalization and to look carefully at error responses.
4. . . . Introduce aspects of the generalization environment into treatment, or introduce aspects of the training environment into the generalization environment in early stages of treatment.
5. . . . Use treatment methods, such as loose training (see below), that have resulted in generalization.
6. . . . Extend treatment across settings or persons, when . . . (generalization does not occur as planned)" (p. 112).

Thompson's suggestions highlight the steps involved in the development of a generalization plan and underscore the importance of having clinicians becoming actively involved in programming generalization. However, as in other areas of clinical practice, we are only beginning to develop an appropriate technology for facilitating generalization. Clinicians, therefore, should incorporate measurement techniques that allow them to evaluate the success of their treatments, so they can objectively determine if, when, and where generalization occurs.

The effectiveness and generality of treatment procedures reviewed below have been examined to varying degrees. This does not, however, relieve the clinician of the responsibility of determining their success for individual clients. Published treatment procedures are rarely sufficiently detailed to permit exact duplication in the clinical arena. Furthermore, clinicians often justifiably modify published treatment programs rather than utilize them exactly as they are presented in the literature. Consequently, the following approaches should be viewed as providing a beginning framework that can be changed, built upon, and expanded to suit individual needs. However, clinicians are responsible for evaluating the effectiveness of the treatment procedures used with their clients.

Generic Treatment Strategies

The term *generic treatment strategy* is used here to refer to intervention approaches that do not target improvement in a single modality, such as verbal production. For example, several authors have suggested that a relatively intact language or communication skill can be used to facilitate performance of a more severely impaired ability (Luria, 1970). This principle can be applied regardless of the specific modality that is being treated.

Kearns et al. (1982), for example, isolated the effects of gestural training on verbal production. They systematically trained two nonfluent subjects to produce individual iconic gestures and examined the facilitation effects of training on subjects' ability to name the trained items. The results of this study demonstrated that gestural training alone did not enhance verbal production. Improved naming was documented, however, once gestural training was accompanied by verbal production training

In addition to using an intact function to "deblock" an impaired ability in therapy, patients can be taught a specific self-cuing strategy as a means of circumventing communicative difficulties. Linebaugh and Lehner (1977), for example, taught self-generated cues to five Broca's patients in an attempt to facilitate word retrieval with a cuing hierarchy treatment program. They organized a series of cues to facilitate confrontation naming and then worked up and down the hierarchy until sufficient progress was attained. Patients were taught to use appropriate self-generated cues to facilitate word retrieval within this program. For example, patients were apparently taught to cue themselves to produce a target noun by trying to say the *function* of the target word. The results of this study demonstrated significant improvement in patients' ability to name treatment stimuli, and generalization of improved naming ability was also reported for untrained word lists.

This study demonstrates the subtle but important difference between simply using an intact skill to deblock an impaired ability during therapy and actually training the patient to consciously utilize those cues. The goal of training a *self*-generated cuing strategy is to teach patients to help themselves when they encounter communicative difficulty. That is, training patients to generate their own cues allows them to become less reliant on the clinician and thereby to communicate more effectively in natural settings when the clinician is not available to provide assistance.

Meuse and Marquardt (1985) describe several strategies used by Broca's patients to maintain communicative effectiveness. These included requests for clarification, verbally eliminating alternative choices, and using alternative forms of verbal communication, such as singing. The astute clinician will observe patients' individualized strategies and determine their clinical utility. Compensatory strategies that enhance communication can be identified, stabilized, and reinforced. Those that are found to interfere with communication efficiency can be extinguished.

Simmons-Mackie and Damico (1995) used ethnographic analyses to identify compensatory strategies used by two nonfluent aphasic women. Their study revealed that *transactional* and *interactional* strategies were used. We are most familiar with the transactional strategies, those that convey information. An example of a transactional compensatory strategy used by subject D.C. was that she selectively wrote key words during conversations in an attempt to enhance the exchange of information. Interactional compensatory strategies served to regulate social exchanges, and these were also observed. An example of this type of strategy was provided for subject N.N., who used utterances such as "Yes yes yes," "Really," and "Wonderful" to regulate and promote social interactions. These politeness markers were signaled to her partner to take the burden of communication and maintain conversational flow. Importantly, the strategies identified were used selectively, and their use was dictated by contextual social constraints. In addition, the subjects preferred some of their own idiosyncratic strategies to those encouraged by the clinician. This important study demonstrates the necessity of observing patients' compensatory strategies, determining how often they are used, in what contexts, and with what degree of success.

One final general treatment approach that may be effective with Broca's patients is PACE therapy (Davis, 2000; Davis & Wilcox, 1985). PACE is an acronym for Prompting Aphasics' Communicative Effectiveness. As the name implies, PACE was designed to incorporate aspects of natural conversation into treatment. PACE therapy was perhaps the first clearly articulated and well-known pragmatic treatment approach for aphasia. It can be easily adapted to patients of varying severity levels because it does not require high-level verbal skills for participation.

Generic treatment strategies, such as deblocking, using treatment hierarchies, self-cuing strategies, and training compensatory strategies that enhance communication can all be incorporated into broader treatment contexts such as that provided by PACE therapy (Carlomango et al., 1991; Pulvermuller and Volkbert, 1991). The treatment principles and turn-taking guidelines of PACE are flexible enough to accommodate individualized patient goals, and this approach can also be readily adapted to small group therapy for aphasia (Davis, 2000; Kearns & Elman, 2000). This malleable treatment format could also conceivably be combined with some of the more specific treatment approaches examined in the following discussion.

Specific Treatment Tasks

Although there is a paucity of structured auditory comprehension treatment programs available, clinicians can utilize the invaluable treatment suggestions of Schuell and her colleagues regarding auditory stimulation treatment procedures (Duffy & Cohelo, 2001; Schuell et al., 1964). One cognitive neuropsychological treatment approach that has been applied to training sentence-level comprehension deficits is mapping therapy (Marshall, 1995; Mitchum & Berndt, 2001; Mitchum et al., 2000; Schwartz et al., 1994). As noted earlier, research by Schwartz and her colleagues (1994; Saffran et al., 1980) led to the conclusion that comprehension deficits in agrammatism were a result of a failure to map grammatically defined sentences constituents (e.g., subject, object) onto thematic roles such as agent, theme, and goal. Agrammatism was not seen as a failure of syntactic analysis, but rather a failure to retrieve verb-specific information about thematic roles and/or correctly merge this semantic information with syntactic information. Mapping therapy addresses agrammatism by targeting the relationship between sentence structure and thematic roles. Subjects are taught the semantic relations of verbs in sentences through a series of tasks that identify the logical subject and object of sentences of varying complexity. Some Broca's aphasic individuals who have undergone mapping therapy have shown generalized improvements in their verbal production skills. The mapping therapy is one of the most widely researched treatment approaches for patients with Broca's aphasia, and it demonstrates the value of applying a neuropsychological model to intervention issues (Mitchum & Berndt, 2001; Mitchum et al., 2000).

As noted earlier, the vast majority of recent treatment studies for Broca's patients have targeted improvements in verbal skills, and many of these studies have examined syntactic abilities. Loverso and his colleagues (1992) developed one of the earliest and most extensively investigated linguistically motivated syntax training programs for aphasia. Commonly known as the Cueing Verb Treatments (CVT) program, these investigators developed a sentence-production training program based on the notion that the verb was the central constituent in sentence structure. Verbs are presented as pivots, and thematic associations (actor-action-object) are elicited using a "wh" cuing strategy. Six hierarchical levels are used to train sentences in this program, which can be individualized to meet patient needs. Single-subject data from a computerized version of the CVT program demonstrated that 18 of 21 subjects acquired target sentences on clinical probes and subsequently generalized their improvement to performance on standardized testing.

Thompson and her colleagues (Thompson, 2001; Thompson and McReynolds, 1986; Thompson and Shapiro, 1994) have conducted a series of well-controlled treatment studies examining the efficacy and generalization of a linguistic specific treatment program for sentence production deficits in Broca's aphasia. Using Chomsky's (1986) theory of government and binding as their conceptual framework, these researchers have developed procedures for targeting the underlying linguistic representations of sentences rather than treating the surface (i.e., word order) representation. Aphasic subjects have been taught to recognize verbs,

arguments, and the arguments' thematic roles in various types of sentences. Instructions are provided regarding the movement of the various sentence constituents that result in the surface form of the target sentences. The general approach of this program is to treat the underlying forms of sentences. The result of this research has been to develop a novel, linguistically based therapy approach that has been carefully researched and shown to be efficacious for Broca's patients (Thompson, 2001).

Helm-Estabrooks and her colleagues described a syntax training program called the Helm Elicited Language Program for Syntax Stimulation (HELPSS; Helm-Estabrooks, 1981; Helm-Estabrooks & Ramsburger, 1986; Helm-Estabrooks et al., 1981). The HELPSS program uses a story completion format to elicit multiple exemplars of 11 different syntactic structures. These structures are then systematically trained at two levels of difficulty until criteria for successful production is achieved. Helm-Estabrooks and Ramsburger (1986) report that six chronic agrammatic patients achieved significant improvement on formal language measures after completing the HELPSS. Other researchers have found that the order of difficulty of the HELPSS syntactic constructions may vary for individual Broca's patients (Salvatore et al., 1983), and that a limited amount of generalization may result from training with the HELPSS (Doyle et al., 1987).

Melodic Intonation Therapy (MIT) is an aphasia treatment approach that uses intoned melodies as a means of improving verbal production (Helm-Estabrooks et al., 1986). The use of melody and intonational contour used in this program is based on the notion that the intact right cerebral hemisphere, which is specialized for melodic functions, can be tapped as a means of facilitating verbal responding. The four levels of MIT are designed to increase patients' ability to independently produce high-probability phrases and sentences. Programmed instruction methods are used, as the amount of cues provided by the clinician are gradually reduced at each step of the MIT program. The program includes a variety of prompts ranging from intoning a melodic line and hand tapping to having the patient answer questions using drilled phrases and sentences. MIT appears to be most effective for highly motivated patients who have suffered a unilateral, left hemisphere lesion involving Broca's area or undercutting Broca's area; poorly articulated, nonfluent, or severely restricted verbal output; moderately preserved auditory comprehension (45th percentile on BDAE Rating Scale); and poor repetition, even for single words ability.

Response elaboration training (RET) is a program that was developed by Kearns and his colleagues to increase the length and information content of verbal responses of nonfluent aphasic patients (Gaddie et al., 1991; Kearns, 1985, 1986, 1989; Kearns & Kirschenbaum, 1994; Kearns & Yedor, 1991, 1993). RET is a "loose training" program that was designed in reaction to treatment programs in which the clinicians treat a narrow range of predetermined patient responses. An important underlying assumption during the development of RET was that overly structured treatment programs may actually inhibit patients from using language creatively and flexibly by severely limiting their response options. Loose training procedures are designed to facilitate generalization by providing a wider variety of stimuli and responses than are encountered within overly didactic treatment approaches (Doyle et al., 1989).

The rationale for RET is consistent with an adaptation agrammatism in Broca's aphasia (Kolk et al., 1985), which claims that patients simplify their speech to communicate more effectively. As Kolk and Heeschen (1990) suggest, treatment programs that encourage patients to produce complex and complete sentences may foster a slow and laborious way of communicating that will not be accepted and carried over to the natural environment. RET encourages clients to scaffold elliptical utterances into longer strings that communicate effectively regardless of the form of the output.

Procedurally, loose training attempts to loosen control over stimuli and responses during therapy in an effort to expose the patient to parameters that occur in naturalistic settings. In particular, RET loosens response parameters by using *patient-initiated* responses as the primary content of therapy rather than restricting responding to a narrow range of clinician-selected target responses. Patients enrolled in RET are encouraged to elaborate on "whatever they are reminded of" when picture stimuli are presented, and they are discouraged from simply describing or naming elements of the stimulus pictures. In fact, RET stimuli consist of line drawings of transitive and intransitive verbs that contain minimal contextual information so that patients cannot simply describe them; instead, they must rely on their personal history and world knowledge to respond. RET stimuli depict individuals involved in everyday activities and sports, and they also include a separate set of related items for probing generalization.

The emphasis in RET is on shaping and chaining spontaneous, patient-initiated responses. RET stimuli serve primarily as a catalyst for clinician-patient interactions around an action concept. Consequently, the patient can rely on the line drawings to "get started," but he or she must provide increasingly elaborate descriptions with minimal assistance from context and with minimal input from the clinician. Unlike clinician-directed approaches, the patient directs the course of therapy in RET because his responses and subsequent elaborations provide the primary focus of treatment. In essence, the patient is required to take the primary burden of communication during RET while the clinician merely ensures that the direction chosen by the patient is properly channeled to maximize his therapeutic gain. The RET program was designed to reinforce novel and varied informational content instead of linguistic form so that highly informative, telegraphic responses are quite acceptable within this protocol. Moreover, it provides a marked contrast to structured syntactic programs that typically target clinician-selected responses such as "The boy is swimming."

The efficacy and generalizability of RET has been examined using a series of single-subject experimental studies, and results have demonstrated that RET facilitates an increase in the amount and variety of information content produced by aphasic patients (Gaddie et al., 1991; Waumbaugh et al., 2001). In addition, a moderate degree of generalization has been reported across stimuli, people, and settings following RET (Kearns, 1985, 1989; Kearns & Yedor, 1991; Yedor et al., 1993). Although originally designed for use with individuals with Broca's aphasia, the effectiveness of RET has been demonstrated with nonfluent and fluent subjects (Kearns, 1989) and with aphasic patients with moderate to severe apraxia (Waumbaugh & Martinez, 2000). RET has also been used to facilitate functional communicative drawing ability with nonverbal aphasic patients (Kearns & Yedor, 1993). Most recently, a computerized version of this treatment paradigm was used to examine the effects on animation on treatment outcomes. Overall, these results, in combination with findings from other aphasia training studies (Doyle et al., 1989), indicate that loose training procedures, such as RET, may provide a potentially effective means of improving the expressive communication abilities of Broca's aphasic patients.

Conclusion

Verbal treatment programs for Broca's patients were reviewed, and representative examples of specific approaches were considered. Treatment approaches have been designed to improve syntactic aspects of verbal impairments (HELPSS) (Helm-Estabrooks & Ramsberger, 1986) and to take advantage of intact right hemisphere processes governing intonation and melody (MIT). In addition, recent programs have attempted to use neurolinguistic and generalization programming principles to develop and research treatment approaches. Further research is needed to fully evaluate the usefulness of these and other treatment approaches for Broca's aphasic patients. It appears, however, that future treatment will utilize combined behavioral linguistic, neurologic stimulation, and pharmacologic approaches to treat Broca's aphasic individuals (Small, 2000).

References

Badecker, W. & Caramazza, A. (1985). On Considerations of Method and Theory Governing the Use of Clinical Categories in Neurolinguistics and Cognitive Neuropsychology: The Case Against Agrammatism. *Cognition, 20*, 97–115.

Benton, A. (1998). Aphasia: Historical Perspectives. In: M.T. Sarno (Ed.), *Acquired Aphasia* (pp. 1–26). New York: Academic Press.

Berman, M. & Peele, L.M. (1967). Self-Generated Cues: A Method for Aiding Aphasic and Apraxic Patients. *Journal of Speech and Hearing Disorders, 32*, 372–376.

Berndt, R.S. (1998). Sentence Processing in Aphasia. In: M.T. Sarno (Ed.), *Acquired Aphasia* (2nd ed., pp. 223–270). New York: Academic Press.

Berndt, R.S. & Caramazza, A. (1980). A Redefinition of the Syndrome of Broca's Aphasia: Implications for a Neuropsychological Model of Language. *Applied Psycholinguistics, 1*, 225–278.

Berndt, R.S., Salasso, A., Mitchum, C.C. & Blumstein, S.E. (1988). The Role of Intonation Cues in Aphasic Patients' Performance on the Grammaticality Judgment Task. *Brain and Language, 34*, 65–97.

Broca, P. (1861). Portee de Ia parole. Ramollissement Chronique et Destruction Partielle du Lobe Anterieur Gauche du Oerveau. *Bulletin Sociologie Anthropologie Paris, 2*, 219.

Broca, P. (1865). Sur le Siege de la Faculte du Langage Articule. *Bulletin Sociologie Anthropologie Paris, 6*, 337–393.

Brookshire, R.H. (1992). *An Introduction to Neurogenic Communication Disorders* (4th ed.). St. Louis: Mosby Year Book.

Brookshire, R.H. & Nicholas, L.E. (1993). *Discourse Comprehension Test*. Tucson, AZ: Communication Skill Builders.

Brookshire, R.H. & Nicholas, L.E. (1994). Test-Retest Stability of Measures of Connected Speech in Aphasia. In: M.L. Lemme (Ed.), *Clinical Aphasiology* (vol. 22, pp. 119–134). Austin, TX: PRO-ED.

Brown, J. (1973). *Aphasia by Arnold Pick*. Springfield, IL: Charles C. Thomas.

Brown, J.W., Chobor, K.L. (1992). Phrenological Studies of Aphasia Before Broca: Broca's Aphasia or Gall's Aphasia? *Brain and Language, 43*, 475–486.

Brown, J.W., Perecman, E. (1986). Neurological Bases of Language Processing. In: R. Chapey (Ed.), *Language Intervention Strategies in Adult Aphasia* (2nd. ed., pp. 12–27). New York: William & Wilkins.

Caramazza, A. & Berndt, R.S. (1985). A Multicomponent Deficit View of Agrammatic Broca's Aphasia. In:

M.L. Kean (Ed.), *Agrammatism* (pp. 27–62). New York: Academic Press.

Carlomango, S., Losanno, N., Emanuelli, S. & Cosadio, P. (1991). Expressive Language Recovery of Improved Communicative Skills: Effects of P.A.C.E. Therapy on Aphasics' Referential Communication and Story Retelling. *Aphasiology, 5*, 419–424.

Chomsky, N. (1986). *Knowledge of Language, Its Nature, Origins and Use*. New York: Praeger.

Crain, S., Shankweiler, D. & Tuller, B. (1984). Preservation of Sensitivity to Closed-Class Items in Agrammatism. Talk presented at the annual Academy of Aphasia meeting, Los Angeles.

Critchley, M. (1964). Dax's Law. *International Journal of Neurology, 4*, 199–206.

Crosson, B. (1985). Subcortical Functions in Language: A Working Model. *Brain and Language, 25*, 257–292.

Dale, A.M. & Halgren E. (2001). Spatiotemporal Mapping of Brain Activity by Integration of Multiple Imaging Modalities. *Current Opinion in Neurobiology, 11*, 202–208.

Damasio, A. (1998). Signs of Aphasia. In: M.T. Sarno (Ed.), *Acquired Aphasia* (pp. 25–40). New York: Academic Press.

Damasio, H. (1998). Neuroanatomic Correlates of the Aphasias. In: M.T. Sarno (Ed.), *Acquired Aphasia* (pp. 43–68). New York: Academic Press.

Davis, A. & Wilcox, M.J. (1985). *Adult Aphasia Rehabilitation: Applied Pragmatics*. San Diego: College-Hill Press.

Davis, G.A. (2000). *Aphasiology: Disorders and Clinical Practice*. Boston: Allyn & Bacon.

Demonet, J. & Thierry, G. (2001). Language and Brain: What Is Up? What Is Coming Up? *Journal of Clinical and Experimental Neuropsychology, 12*, 49–73.

DeRenzi, E. & Vignolo, L. (1962). The Token Test: A Sensitive Test to Detect Receptive Disturbances in Aphasia. *Brain, 85*, 556–678.

DeRenzi, F. & Faglioni, P. (1978). Normative Data and Screening Power of a Shortened Version of the Token Test. *Cortex, 14*, 41–49.

Doyle, P., Goldstein, H. & Bourgeois, M.S. (1987). Experimental Analysis of Syntax Training in Broca's Aphasia: A Generalization and Social Validation Study. *Journal of Speech and Hearing Disorders, 52*, 143–155.

Doyle, P., Goldstein, H., Bourgeois, M. & Nakles, K. (1989). Programming "Loose Training" as a Strategy to Facilitate Generalization of Questioning in Broca's Aphasic Subjects. *Journal of Applied Behavior Analysis, 22*, 157–170.

Duffy, J.R. (1995). *Motor Speech Disorders: Substrates, Differential Diagnosis and Management*. St. Louis: Mosby.

Duffy, J.R. & Cohelo, C. (2001). Schuell's Stimulation Approach to Rehabilitation. In: R. Chapey (Ed.), *Language Intervention Strategies in Adult Aphasia* (4th ed., pp. 341–382). Baltimore: William & Wilkins.

Duffy, R. & Duffy, J. (1984). *The New England Pantomime Test*. Tigard, OR: C.C. Publications.

Frattali, C., Thompson, C., Holland, A., Wohl, C. & Ferketic, M. (1995). *American Speech-Language-Hearing Association Functional Assessment of Communication Skills for Adults*. Rockville, MD: ASHA.

Freedman, M., Alexander, M.P. & Naeser, M.A. (1984). Anatomical Basis of Transcortical Motor Aphasia. *Neurology, 34*, 409–417.

Gaddie, A., Kearns, K.P. & Yedor, K. (1991). A Qualitative Analysis of Response Elaboration Training Effects. In: T.E. Prescott (Ed.), *Clinical Aphasiology* (vol. 19, pp. 171–184). San Diego: College-Hill Press.

Goodglass, H. (1993). *Understanding Aphasia*. San Diego: Academic Press.

Goodglass, H., Kaplan, E. & Barresi, B. (2001). *The Assessment of Aphasia and Related Disorders* (3rd ed.). Philadelphia: Lippincott, Williams & Wilkins.

Goodglass, H. & Menn, L. (1985). Is Agrammatism a Unitary Phenomenon? In: M.L. Kean (Ed.), *Agrammatism* (pp. 1–25). New York: Academic Press.

Grodzinsky, Y. (1990). *Theoretical Perspectives on Language Deficits*. Cambridge, MA: MIT Press.

Hanson, W.R., Metter, E.J., Riege, W.H., et al. (1984). Positron Emission Tomography. In: R.H. Brookshire (Ed.), *Clinical Aphasiology* (pp. 14–23). Minneapolis: BRK.

Head, H. (1963). *Aphasia and Kindred Disorders of Speech* (vol. 1). New York: Hafner.

Heeschen, C. (1985). Agrammatism Versus Paragrammatism: A Fictitious Opposition. In: M.L. Kean (Ed.), *Agrammatism* (pp. 207–248). New York: Academic Press.

Helm-Estabrooks, N. (1981). *Helm Elicited Language Program for Syntax Stimulation*. Austin, TX: PRO-ED.

Helm-Estabrooks, N. (1992). *Aphasia Diagnostic Profiles (ADP)*. Austin, TX: PRO-ED.

Helm-Estabrooks, N. & Albert, M.L. (1991). *Manual of Aphasia Therapy*. Austin, TX: PRO-ED.

Helm-Estabrooks, N., Fitzpatrick, P.M. & Barresi, B. (1981). Response of an Agrammatic Patient to a Syntax Stimulation Program for Aphasia. *Journal of Speech and Hearing Disorders, 46*, 422–427.

Helm-Estabrooks, N., Nicholas, M. & Morgan, A. (1989). *Melodic Intonation Therapy Program*. Austin, TX: PRO-ED.

Helm-Estabrooks, N. & Ramsberger, G. (1986). Treatment of Agrammatism in Long-Term Broca's Aphasia. *British Journal of Communication Disorders, 21*, 39–45.

Hillis, A.E., Kane, A., Barker, P., Beauchamp, N., Gordon, B. & Wityk, R. (2001). Neural Substrates of the Cognitive Processes Underlying Reading: Evidence from Magnetic Resonance Perfusion Imaging in Hyperactive Stroke. *Aphasiology, 15*, 919–931.

Hillis, A.E., Wang, P., Barker, P., Beauchamp, N., Gordon, B., & Wityk, R. (2000). Magnetic Resonance Perfusion Imaging: A New Method for Localizing Regions of Brain Dysfunction Associated with Specific Lexical Impairments? *Aphasiology, 14*, 471–483.

Holland, A. (1980). *Communicative Abilities in Daily Living*. Austin, TX: PRO-ED.

Holland, A. (1994). Cognitive Neuropsychological Theory and Treatment for Aphasia: Exploring the Strengths and Limitations. In: M.L. Lemme (Ed.), *Clinical Aphasiology* (vol. 22, pp. 275–282). Austin, TX: PRO-ED.

Jackson, H. (1915). Selected Writings of J. Hughlings Jackson. *Brain, 38*, 1–90.

Jakobson, R. (1952). Aphasia as a Linguistic Topic. Clarke University Monographs on Psychology and Related Disciplines. Worcester. Reprinted in R. Jakobson. *Selected Writings* (vol. 2): *Words and Language*. The Hague: Mouton.

Jakobson, R. & Halle, M. (Eds.) (1956). *Fundamentals of Language*. The Hague: Mouton.

Kagan, A., Black, S.E., Duchan, J.F., Simmons-Mackie, N. & Square, P. (2001). Training Volunteers as Conversation Partners Using "Supported Conversation for Adults with Aphasia" (SCA): A Controlled Trial. *Journal of Speech, Language, and Hearing Research, 44,* 624–638.

Kaplan, E., Godglass, H. & Weintraub, S. (1983). *The Boston Naming Test.* Philadelphia: Lea & Febiger.

Katz, R.C. & Wertz, R.T. (1997). The Efficacy of Computer-Provided Reading Treatment for Chronic Aphasics. *Journal of Speech, Language, and Hearing Research, 40,* 493–507.

Kay, J., Lesser, R. & Coltheart, M. (1992). *Psycholinguistic Assessment of Language Production in Aphasia.* East Sussex, UK: Lawrence Erlbaum.

Kean, M.L. (1985). *Agrammatism.* New York: Academic Press.

Kearns, K.P. (1985). Response Elaboration Training for Patient Initiated Utterances. In: R.H. Brookshire (Ed.), *Clinical Aphasiology Conference Proceedings* (pp. 196–204). Minneapolis: BRK.

Kearns, K.P. (1986). Systematic Programming of a Pragmatic Approach to Aphasia Management. In: R.C. Marshall (Ed.), *Case Studies in Aphasia Rehabilitation* (pp. 225–244). Austin, TX: PRO-ED.

Kearns, K.P. (1989). Methodologies for Studying Generalization. In: L.V. McReynolds & J. Spradlin (Eds.), *Generalization Strategies in the Treatment of Communication Disorders* (pp. 13–30). Lewiston, NY: BC Decker.

Kearns, K.P. (2000). Single-Subject Experimental Designs in Aphasia. In: S. Nadeau, L. Gonzalez-Rothi, & B. Crosson (Eds.), *Aphasia and Language: Theory to Practice.* New York: Guilford Press.

Kearns, K.P. & Elman, R. (2001). Group Therapy for Aphasia: Theoretical and Practical Considerations. In: R. Chapey (Ed.), *Language Intervention Strategies in Adult Aphasia* (4th ed., pp. 316–340). Baltimore: Williams & Wilkins.

Kearns, K.P. & Kirschenbaum, L. (1994). An Examination of Animation: A Computerized Treatment Program for Aphasia. Presented at the Clinical Aphasiology Conference, Traverse City, MI.

Kearns, K.P. & Potechin-Scher, G. (1988). The Generalization of Response Elaboration Training Effects. In: T.E. Prescott (Ed.), *Clinical Aphasiology* (pp. 223–246). Austin, TX: PRO-ED.

Kearns, K.P. & Potechin-Scher, G. (1989). The Generalization of Response Elaboration Training Effects. In: T.E. Prescott (Ed.), *Clinical Aphasiology* (vol. 18, pp. 223–246). San Diego: College-Hill.

Kearns, K.P. & Salmon, S.J. (1984). An Experimental Analysis of Auxiliary and Copula Verb Generalization in Aphasia. *Journal of Speech and Hearing Disorders, 49,* 152–163.

Kearns, K.P., Simmons, N. & Sisterhen, C. (1982). Gestural Sign (Am-Ind) as a Facilitator of Verbalization in Patients with Aphasia. In: R.H. Brookshire (Ed.), *Clinical Aphasiology Conference Proceedings* (pp. 183–191). Minneapolis: BRK.

Kearns, K.P. & Yedor, K. (1991). An Alternating Treatments Comparison of Loose Training and a Convergent Treatment Strategy. In: T.E. Prescott (Ed.), *Clinical Aphasiology* (vol. 20, pp. 223–238). Austin, TX: PRO-ED.

Kearns, K.P. & Yedor, K. (1993). Artistic Activation Therapy: Drawing Conclusions. Presented at the Clinical Aphasiology Conference, Sedona, AZ.

Kertesz, A. (1979). *Aphasia and Associated Disorders: Taxonomy, Localization, and Recovery.* New York: Grune and Stratton.

Kertesz, A. (1982). *Western Aphasia Battery.* New York: Grune and Stratton.

Kertesz, A., Harlock, W. & Coates, R. (1979). Computer Tomographic Localization, Lesion Size and Prognosis in Aphasia and Nonverbal Impairment. *Brain and Language, 8,* 34–50.

Knopman, D.S., Selnes, G.A., Niccum, N.D., et al. (1983). A Longitudinal Study of Speech Fluency in Aphasia: CT Correlates of Recovery and Persistent Nonfluency. *Neurology, 33,* 1170–1178.

Kolk, H. & Heeschen, C. (1990). Adaption Symptoms and Impairments in Broca's Aphasia. *Aphasiology, 4,* 4221–4231.

Kolk, H. & Heeschen, C. (1992). Agrammatism, Paragrammatism and the Management of Language. *Language and Cognitive Processes, 7,* 89–129.

Kolk, H.H.J., Van Grunsven, M.J.F. & Keyser, A. (1985) On Parallelism Between Production and Comprehension in Agrammatism. In: M.L. Kean (Ed.), *Agrammatism* (pp. 165–206). New York: Academic Press.

LaPointe, L.L. & Horner, J. (1978). The Functional Auditory Comprehension Task (FACT): Protocol and Test Format. *FL. ASHA Journal,* Spring, 27–33.

LaPointe, L.L. & Horner, J. (1998). *Reading Comprehension Battery for Aphasia* (2nd ed.) Austin, TX: Pro-Ed.

Lichtheim, L. (1885). On Aphasia. *Brain, 7,* 433–484.

Linebaugh, C. & Lehner, L. (1977). Cueing Hierarchies and Word Retrieval: A Therapy Program. In: R.H. Brookshire (Ed.), *Clinical Aphasiology Conference Proceedings* (pp. 19–31). Minneapolis: BRK.

Loverso, F.L., Prescott, T.E. & Selinger, M. (1992). Microcomputer Treatment Application in Aphasiology. *Aphasiology, 6,* 155–163.

Luria, A. (1970). *Traumatic Aphasia.* The Hague: Mouton.

Lyon, J.G. (1992). Communication Use and Participation in Life for Adults with Aphasia in Natural Settings: The Scope of the Problem. *American Journal of Speech-Language Pathology, 1,* 7–14.

Lyon, J.G. (1995). Drawing: Its Value as a Communication Aid for Adults with Aphasia. *Aphasiology, 9,* 33–94.

Marshall, J. (1995). The Mapping Hypothesis and Aphasia Therapy. *Aphasiology, 9,* 517–539.

McNeil, M. & Prescott, T. (1978). *Revised Token Test.* Baltimore: University Park.

Menn, D. & Obler, L.K. (1990) *Agrammatic Aphasia.* Amsterdam: Benjamins.

Metter, E.J., Jackson, C.A., Kempler, D. & Hanson, W.R. (1992). Temporoparietal Cortex and Recovery of Language Comprehension in Aphasia. *Aphasiology, 6,* 349–358.

Metter, E.J., Kempler, D., Jackson, C.A., et al. (1986). Cerebral Glucose Metabolism: Differences in Wernickes' Broca's Conduction Aphasia. In: R.H. Brookshire (Ed.), *Clinical Aphasiology* (pp. 97–104). Minneapolis: BRK.

Metter, E.J., Kempler, D., Jackson, C.A., et al. (1987). A Study of Broca's Aphasia by Fluorodeoxyglucose Positron Emission Tomography. *Annals of Neurology*, 134.

Metter, E.J., Riege, W.H., Hanson, W.R., et al. (1988). Subcortical Structures in Aphasia: An Analysis Based on (F-18) Fluorodeoxyglucose, Positron Emission Tomography, and Computer Tomography. *Arch Neurology*, 45, 1229–1234.

Meuse, S. & Marquardt, T.P. (1985). Communicative Effectiveness in Broca's Aphasia. *Journal of Communication Disorders*, 18, 21–34.

Mitchum, C. & Berndt, R.S. (2001). Cognitive Neuropsychological Approaches to Diagnosing and Treating Language Disorders: Production and Comprehension of Sentences. In R. Chapey (Ed.), *Language Intervention Strategies in Aphasia* (4th ed.). Baltimore: Williams & Wilkins.

Mitchum, C.C., Greenwald, M.L. & Berndt, R.S. (2000). Cognitive Treatments of Sentence Processing Disorders: What Have We Learned? *Neuropsychological Rehabilitation*, 10, 311–336.

Mlcoch, A. & Metter, J. (2001). Medical Aspects of Stroke Rehabilitation. In: R. Chapey (Ed.), *Language Intervention Strategies in Aphasia and Related Neurogenic Disorders* (4th ed.). Philadelphia: Lippincott Williams & Wilkins.

Mohr, J.P. (1980). Revision of Broca's Aphasia and the Syndrome of Broca's Area Infarction and Its Implication in Aphasia Theory. *Clinical Aphasiology Conference Proceedings* (pp. 1–16) Minneapolis: BRK.

Mohr, J., Pessin, M., Finkelstein, S., Funkenstein, H., Duncan, G.W. & Davis, K.R. (1978). Broca's Aphasia: Pathological and Clinical. *Neurology*, 28, 311–324.

Naeser, M.A., Palumbo, C.L., Helm-Estabrooks, N., et al. (1986). Severe Non-Fluency in Aphasia: Role of the Medical Subcallosal Fasciculus Plus Other White Matter Pathways in Recovery of Spontaneous Speech. Presented at the Annual Academy of Aphasia Meeting, October, Nashville, TN.

Naeser, M.X. & Hayward, R.W. (1978). Lesion Localization in Aphasia with Cranial Computed Tomography and the Boston Diagnostic Aphasia Exam. *Neurology*, 28, 545–551.

Nespoulous, J., Dordain, M., Perron, C., et al. (1988). Agrammatism in Sentence Production Without Comprehension Deficits: Reduced Availability of Syntactic Structures and/or of Grammatical Morphemes? A case study. *Brain and Language*, 33, 273–295.

Nicholas, L.E. & Brookshire, R.H. (1993). A System for Quantifying the Informativeness and Efficiency of the Connected Speech of Adults with Aphasia. *Journal of Speech and Hearing Research*, 36, 338–350.

Nikels, L. & Best, W. (1996). Therapy for Naming Disorders (Part I): Principles, Puzzles, and Progress. *Aphasiology*, 10, 21–48.

Petocz, A. & Oliphant, G. (1988). Closed-Class Words as First Syllables Do Interfere with Lexical Decisions for Nonwords: Implications for Theories of Agrammatism. *Brain and Language*, 34, 127–146.

Pick, A. (1931). *In the Handbuch der Normalen und Pathologischen Physiologie* (vol. 15). Heidelberg: Springer-Verlag.

Prescott, T., Selinger, M. & Loverso, F. (1982). An Analysis of Learning, Generalization and Maintenance of Verbs by an Aphasic Patient. In: R.H. Brookshire (Ed.), *Clinical Aphasiology Proceedings* (pp. 178–182). Minneapolis: BRK.

Pulvermuller, F. & Volkbert, M.R. (1991). Communicative Aphasia Treatment as Further Development of P.A.C.E. Therapy. *Aphasiology*, 5, 39–50.

Raven, J.C. (1962). *Coloured Progressive Matrices*. London: HK, Lewis.

Rogers-Warren (Eds.), *Teaching Functional Language* (pp. 197–224). San Diego: College-Hill.

Rosenbek, J.C. & Shimon, D. (1984). Computerized Axial Tomography in Aphasiology. In: R.H. Brookshire (Ed.), *Clinical Aphasiology Conference Proceedings 1986* (pp. 1–6). Minneapolis: BRK.

Roth, H.L. & Heilman, K. (2000). Aphasia: A Historical Perspective. In: S.E. Nadeau, R.L. Gonzalez & B. Crosson (Eds.), *Aphasia and Language Theory and Practice*. New York: Guilford Press.

Saffran, E., Schwartz, M. & Marin, O. (1980). The Word Order Problem in Agrammatism I: Comprehension. *Brain and Language*, 10, 249–262.

Salvatore, A.P., Trunzo, M.G., Holtzapple, P., et al. (1983). Investigation of the Sentence Hierarchy of the Helm Elicited Language Program for Syntax Stimulation. In: R.H. Brookshire (Ed.), *Clinical Aphasiology Conference Proceedings* (pp. 73–84). Minneapolis: BRK.

Schuell, H., Jenkins, J.J. & Jimenez-Pabon, E. (1964). *Aphasia in Adults: Diagnosis, Prognosis and Treatment*. New York: Harper & Row.

Schwartz, M.F., Linebarger, M.C. & Saffran, E.M. (1985). The Status of the Syntactic Deficit Theory of Agrammatism. In: M.L. Kean (Ed.), *Agrammatism* (pp. 83–124). New York: Academic Press.

Schwartz, M.F., Saffran, M., Fink, R., Myers, J. & Martin, N. (1994). Mapping Therapy: A Treatment Programme for Agrammatism. *Aphasiology*, 8, 19–54.

Shapiro, L.P. & Thompson, C. (1994). The Use of Linguistic Theory as a Framework for Treatment Studies in Aphasia. In: M.L. Lemme (Ed.), *Clinical Aphasiology* (vol. 22, pp. 291–306). Austin, TX: PRO-ED.

Shewan, C.M. (1979). *Auditory Comprehension Test for Sentences*. Chicago: Biolinguistics Clinical Institutes.

Shuell, H., Jenkins, J. & Jimenez-Pabon, E. (1964). *Aphasia in Adults*. New York: Harper and Row.

Simmons, N.N., Kearns, K.B. & Potechin, G. (1987). Treatment of Aphasia Through Family Member Training. In: R.H. Brookshire (Ed.), *Clinical Aphasiology* (vol. 17, pp. 106–116). Minneapolis: BRK.

Simmons-Mackie, N.N. & Damico, J.S. (1995). Communicative Competence in Aphasia: Evidence from Compensatory Strategies. In: M.L. Lemme (Ed.), *Clinical Aphasiology* (vol. 23, pp. 95–106). Austin, TX: PRO-ED.

Small, S. (2000). The Future of Aphasia Therapy. *Brain and Language*, 71, 227–232.

Thompson, C.K. (1989). Generalization in the Treatment of Aphasia. In: L.V. McReynolds & J. Spradlin (Eds.), *Generalization Strategies in the Treatment of Communication Disorders* (pp. 82–115). Toronto: BC Decker.

Thompson, C.K. (2001). Treatment of nonfluent Broca's aphasia. In: R. Chapey (Ed.), *Language Intervention Strategies in Aphasia* (3rd ed.). Baltimore: Williams & Wilkins.

Thompson, C.K., Ballard, K.L. & Shapiro, L.P. (1998). The Role of Syntactic Complexity in Training Wh-Movement Structures in Agrammatic Aphasia: Optimal Order for Promoting Generalization. *Jour-*

nal of the International Neuropsychological Society, 4, 661–674.

Thompson, C.K. & McReynolds, L.V. (1986). *Wh* Interrogative Production in Agrammatic Aphasia: An Experimental Analysis of Auditory-Visual Stimulation and Direct-Production Treatment. *Journal of Speech and Hearing Research, 29,* 193–206.

Thompson, C.K. & Shapiro, L. (1994). A Linguistic-Specific Approach to Treatment of Sentence Production Deficits in Aphasia. In: M.L. Lemme (Ed.), *Clinical Aphasiology* (vol. 22, pp. 307–323). Austin, TX: PRO-ED.

Wambaugh, J.L. & Martinez, A.L. (2000). Effects of Modified Response Elaboration Training with Apraxic and Aphasic Speakers. *Aphasiology, 15,* 603–617.

Wambaugh, J.L., Martinez; A.L. & Alegre, M.N. (2001). Qualitative Changes Following Application of Modified Response Elaboration Training with Apraxic-Aphasic Speakers. *Aphasiology, 15,* 965–976.

Warburton, E., Wise, R.J., Price, C.J., Weiller, C., Hadar, U., Ramsay, S. & Frackowaik, R.S. (1996). Noun and Very Retrieval by Normal Subjects. Studies with PET. *Brain, 119,* 159–179.

Wernicke, C. (1874). *Der Aphasische Symptomenkomplex.* Breslau: Cohn and Weigert.

Wertz, R.T., Deal, J.L. & Robinson, A.J. (1984). Classifying the Aphasias: A Comparison of the Boston Diagnostic Aphasia Examination and the Western Aphasia Battery. In: R.H. Brookshire (Ed.), *Clinical Aphasiology Conference Proceedings* (pp. 40–47). Minneapolis: BRK.

Wertz, R.T., LaPointe, L.L. & Rosenbek, J.C. (1984). *Apraxia of Speech in Adults: The Disorder and Its Management.* New York: Grune & Stratton.

Yedor, K., Conlon, K. & Kearns, K.P. (1993). Measurements Predictive of Response Elaboration Training.

In: M.L. Lemme (Ed.), *Clinical Aphasiology* (vol. 21, pp. 213–224). Austin, TX: PRO-ED.

Suggested Readings

Berndt, R. S. (1998). Sentence Processing in Aphasia. In: M.T. Sarno (Ed.), *Acquired Aphasia* (3rd ed., pp. 229–268). New York: Academic Press.

Goodglass, H. (1993a). *Aphasic Agrammatism: Underlying Causes and Overt Manifestations.* National Center for Neurogenic Communication Disorders, Telerounds No. 10, University of Arizona, Tucson, AZ.

Goodglass, H. (1993b). *Understanding Aphasia.* San Diego: Academic Press.

Kearns, K.P. (2000). Single-Subject Experimental Designs in Aphasia. In: S. Nadeau, L. Gonzalez-Rothi, & B. Crosson (Eds.), *Aphasia and Language: Theory to Practice.* New York: The Guilford Press.

Kearns, K.P. & Elman, R. (2001). Group Therapy for Aphasia: Theoretical and Practical Considerations. In: R. Chapey (Ed.), *Language Intervention Strategies in Adult Aphasia* (3rd ed.). Baltimore: Williams & Wilkins.

Mitchum, C. & Berndt, R.S. (2001). Cognitive Neuropsychological Approaches to Diagnosing and Treating Language Disorders: Production and Comprehension of Sentences. In: R. Chapey (Ed.), *Language Intervention Strategies in Aphasia* (4th ed.). Baltimore: Williams & Wilkins.

Thompson, C.K. (2001). Treatment of Underlying Forms: A Linguistic Specific Approach to Sentence Production Deficits in Agrammatic Aphasia. In: R. Chapey (Ed.), *Language Intervention Strategies in Aphasia* (3rd ed.). Baltimore: Williams & Wilkins.

9

Wernicke's Aphasia

ISABELLE CASPARI

Carl Wernicke, the man whose 1874 treatise leads us to this discussion, died tragically when his bicycle fell under an oxcart (Wernicke, 1977). He was more fortunate in developing his thoughts on aphasia. Crystallizing in one chapter the genesis and current status of thought on Wernicke's aphasia since his time is a challenge. Some clinicians have yet to find a definitive case of Wernicke's aphasia. Essentially identical aphasia syndromes have been called sensory aphasia, receptive aphasia, central aphasia, and many other names. Although the debate over the specifics of Wernicke's aphasia continues, the constellation of behaviors associated with it tends to be the same. For a moment in time, during the evolution of the aphasic condition, Wernicke's aphasia may appear as an identifiable type. Often a patient's recovery and/or rehabilitation may take him on a course that starts with classic Wernicke's symptomatology and brings him into the more general "fluent type" classification. For a clinically useful description, we must settle on a set of behaviors associated with a generally similar lesion. Despite the controversy that exists over the condition, it is firmly entrenched in many quarters as a concept and a clinical reality. Thus an understanding of the suggested underlying mechanisms and the possibilities for remediation is essential to the clinician.

History/Pathophysiology

Until Carl Wernicke's paper (1874), aphasic behaviors had been localized and delineated most notably by Paul Broca (1861). Broca had described the location and characteristics for frontal motor aphasia, or "aphemia" as he called it. He identified the source of defect as anterior to the central sulcus, whose location as a division for motor and sensory functions was known at the time. It was left to Wernicke to describe those aphasias apparent in individuals whose frontal lobes remained intact. Wernicke's work, "The Aphasia Symptom-Complex: A Psychological Study on an Anatomical Basis" described the existence of sensory aphasia and provided postmortem evidence of this new localization at or around the Sylvian fissure. Following the logic of his teacher and mentor, Meynart (who had suggested that the acoustic pathways would end near the Sylvian fissure), Wernicke postulated that traces of words would be stored near this zone, where interruption would result in loss of comprehension. The landmark of sensory aphasia, later to become Wernicke's aphasia, was thus described by Wernicke as the result of a lesion in the dominant first temporal gyrus, the area first postulated by Meynert and subsequently named Wernicke's area for its descriptor.

The primary deficit in sensory aphasia, according to Wernicke, was an interruption of the central auditory projection area, or "klangfeld" (sound field). Wernicke explained that, as Broca's areas must be the center for representation of memory images of movement of the mouth and tongue, so the sound field at the first temporal gyrus must be the center for representation of sounds. Given that the primary deficit is auditory comprehension loss, Wernicke maintained there would exist corresponding losses in the ability to understand written language, or produce it oneself. He felt these losses were a consequence of learning reading and writing in indivisible association with sounds. Obviously, without auditory comprehension, the ability to repeat also would be lost. Speech movements would be preserved as a function of the anterior system, and quality would be fluent, perhaps even rapid. However, speech content would be paraphasic due to loss of the internal correction of the motor process ordinarily overseen by the receptive speech zone. This paraphasic speech pattern would go unnoticed by the speaker because of impaired auditory monitoring. Owing to the posterior lesion and the location of motor function in the frontal lobes, the individual would demonstrate no obvious hemiplegia.

As a formal definition of Wernicke's aphasia, these original findings on localization and behavioral hallmarks have stood the test of time. Currently, the behaviors associated with this syndrome are still considered a result of injury to the posterior region of the left superior temporal gyrus. The resulting associated behaviors include (a) fluent but paraphasic speech; (b) defective auditory comprehension; (c) defective repetition of words and sentences; (d) both reading and writing usually disturbed; and (e) infrequent hemiparesis.

Wernicke originally asserted that sensory aphasia resulted from lesion to the dominant superior temporal gyrus. Hannah Damasio (2001) summarized recent research pertaining to Wernicke's aphasia as well as other fluent aphasias. She states that Wernicke's original description of the underlying brain damage resulting in Wernicke's aphasia (Wernicke, 1886)" is consonant with contemporary investigations" (p. 26). The core location for the lesion remains in the posterior portion of the superior temporal gyrus, the auditory association area, or Wernicke's area, contained in the Sylvian fissure. In fact, Kertesz (1993) suggested that a superior posterior temporal lesion is obligatory for Wernicke's aphasia. In support, Chapman et al. (1989) presented preliminary findings that point to damage in the dominant superior temporal gyrus as a common factor among patients who are deemed most seriously impaired by their aphasia.

Naesar et al. (1987) found significant correlations between comprehension loss and the amount of temporal lesion in Wernicke's area. However, they found no correlation between comprehension loss and total temporoparietal lesion size. In another study utilizing CT scans, Kertesz et al. (1993) determined that persisting Wernicke's aphasia usually involves the supramarginal and angular gyri in addition to the superior temporal area. They reported also that the supramarginal and angular gyri appear to be important structures in recovery, especially for compensation of the accompanying comprehension deficit.

Many have long felt that Wernicke's aphasia is particularly resistant to recovery of function. However, new evidence suggests that recovery of function in Wernicke's aphasia may be accompanied by a redistribution of activity within both cerebral hemispheres, but particularly the right hemisphere. Recently, Weiller et al. (1995) used positron emission tomography (PET) to investigate changes in the organization of the brain after recovery from aphasia. They measured increases in regional cerebral blood flow (rCBF) during the repetition of pseudowords and during verb generation in healthy controls and patients with damage to Wernicke's area. In the healthy controls there was evidence of strong rCBF activation in Wernicke's and Broca's areas, with weak activation of the right hemisphere. While, in the patients, there was clear right hemisphere activation in zones, homotopic to the left hemisphere language zones. The researchers argued that the redistribution of activation might be a central mechanism in functional reorganization of the language system after stroke.

Thurlborn et al. (1999) provide further support for the theory of functional reorganization of language after stroke. They obtained functional magnetic resonance imaging (fMRI) data during a simple sentence reading task for a patient who had sustained damage to Wernicke's area. Interestingly, fMRI data were available prior to the stroke for this patient. Not surprisingly, there was strong, left hemisphere activation of Wernicke's area before to the stroke. Functional MRI results recorded at 3 and 9 months poststroke, however, indicated a change from left hemisphere activation to weak right hemisphere activation in Wernicke's area that became progressively stronger over time. These results support the position that clinical recovery is associated with a redistribution of function to the right hemisphere (Cherney & Robey, 2001).

Nature and Differentiating Features

Wernicke's aphasia is differentiated primarily from the anterior, nonfluent aphasias. Once a diagnosis of fluent aphasia has been made, a person may be classified into one of three major posterior, fluent syndromes: Wernicke's aphasia, conduction aphasia, or transcortical sensory aphasia. The behavioral patterns of the three aphasia types not only overlap, but in some cases, mimic each other exactly. Table 9–1 outlines the behavioral hallmarks for each of these syndromes. However, successful differential diagnosis requires that the clinician be familiar with the characteristics and behavioral correlates of all the fluent aphasias well beyond the range of the table.

The comprehension deficit in Wernicke's aphasia is likely the most debilitating aspect of the disorder (Davis, 1993; Goodglass, 1993; Marshall, 2001; Schuell, 1953). A person with Wernicke's aphasia may be incapable of processing input of any kind. Schuell maintained that an important factor in the prognosis of recovery from any aphasia was the degree of residual auditory comprehension ability, specifically for individual words. She posited that damage to the temporal lobe would not produce isolated symptoms, but rather patterns of deficit based on the dissolution of established neural interconnections. This was the premise of Wernicke as well in his postulate that higher functions were managed by the associative tracts instead of each function being handled by a discrete area of brain. The severity of comprehension deficit varies in Wernicke's aphasia from inability to understand any spoken language to a less obvious shutter-effect type comprehension disorder, where some stimuli are processed adequately but others remain unprocessed. The exact quality of the deficit is not well under-

Table 9–1. Behavioral Patterns of Types of Aphasia

	Wernicke's	*Conduction*	*Transcortical Sensory*
Auditory comprehension	Severely impaired	Slightly impaired	Severely impaired
Repetition	Impaired	Impaired	Intact
Speech	Fluent, paraphasic	Paraphasic	Fluent, paraphasic
Reading	Impaired	Intact	Impaired
Writing	Impaired	Impaired	Impaired

stood, as comprehension does not disintegrate predictably along defined lines. Nor do we have adequate precision in our measurement tools or even an adequate understanding of the nature of comprehension in healthy individuals to precisely delineate the nature of the deficit.

Fluent, but paraphasic speech (phonemic and semantic substitutions) is another hallmark of Wernicke's aphasia. Often, the words of the fluent aphasic speaker are supplemented with extra syllables or are even fabricated anew (neologisms). The term "jargon aphasia" frequently is used to describe the semantically anomalous sentence production observed in Wernicke's aphasia (Davis, 1993, 2000). Sentences tend to be grammatically tangled and characterized by unsystematic substitutions or omissions of grammatical morphemes (paragrammatisms) and lexical words (nouns, verbs, and adjectives) (Goodglass, 1993; Goodglass et al., 2000). Patients demonstrate little awareness of their expressive deficits that are exacerbated by the confounding factor of "press of speech." Also termed logorrhea, this behavior is characteristic of Wernicke's aphasia, although arguably it may exist with other syndromes, notably transcortical sensory aphasia. Press of speech manifests itself not so much in rate, although that is possible, but rather in the irrepressible intention of the speaker to continue in his monologue, often to the point where he must be forcibly stopped by physical gesture or insistent interruption by the listener. Wernicke explained this phenomenon as resulting from the lack of correction over output normally exercised by the sensory areas. This theory has been widely accepted, or at least not directly refuted, and the emphasis in treatment on having the patient monitor his output lends credence to our belief in Wernicke's explanation as a credible underlying cause.

Reading comprehension also is affected in Wernicke's aphasia. Patients may demonstrate difficulty in associating written words with their sounds or their meanings. They may even have difficulty in matching letters or recognizing letters by name. Goodglass (1993) refers to this generalized loss of meaning and sound associations to written symbols as "aphasic alexia," which he considers secondary to the loss of oral language. Wernicke's original explanation of this problem was based on the assumption that reading is learned in such a way as to be tied inexorably to auditory comprehension. He argued that each of us auditorizes what we process visually, and in the absence of an ability to do that, reading is no longer possible. Goodglass reports that the more the lesion extends posteriorly, encroaching on the region of the angular gyrus (thought to be the location for reading abilities), the more severe the alexia. It is important for the clinician to distinguish between disabilities in oral reading and reading comprehension (Webb & Love, 1994). There may be cases of intact oral reading accompanied by impaired comprehension; whereas errors in oral reading may mask adequate comprehension (Goodglass, 1993)

Writing deficits also contribute to the mosaic of Wernicke's aphasia. The writing deficits consequent to posterior damage are strikingly dissimilar from those evidenced in anterior lesions. Whereas the person with Broca's aphasia struggles valiantly over the production of a single legible word or letter, the person with Wernicke's aphasia may write easily and voluminously. Unfortunately, while letter formation may be appropriate and there may be occasional breaks in the letter strings to symbolize words, spelling may be significantly impaired. Individuals with Wernicke's aphasia often produce fluent paragraphic written jargon that has a similar linguistic structure to their speech (Davis, 1993). Overall, the writing disorder tends to be commensurate with the severity of the speech output disorder. Of interest is the fact that there is an apparent lack of awareness or concern by the individual with Wernicke's aphasia for the nonsense that he has just distributed across the page. Explanations for this phenomenon parallel those offered for press of speech. Barring any monitoring ability, the patient is left with only the preserved anterior abilities to produce, but without the pivotal abilities to monitor and correct.

The overview of the characteristics most cited as hallmarks of Wernicke's aphasia have been completed. Important as well are some of the ancillary behaviors that arise, not from the lesion itself, but from the behavioral profile it causes. Some of these fall into the area of disorders of mood or emotion. Although depression remains the major psychological reaction to stroke, its identification is complicated by cognitive, language, and functional impairments (Gupta et al., 2002). Researchers, Turner-Stokes and Hassan (2002) suggest that it can hinder rehabilitation and may be responsible for poor outcomes and increased length of stays. According to the National Mental Health Association fact sheet (2002), depression occurs in 10 to 27% of stroke survivors and usually lasts about one year. Aben and colleagues (2002) conducted a one-year prospective follow-up study on the incidence of depression as a sequela of stroke. They found that there was a cumulative incidence of depression of 37.8%. Wahrborg (1991) categorizes depression following stroke either as "major post stroke depression," which is associated with the proximity of the lesion to the frontal lobe, or as "reactive post stroke depression," which is related to the ability to cope with the challenges of stroke and aphasia. Lubinsky (2001) reports that in aphasia, depressive symptoms may be multiple ranging from sadness, dependency, and indecisiveness with the most extreme symptom being suicide. She notes further that aphasic individuals with depression are in "double jeopardy" because of their increased difficulty in verbally expressing their feelings.

The apparent lack of concern in the person with Wernicke's aphasia is often short lived following initiation of treatment, and occasional reports of attempted suicide are heard. The potential for alienation in severe cases of Wernicke's or any aphasia should be taken seriously by all health-care providers and explained carefully to the family. Lubinsky (2001) suggests that speech-language pathologists (SLP) have an important role in identifying affective symptoms and making appropriate referrals for accurate differential diagnosis and medical, psychiatric, or pharmaceutical intervention. Moreover, SLPs are in a unique position to deal directly with the psychological reactions of aphasic individuals to ensure that therapy is functional and effective. The psychosocial consequences of cerebral damage together with the SLP's role in management are addressed elsewhere in this book.

The final note on correlates of Wernicke's aphasia actually concerns a condition usually not present. As mentioned previously, obvious paralysis is a rare accompaniment of Wernicke's aphasia. Because of this, a lesion causing Wernicke's symptomatology may well go unnoticed in the standard, non-radiographic neurological examination. In the words of Carl Wernicke, "thoroughly experienced and intelligent physicians regard this condition as a confusional state, as I myself have had the opportunity to experience." (Geschwind, 1967, p. 290). Unfortunately, the same error is possible today and is best countered by a complete language examination, especially examination of the auditory system.

Evaluation

Appraisal of aphasia ideally begins upon first hearing of the patient. Anything shown, told, or reported to us becomes part of the appraisal information bank. Typically, initial evaluation occurs at bedside after the clinician has received an order to evaluate. Initially, an informal screen may be conducted. Holland and Fridriksson (2001) recommend that acute care clinicians forgo formal screening in favor of very careful observations and documentation of patients' language strengths and weaknesses during multiple daily communication exchanges.

Formal screening or bedside tests of aphasia are useful for determining the presence or absence of aphasia. They are particularly helpful for those patients whose hospital stays may be short or for those who may be medically stable, but lack the stamina to complete a lengthy examination (Murray & Chapey, 2001). Some of the more recently developed bedside tests include the Bedside Evaluation Screening Test, Second Edition (BEST-2; Fitch-West & Sands, 1998), the Aphasia Screening Test (AST; Whurr, 1996), and the Quick Assessment for Aphasia (Tanner & Culbertson, 1999).

When there are no constraints of time, or a more comprehensive evaluation of aphasia is desirable, the clinician can administer one of the standardized aphasia test batteries. Tests such as the Boston Diagnostic Aphasia Examination–3 (BDAE-3; Goodglass et al., 2000), the Porch Index of Communicative Abilities (PICA; Porch, 1981) and the Western Aphasia Battery (WAB; Kertesz, 1982), are popular choices. They indicate type and severity of aphasia, and to some extent, point the clinician in the direction to take in further testing or treatment. Individuals with Wernicke's aphasia who frequently demonstrate severely compromised linguistic systems may profit from a more pragmatic approach to assessment that emphasizes the evaluation of all forms of communication—both verbal and nonverbal—in a variety of real-life situations (Worrall, 1995). Such an approach lays the foundation for the type of intervention that ultimately promotes progress in activities essential for daily living (Davis, 2000). In point of fact, a recent review of the literature on assessment suggests that there has been a shift in emphasis regarding appraisal of the aphasic condition. Acceptance of the recent World Health Organization's (WHO) healthcare initiative that emphasizes quality of life through its "Body Structure and Function, Activity and Participation" Framework (ICIDH-2, 1999) has led clinicians to recognize the importance of determining the functional abilities of their clients. What is of importance today is evaluating the level of communicative independence their clients demonstrate in a variety of daily social activities. Indeed, prevailing healthcare legislation and standards mandate that SLPs show clear evidence of useful functional outcomes in order for treatment to be considered effective (Fratalli, 1998). In fact, reimbursement for treatment may depend on demonstrating functional progress to third party payors. (Frattali, 1998; Holland, 1998). A number of structured tests of functional ability have been developed to assist the clinician in evaluating functional performance. These include the Assessment of Language Related Functional Abilities (Baines et al., 1999), the Communication Activities of Daily Living–2 (Holland et al., 1999), and the Amsterdam-Nijmegen Everyday Language Test (ANELT; Blomert et al., 1994). The latter test identifies pragmatic verbal sensibilities for 15 scenarios of everyday life.

Another method of assessing functional communication skills in individuals with aphasia and their significant caregivers is to rate communication behavior on a scale. There are several rating scales available for profiling functional change over time. The American Speech-Language-Hearing Association (ASHA) Functional Assessment of Communicative Skills (FACS) for Adults (Frattali et al., 1995) provides an easy and efficient way to keep track of a patient's progress in a wide range of domains. Lomas et al. (1989) developed the Communicative Effectiveness Index (CETI), a questionnaire for rating communicative abilities in daily living of aphasic individuals by significant caregivers. Worrall's (1992) Everyday Communication Needs Assessment can be used to determine a hierarchy of needs. The Functional Communication Measures (FCM; ASHA, 1995) was developed specifically to measure functional progress consequent to treatment as perceived by the clinician. In a recent treatment study, Caspari and Katz (2001) found a high correlation between the CETI and the FCM consequent to functionally based aphasia treatment.

Supplemental Tests

Among the most important tasks in diagnosing Wernicke's aphasia is thorough testing of auditory comprehension. Although several comprehension tests exist, none can be said to provide a completely adequate indication of the person's status. The clinician should always be aware that because auditory comprehension is not an openly observable ability, our estimates of its status are only as good as our means of inference and prediction. Typically, off-line procedures, such as picture pointing or forced choice tasks, are used to assess processing abilities of syntactic and/or semantic attributes of language at the word, sentence, or discourse level (Davis, 1993). Not surprisingly, off-line tasks do not measure comprehension during spontaneous conversation or as it occurs on-line. Although it may be advantageous to assess on-line processing, few measurement techniques are available at this time (but see Tyler et al., 1992).

Clinicians can select the Token Test (De Renzi and Vignolo, 1962) or the Revised Token Test (McNeil and Prescott, 1978) to more thoroughly assess auditory comprehension in aphasia. These tests focus on auditory comprehension ability in the absence of linguistic redundancy or environmental cues. However, as alluded to previously, a more functional approach to the assessment of comprehension is emerging. Although the correlates of natural language remain elusive, we can say that most communication contains heavily redundant and largely predictable information. With this in mind, clinicians should try to assess their patients' abilities to comprehend information in context or in the presence of multiple linguistic and nonlinguistic cues (Marshall, 2001). Observation of functional behaviors in several different natural settings provides a means of identifying an individual's communicative strengths and weaknesses (Carlomagno, 1994). More than 25 years ago LaPointe and Horner (1978), recognizing the importance of investigating functional comprehension abilities, developed the Functional Auditory Comprehension Test (FACT). It is a test with everyday relevance that utilizes stimulus items and directions related to daily living. Brookshire and Nicholas (1997) developed the Discourse Comprehension Test because

they determined that comprehension ability improved when information was provided in paragraph form, or contained information that was of personal interest to their subjects. These and other researchers (Marshall, 1994; Wilcox et al., 1978) remind us that our evaluations need to incorporate information about comprehension in real-life contexts. The potential difference in comprehension estimates is illustrated by two patients in the Wilcox et al. study who scored at 58% and 49% levels in standard testing, yet achieved 100% and 93% when tested in real-life situations.

Supplemental language production tests range in specificity from single-word naming to picture descriptions. Clinicians should collect samples not only during structured tasks, which have the obvious advantage of duplication over time, but also during unstructured tasks. Sampling and analyzing the spontaneous speech of the person with Wernicke's aphasia provides a means of quantifying natural discourse production (Davis, 1993) and measuring subtle progress over time. The Systematic Analysis of Language Transcripts (SALT), originally developed by Miller and Chapman (1991) and adapted for analysis of adult–adult interaction by Holland et al. (1985), facilitates analysis by combining linguistic description and measurement. Language sampling and analysis can assist in the development of a linguistically based intervention program.

There are number of supplemental tests for assessing reading. Perhaps the most widely known of these is the Reading Comprehension Battery for Aphasia–2 (RCBA-2; LaPointe and Horner, 1998), in which tasks range from relating symbols to sounds, comprehending single words, to comprehending sentences and "functional" tasks. The Nelson Reading Skills Test (NRST; Hanna et al., 1977) contains paragraphs with high passage dependency. That is, the client must read the passage to answer the questions. Other reading tests include the John Hopkins University Dyslexia Battery (Goodman and Caramazza, 1986a), the New Adult Reading Test (NART; Nelson, 1984), and the Test of Reading Comprehension (Brown et al., 1995).

Any suspected writing deficit requires further investigation. Writing appraisal tools of interest include the John Hopkins Dysgraphia Battery developed by Goodman and Caramazza (1986b) for use with individuals with aphasia, and McNeil and Tseng's (1990) Experimental Neurogenic Dysgraphia Battery for the evaluation of writing competence. The Test of Written Language–3 (Hammill and Larsen, 1996) explores writing deficits in vocabulary, spelling, word usage, and story-writing skill in high-functioning individuals with aphasia. Amster and Amster (1994) used informal assessment procedures to evaluate the writing skills of higher-functioning individuals. These explore the patients' ability to recognize and formulate letters, to write a variety of words, and to string words together in meaningful constructions. Accuracy, content, and organization are also evaluated.

For supplemental tasks in both reading and writing Murray and Chapey (2001) report that for some tests the normative data are provided in the test manual, allowing the patient's performance to be compared with that of other brain-damaged patients. For other tests, the normative data must be sought in the empirical literature.

Although our concept of aphasia may evolve and change over time, which may, in turn, influence the way we set about appraising and treating the aphasic condition, the purpose of assessment remains essentially unchanged. The goal of assessment is to provide a road map for treatment.

General Treatment Principles

Often, severely impaired individuals with Wernicke's aphasia, with no predictable reason for being so, are either quite lucid or flamboyantly incomprehensible. Their euphoric outlook and reduced awareness of deficit contribute to the challenge of formulating an effective intervention program (Schuell, 1953). Ultimately, the patient with Wernicke's aphasia retains the hope that his problem will "go away," or at least that somebody will help him understand and adapt. Designing effective treatment in quest of addressing that hope is what motivates many clinicians.

Careful analysis of the initial exchanges with the clinician often will yield useful information for therapy. Although any positive exchanges should be replicated and expanded upon, the clinician should keep in mind that the key to clinical success may be elusive and may take several sessions to establish.

Development of a treatment plan begins with information from interviews, chart review, and an accumulation of test results. Unfortunately, it is not possible to make a classification of aphasia type and then turn to page "Wernicke" in the "Book of Therapy." Auditory comprehension deficits and poor self-monitoring must be dealt with in the beginning because their presence affects all interactions. The problem should be addressed within the confines of many selected treatment tasks and not approached as though manageable in a task or two. The initial responsibility of the clinician is to create a therapeutic set—a cooperative attitude (Davis, 1993, 2000). The individual with Wernicke's aphasia often does not appear to understand or appreciate the reasons for therapy. As Davis suggests, such a patient must be almost forced into a mode of cooperating with the clinician and of responding to specific stimuli. The patient may require specific training in listening to simple instructions and pointing to an object or picture in response. Once reliable responding is established, the clinician can introduce more demanding comprehension tasks.

Almost immediately, the clinician needs to confront the problem of press of speech. Wernicke's patients prefer to talk rather than listen, especially during comprehension training; therefore, their attention should be directed toward listening. Press of speech is most often addressed with a stop technique, wherein the clinician quite literally stops the patient, usually by means of gesture (Davis, 1993). The idea, says Davis, is to alert or remind the patient to stop talking while listening to a stimulus. Improved listening leads to improved comprehension and ultimately to improved verbalization.

It is well known that reducing the rate of speech improves comprehension for the aphasic listener when that reduction is achieved through pauses between meaningful segments (Nicholas and Brookshire, 1986). Here, clinical research is buttressed by comments from our patients, "Why does everybody talk so fast?" "You know, your words are on top of each other!" In addition to slowing rate, some clinicians alert a patient to incoming information nearly automatically ("Hey, Mr. Green, here's the next one"), a technique confirmed to enhance attention (Loverso and Prescott, 1981). The patient is also encouraged to slow down and monitor his excessive rate of speech. The clinician literally stops the patient, usually by means of a gesture, and then indicates that the patient should slow down to listen to himself and monitor his output. "The improvement in self-monitoring," argues Davis (1993), "must be a goal when considering verbal expression of the Wernicke's patient because verbal expression can only be modified when a patient can recognize difficulties." Doyle and Holland (1982) report on a patient with severe press of speech who achieved an immediate reduction of rate and extraneous speech through the use of a pacing board. They suggest transfer of this technique to a less cumbersome method for functional use.

All methods for enhancing comprehension and controlling speech output should be incorporated by the clinician into strategies that can be generalized to communication outside the clinic. Moreover, explanation and modeling of these techniques for family members is an effective first step in environmental therapy.

Treatment Planning

The purpose of effective treatment, states Marshall (2001), is to foster maximum success in sending and receiving information, however possible. He suggests some practical ways to accomplish this objective during each therapy session. He proposes that messages should be context-dependent to maximize patent and latent processing abilities. He suggests further, that messages should be

salient and short, and that message redundancy should be increased because redundancy facilitates comprehension. As a final point, he contends that communication partners should exaggerate facial expression and gesture to increase understanding.

One way to develop a preliminary treatment outline based on successes and failures in evaluation is simply to sit down with accumulated tests and notes and begin writing. These notes on possible remedial techniques and their effectiveness during treatment trials form the groundwork for a strong intervention program. Here are samples of preliminary treatment development notes taken from a Wernicke's patient's chart over several sessions:

> Counting is good when the items are ordered for him . . . he's somewhat messy; did not organize cards logically for him to count, but usually got them once started. Automatic language tasks are starters? Surprised me! He was related on naming today—table for chair, truck for car (dismal in testing); got some outright. Slight tendency to perseverate . . . especially on error response. Some bizarre responses ("piano toast" for "butter"). Semantic cues helpful?
>
> Asked repeatedly for nail polish for sore finger . . . even when confronted with nail polish. Never did realize error. Has tendency to go off task, perseverates on his own conversations. Self-monitoring seems like it could come around. Once or twice he corrected errors and knew it. Add monitoring component to tasks at start.
>
> Talk to family and NURSES. Begin yes/ no personal questions.

Writing these notes at the beginning of treatment development reinforces the observation that even within major deficit parameters, each aphasic individual behaves differently and will respond to treatment based only on his or her own idiosyncrasies.

Family Inclusion

The success of any treatment approach likely depends on the inclusion of family members in treatment. Participation in therapy by those who communicate most often with the client is a critical aspect of treatment with any aphasic person. With the often-confusing behaviors of the person with Wernicke's aphasia, the family members benefit particularly well from understanding their part in successful communication. An excellent assessment of communication between partners can be made with Flowers and Peizer's "Strategies for Obtaining Information from Aphasic Persons" (1994). The requisites of conversation for the aphasic person and the speaking partner are outlined and can be addressed by the clinician. No treatment plan can succeed unless family members are taught how to adjust their own expectations and how to support their loved one during conversational exchanges. Increasing the communicative skills of caregivers is an important goal (Simmons-Mackie and Kagan, 1999).

Specific Treatment Methodologies

There are several approaches to the treatment of aphasia cited in the literature that facilitate improvement in communication in individuals with Wernicke's aphasia. Schuell's stimulation approach to rehabilitation in aphasia is perhaps the best known and the one that for the time being, at least, is the most efficacious (Robey, 1998). The cornerstone of this approach is the employment of strong, controlled, and intensive auditory stimulation. Its proponents, Schuell et al., (1964), Darley (1982), and Duffy and Coelho (2001), posit that immersion in language through intensive sensory stimulation could increase neuronal firing, thereby effecting an increase in neural activation. The approach is seen as the primary tool to facilitate and maximize the patient's reorganization and recovery of language (Duffy and Coelho, 2001).

The social approach to rehabilitation in aphasia is gaining acceptance. With the focus on functional improvement, health-care professionals are seeking ways of optimizing functional outcomes (Simmons-Mackie, 2001). Worrall and Fratalli (2000) propose that speech-language professionals and clients collaborate on determining and prioritizing personal goals of therapy in accordance with the everyday needs expressed by the client. Therapy is directed at accomplish-

ing these goals, and performance is periodically evaluated and goals modified as needed. An initial goal in therapy might focus on improving conversational skills.

Perhaps the most common complaint from spouses or caregivers of individuals with aphasia is that "friends simply stop coming around because they don't know what to say or how to maintain a conversation" with the affected family member. Holland and Fridriksson (2001) advocate a conversational approach even in the early acute phase of treatment. They argue that conversation can provide authentic opportunities for patients and caregivers to develop effective strategies for overcoming potential obstacles to communication. Simmons-Mackie (2001) suggests that expanding conversational skills and increasing confidence in the conversational arena is an appropriate goal for therapy. She advocates direct conversational therapy involving planned intervention that is explicitly designed to enhance conversational abilities.

Other approaches for improving conversation include conversational coaching, supported conversations, and partner training. Conversational coaching (Holland, 1988) requires that individuals with aphasia practice communicative scenarios with the guidance of the speech-language pathologist who serves as coach. Intervention involves determining a scenario (e.g., ordering drinks at a restaurant), planning what is needed, developing a script, and practicing with the coach as needed. Finally, the scenario is performed in real life and the outcome is evaluated.

Supported conversation (Kagan, 1999) is yet another method of enhancing communication exchanges between family and friends. This method employs scaffolding techniques in which the communicative partner provides cues or facilitators within the natural flow of communication. For example, the communication partner might write down key words or provide subtle gestural cues to support the client during a communicative exchange. Kagan and Gailey (1993) promote the idea that the conversation skills of the individuals with aphasia could be improved if the communication partners were trained to support conversation with persons with aphasia. Recent research provides experimental support for the efficacy of training volunteers as conversation partners in supported conversation (Kagan et al., 2001).

Promoting Aphasics Communicative Effectiveness (PACE) is likely one of the most popular therapies for aphasia. It is a versatile treatment method that can be modified to support the prevailing conceptualization of aphasia. Originated by Davis and Wilcox (1985), it is described as a method of encouraging more "real-world" conversations in the clinic. According to Carlomagno (1994), what sets PACE apart from other functional or linguistically based treatment protocols is the introduction of several innovative procedures into the therapeutic set. Among its unique qualities are the emphases on free choice of communicative modality, and equal opportunity to send and receive messages for the client and the clinician or other partner. Another feature of the method is that the information passing between the two participants must be novel. This aspect of the program departs radically from traditional approaches, where the clinician quite literally gets to hold all the cards. The method is highly reinforcing for the client and is usually equally reinforcing for the clinician. PACE therapy easily can incorporate techniques developed in more structured therapy, such as intentional pause before speaking, use of a pacing board, and requests for repeats. The effectiveness of PACE therapy has been examined by several specialists, some of whom have modified and extended its use (Carlomagno, 1994). Some contemporary approaches to treatment have been described. For a more comprehensive review see Chapey (2001).

A Final Note

An effective treatment program needs to incorporate numerous styles of communication, all of which might be suggested by the aphasic person's characteristics and responses to treatment. Perhaps because the direction of therapy follows the many paths

of the client, work with a person with Wernicke's aphasia is much less predictable in its course than that with behaviors associated with more anteriorly placed lesions. This necessitates use of a much more comprehensive variety of clinical tasks and strategies. Treatment of the person with Wernicke's aphasia is never easy, and sometimes may demand a greater degree of creativity and tolerance than treatment with our quieter, more plodding clients. With the extroverted, excessive, exceptionally off-task, and occasionally exhausting client, we may see ourselves more in a struggle to keep up and perhaps out of the way than in our preferred position as director of production. For our clinical science to advance, we must continue our attempts to understand change in all our clients. We must continue to discover and establish the validity of whatever makes a difference using the best of our knowledge, techniques, and creativity, regardless of the limitations of our insight as to precisely when and where we are able to influence meaningful change in this most puzzling but fascinating condition.

References

Aben, I., Denollet, J., Lousberg, R., Verhay, F., Wojciechowski, F. & Honig A. (2002). Personality and Vulnerability to Depression in Stroke Patients: A 1-Year Prospective Follow-Up Study. *Stroke, 33,* 2391–2395.

American Speech-Language-Hearing Association. (1995). *Functional Communication Measures.* Rockville, MD: ASHA.

Amster, W.W. & Amster, J.B. (1994). Treatment of Writing Disorders in Aphasia. In: R. Chapey (Ed.), *Language Intervention Strategies in Adult Aphasia* (3rd ed., pp. 458–466). Baltimore: Williams & Wilkins.

Baines, K.A., Martin, A.W. & Heeringa, H.M. (1999). *Assessment of Language-Related Functional Activities.* Austin, TX: Pro-Ed.

Blomert, L., Kean, M.L., Koster, C., & Schokker, J. (1994). The Amsterdam-Nijmegen Everyday Language Test (ANELT): construction, reliability and validity. *Aphasisology, 8,* 381–407.

Broca, P. (1861). Portee de la Parole: Ramollisement Chroniqueet Destruction Partielle du Lobe Anterieur Gauche du Oerveau. *Bulletin Sociologie Anthropologie Paris, 2,* 219.

Brookshire, R.H. & Nicholas, L. (1997). *The Discourse Comprehension Test* (rev. ed.). Minneapolis: BRK.

Brown, V.L., Hammill, D.D. & Wiederholt, J.L. (1995). *Test of Reading Comprehension* (3rd ed.). Austin: Pro-Ed.

Carlomagno, S. (1994). *Pragmatic Approaches to Aphasia Therapy: Promoting Aphasics' Communicative Effectiveness.* London: Whurr.

Caspari, I. & Katz, R.C. (2001). *Comparative Effects of Ten or Twenty Hours of Treatment on Treatment Effectiveness in Aphasia.* Poster presented at the Clinical Aphasiology Conference, Santa Fe, New Mexico.

Chapman, S.B., Pool, K.D., Finitzo, T. & Hong, C.T. (1989). Comparison of Language Profiles and Electrocortical Dysfunction in Aphasia. In: T.E. Prescott (Ed.), *Clinical Aphasiology* (vol. 18, pp. 41–59). Boston: College Hill Press.

Chapey, R. (Ed.) (2001). Language Intervention Strategies in Aphasia and Related Neurogenic Communication Disorders (4th ed.). Baltimore: Lippincott Williams & Williams.

Cherney, L.R. & Robey, R.R. (2001). Aphasia Treatment: Recovery, Prognosis and Clinical Effectiveness. In: R. Chapey (Ed.), *Language Intervention Strategies in Aphasia and Related Neurogenic Communication Disorders* (4th ed., pp. 148–172). Baltimore: Lippincott Williams & Williams.

Damasio, H. (2001). Neural Basis of Language Disorders. In: R Chapey (Ed.), *Language Intervention Strategies in Aphasia and Related Neurogenic Communication Disorders* (4th ed., pp. 18–36). Baltimore: Lippincott Williams & Wilkins.

Darley, F. (1982). *Aphasia.* Philadelphia: WB Saunders.

Davis, G.A. (1993). *A Survey of Adult Aphasia and Related Language Disorders.* Englewood Cliffs, NJ: Prentice-Hall.

Davis, G.A. (2000). *Aphasiology: Disorders and Clinical Practice.* Boston: Allyn and Bacon.

Davis, G.A. & Wilcox, J.M. (1985). *Adult Aphasia Rehabilitation: Applied Pragmatics.* San Diego: Singular.

DeRenzi, E. & Vignolo, L.A. (1962). The Token Test: A Sensitive Test to Detect Receptive Disturbances in Aphasics. *Brain, 85,* 665–678.

Doyle, R. & Holland, A.L. (1982). Clinical Management of a Patient with Pure Word Deafness. In: R.H. Brookshire (Ed.), *Clinical Aphasiology: Conference Proceedings* (pp. 138–146). Minneapolis: BRK.

Duffy, J.R. & Coelho, C.A. (2001). Schuell's Stimulation Approach to Rehabilitation. In: R. Chapey (Ed.), *Language Intervention Strategies in Aphasia and Related Neurogenic Communication Disorders* (4th ed., pp. 341–382). Baltimore: Lippincott Williams & Williams.

Fitch-West, J. & Sands, E.S. (1998). *Bedside Evaluation Screening Test* (2nd ed., BEST-2). Austin: Pro-Ed.

Flowers, C.R. & Peizer, E.R. (1994). Strategies for Obtaining Information from Aphasic Persons. In: R.H. Brookshire (Ed.), *Clinical Aphasiology: Conference Proceedings* (pp. 106–113). Minneapolis: BRK.

Frattali, C.M. (1998). Measuring Modality Specific Behaviors, Functional Abilities, and Quality of Life. In: C.M. Frattali (Ed.), *Measuring Outcomes in Speech-Language Pathology* (pp. 55–88). New York: Thieme.

Frattali, C.M., Thompson, C.K., Holland, A.L., Wall, C. & Ferkedic, M. (1995). *Functional Assessment of Communication Skills for Adults* (ASHA FACS). Rockville, MD: ASHA.

Geschwind, N. (1967). Wernicke's Contribution to the Study of Aphasia. *Cortex, 3,* 449–463.

Goodglass, H. (1993) *Understanding Aphasia.* San Diego: Academic Press.

Goodglass, H., Kaplan, E. & Barresi, B. (2000). *Boston Diagnostic Aphasia Examination.* Philadelphia: Lea and Febiger.

Goodman, R.A. & Caramazza, A. (1986a). *The John Hopkins University Dyslexia Battery.* Baltimore: John Hopkins University.

Goodman, R.A. & Caramazza, A. (1986b). *The John Hopkins University Dysgraphia Battery.* Baltimore: John Hopkins University.

Gupta, A., Pansari, K. & Shetty, H. (2002). Post Stroke Depression. *International Journal of Clinical Practice, 56,* 531–537.

Hammill, D.D. & Larsen, S. (1996). *The Test of Written Language* (3rd ed.). Austin: Pro-Ed.

Hanna, G., Schell, L.M. & Schreiner, R. (1977). *The Nelson Reading Skills Test.* Chicago: Riverside.

Holland, A.L. (1988). *Conversational Coaching in Aphasia.* Paper presented at the Deep South Conference on Communication Disorders, Baton Rouge, LA.

Holland, A.L. (1998). Functional Outcome Assessment of Aphasia Following Left Hemisphere Stroke. In: C. Frattali (Ed.), *Seminars in Speech and Language, 19,* 249–260.

Holland, A.L, Frattali, C.M. & Fromm, D. (1999). *Communication Activities of Daily Living* (2nd ed.). Austin: Pro-Ed.

Holland, A.L. & Fridriksson, J. (2001). Aphasia Management During the Early Phases of Recovery Following Stroke. *American Journal of Speech-Language Pathology, 10,* 19–28.

Holland, A.L., Miller, J., Reinmuth, O.M., Bartlett, C., Fromm, D., Pashek, G.V., et al. (1985). Rapid Recovery from Aphasia: A Detailed Language Analysis. *Brain and Language, 24,* 156–173.

Kagan, A. (1999). *Supported Conversation for Adults with Aphasia: Methods and Evaluation.* Unpublished dissertation, University of Toronto.

Kagan, A., Black, S.E., Duchan, J.F., Simmons-Mackie, N. & Square, P. (2001). Training Volunteers as Conversation Partners Using "Supported Conversation for Adults with Aphasia" (SCA): A Controlled Trial. *Journal of Speech, Language and Hearing Research, 44,* 624–638.

Kagan, A. & Gailey, G.F. (1993). Functional is Not Enough: Training Conversational Partners for Aphasic Adults. In: A.L. Holland & M.M. Forbes (Eds.), *Aphasia Treatment: World Perspectives* (pp. 199–225). San Diego: Singular.

Kertesz, A. (1982). *Western Aphasia Battery.* New York: Grune & Stratton.

Kertesz, A. (1993). Clinical Forms of Aphasia. *Acta Neurochirurgica Supplementum Wein, 56,* 52–58.

Kertesz, A., Lau, W.K. & Polk, M. (1993). The Structural Determinants of Recovery in Wernicke's Aphasia. *Brain and Language, 44,* 153–164.

LaPointe, L.L. & Horner, J. (1978, Spring). The Functional Auditory Comprehension Task (FACT): Protocol and Test Format. *FLASHA Journal,* 27–33.

LaPointe, L.L. & Horner, J. (1998). *Reading Comprehension Battery for Aphasia* (2nd ed.). Austin, TX: Pro-Ed.

Lomas, J., Pickard, L., Bester, S., Elbard, H., Finlayson, A. & Zoghaib, C. (1989). The Communicative Effectiveness Index: Development and Psychometric Evaluation of a Functional Communication Measure for Adult Aphasia. *Journal of Speech and Hearing Disorders, 54,* 113–124.

Loverso, F.L. & Prescott, T.E. (1981). The Effect of Alerting Signals on Left Brain Damaged (aphasic) and Normal Subjects' Accuracy and Response Time to Visual Stimuli. In: R.H. Brookshire (Ed.),

Clinical Aphasiology: Conference Proceedings (pp. 55–67). Minneapolis: BRK.

Lubinsky, R. (2001). Environmental Systems Approach to Adult Aphasia. In: R Chapey (Ed.), *Language Intervention Strategies in Aphasia and Related Neurogenic Communication Disorders* (4th ed., pp. 269–296). Baltimore: Lippincott Williams & Williams.

Lyons, J. (1998). *Coping with Aphasia.* San Diego: Singular.

Marshall, R.C. (1994). Management of Fluent Aphasic Clients. In: R. Chapey (Ed.), *Language Intervention Strategies in Adult Aphasia* (3rd ed., pp. 389–406). Baltimore: Williams & Wilkins.

Marshall, R.C. (2001). Management of Wernicke's Aphasia: A Context-Based Approach. In: R. Chapey (Ed.), *Language Intervention Strategies in Aphasia and Related Neurogenic Communication Disorders* (4th ed., pp. 435–456). Baltimore: Lippincott Williams & Williams.

McNeil, M.R. & Prescott, T.E. (1978). *Revised Token Test.* Baltimore: University Park Press.

McNeil, M.R. & Tseng, C.H. (1990). Acquired Neurogenic Dysgraphias. In: L.L. LaPointe (Ed.), *Aphasia and Related Neurogenic Language Disorders* (pp. 147–176). New York: Thieme.

Miller, J. & Chapman R. (1991). *Systematic Analysis of Language Transcripts* (SALT). Madison: University of Wisconsin Press.

Murray, L.L. & Chapey, R. (2001). Assessment of Language Disorders in Adults. In: R. Chapey (Ed.), *Language Intervention Strategies in Aphasia and Related Neurogenic Communication Disorders* (4th ed., pp. 55–126). Baltimore: Lippincott Williams & Williams.

Naeser, M.A., Helm-Estabrooks, N., Haas, G., Auerbach, S. & Srinivasan, M. (1987). Relationship Between Lesion Extent in "Wernicke's Area" on Computed Tomographic Scan and Predicting Recovery of Comprehension in Wernicke's Aphasia. *Archives of Neurology, 44,* 73–82.

National Mental Health Association. (2002). Depression: Co-occurrence of Depression with Medical Psychiatric, and Substance Abuse Disorders. *http://www.nmha.org/infoctr.factsheets.28.cfm.*

Nicholas, L.E. & Brookshire, R.H. (1986). Consistency of the Effects of Rate of Speech on Brain Damaged Subjects' Comprehension of Information in Narrative Discourse. In: R.H. Brookshire (Ed.), *Clinical Aphasiology: Conference Proceedings* (pp. 262–271). Minneapolis: BRK.

Nelson, H.E. (1984). *New Adult Reading Test* (NART). Windsor, England: NFER-Nelson.

Porch, B.E. (1981). *Porch Index of Communicative Ability,* vol. 11: *Administration, Scoring and Interpretation* (rev. ed.). Palo Alto, CA: Consulting Psychologists Press.

Robey, R.R. (1998). A Meta-Analysis of Clinical Outcomes in the Treatment of Aphasia. *Journal of Speech, Language and Hearing Research, 41,* 172–187.

Schuell, H. (1953). Aphasic Difficulties Understanding Spoken Language. *Neurology, 3,* 176–184.

Schuell, H.H., Jenkins, J.J. & Jimenez-Pabon, E. (1964). *Aphasia in Adults.* New York: Harper and Row.

Simmons-Mackie, N. (2001). Social Approaches to Aphasia Intervention. In: R. Chapey (Ed.), *Language Intervention Strategies in Aphasia and Related Neurogenic Communication Disorders* (4th ed., pp. 246–266). Baltimore: Lippincott Williams & Williams.

Simmons-Mackie, N., & Kagan, A. (1999). Communication strategies used by "good" versus "poor" speaking partners of individuals with aphasia. *Aphasiology, 13,* 807–820.

Tanner, D.C. & Clubertson, W. (1999). *Quick Assessment for Aphasia.* Oceanside, CA: Academic Communication Associates.

Thurlborn, K.R., Carpenter, P. & Just, M.A. (1999). Plasticity of Language-Related Brain Function During Recovery from Stroke. *Stroke, 30,* 749–754.

Turner-Stokes, L. & Hassan, N. (2002). Depression After Stroke: A Review of the Evidence Base to Inform the Development of an Integrated Care Pathway. Part 1: Diagnosis, Frequency and Impact. *Clinical Rehabilitation, 16,* 231–247.

Tyler, L.K., Cobb, H. & Graham, N. (1992). *Spoken Language Comprehension: An Experimental Approach to Disordered and Normal Processing.* Cambridge, MA: MIT Press.

Wahrborg, P. (1991). *Assessment and Management of Emotional and Psychological Reactions to Brain Damage and Aphasia.* San Diego: Singular.

Webb, W.E. & Love, R. (1994), Treatment of Acquired Reading Disorders. In: R. Chapey (Ed.), *Language Intervention Strategies in Adult Aphasia* (3rd ed., pp. 446–457). Baltimore: Williams & Wilkins.

Weiller, C., Isensee, C., Rijntjes, M., Huber, W., Muller, S., Bier, D., et al. (1995). Recovery from Wernicke's Aphasia: A Positron Emission Tomographic Study. *Annals of Neurology, 37,* 723–732.

Wernicke, C. (1874). *Der Aphasische Symptomkomplex.* Breslau: Kohn & Neigart

Wernicke, C. (1977). The Aphasia Symptom Complex: A Psychological Study on an Anatomic Basis. In: G.H. Eggert (Ed., trans.), *Wernicke's Work on Aphasia: A Sourcebook and Review* (pp. 91–145). The Hague, Netherlands: Mouton.

Wernicke, C. (1886). Einige Neuere Arbeiten uber Aphasic. *Fortschritte der Medizin, 4,* 377–463.

Whurr, R. (1996). *The Aphasia Screening Test* (2nd ed.). San Diego, CA: Singular.

Wilcox, M.J., Davis, G.A. & Leonard, L.L. (1978). Aphasics' Comprehension of Contextually Conveyed Meaning. *Brain and Language, 6,* 362–377.

World Health Organization. (1999). ICIDH-2: International Classification of Impairments, Activities and Participation: A manual of dimensions of disability and health. *http://www.who.int/msa/mnh/ems/icidh/introduction.htm.*

Worrall, L. (1992). *Everyday Communicative Needs Assessment.* Queensland, Australia: Department of Speech and Hearing, University of Queensland.

Worrall, L.E. (1995). The Functional Communication Perspective. In: C. Code & D.J. Muller (Eds.), *The Treatment of Aphasia: From Theory to Practice* (pp. 47–69). San Diego, CA: Singular.

Worrall, L., & Fratalli, C. (2000). *Neurogenic Communication Disorders: A Functional Approach.* New York: Thieme Medical Publishers.

10

Conduction Aphasia

NINA SIMMONS-MACKIE

In 1874, Carl Wernicke (1977) suggested the existence of a distinct type of aphasia based on his neuroanatomic model of language localization in the brain. Thus, began the concept of conduction aphasia as a predicted outcome of a lesion that disconnects the two primary speech centers. Several years later, Lichtheim (1885) elaborated on Wernicke's model and suggested for the first time the potential for disrupted verbal repetition in conduction aphasia based on the hypothetical disconnection model (see historical reviews by deBleser et al., 1993, and Henderson, 1992). Such hypothetical arguments prompted one historian to describe conduction aphasia as "the quintessential aphasic syndrome derived from diagrammatic schemes" (Henderson, 1992, p. 23). Debate continues over the anatomic model and underlying mechanisms responsible for conduction aphasia. Fortunately, however, there appears to be agreement on the signs and symptoms that define conduction aphasia. A major differentiating feature is a significant impairment of verbal repetition, which is disproportionate to the fluency of spontaneous speech (Table 10–1). In addition, phonemic paraphasias and word-retrieval problems appear in the context of the fluent, melodic speech, and auditory comprehension is relatively good. The condition is considered rare relative to other aphasia types. Benson and colleagues (1973) estimated that between 5% and 10% of new aphasic patients admitted to their

facility fit the classification of conduction aphasia.

Pathophysiology

The localization of the brain lesion associated with conduction aphasia has received substantial attention. Neuroanatomic lesions have been associated most frequently with the postrolandic areas of the left hemisphere (Axer et al., 2001; Palumbo et al., 1992). Conduction aphasia has also been distinguished from Broca's and Wernicke's aphasia by left hemisphere parietal metabolic abnormalities (Metter et al. 1989). In addition, there are reports of lesions compromising deep structures (Palumbo et al. 1992). The two lesion sites most often associated with conduction aphasia are (1) the left hemisphere supramarginal gyrus and the arcuate fasciculus, and (2) the insula, contiguous auditory cortex, and underlying white matter of the left hemisphere. Disruption in Wernicke's area has produced conduction aphasia (Anderson et al. 1999), but when Wernicke's area is involved the lesion size appears smaller than that associated with Wernicke's aphasia. However, conduction aphasia is not a "mild" form of Wernicke's aphasia; rather, the more anterior and inferior lesions (i.e., anterior supramarginal gyrus, underlying white matter, angular gyrus, and insular cortex) are deemed responsible for the phonologic output problems in conduction aphasia, whereas overlap into Wernicke's area would account

Table 10–1. Comparison of Characteristics of Broca's Aphasia and Apraxia of Speech with Conduction Aphasia

Broca's Aphasia/Apraxia of Speech	Conduction Aphasia
Nonfluent	Fluent
Dysprosody	Intact prosody (with self-corrections and word search)
Agrammatic	Preserved grammar or paragrammatic
Comprehension relatively good	Comprehension relatively good
Repetition impaired proportionate to other verbal tasks	Repetition disproportionately impaired
Error recognition	Error recognition
Probably anomic	Probably anomic

for auditory and lexical/semantic problems (Palumbo et al., 1992).

Disconnection Model

Wernicke's original hypothesis described conduction aphasia as a disconnection between the auditory "comprehension" region (Wernicke's area) and the speech "production" region (Broca's area). Based on traditional conceptions, the arcuate fasciculus has been deemed the probable site of damage for conduction aphasia (Geschwind, 1965). This fiber tract connects Wernicke's area in the left temporal lobe with Broca's area in the left frontal lobe. An interruption in these connecting fibers might inhibit information received in an intact Wernicke's area from being transported anteriorly to an intact Broca's area. The sparing of Wernicke's and Broca's areas would account for relatively intact auditory comprehension and fluent, melodic speech production. On the other hand, the disconnection of these centers would result in a disproportionate impairment in activities requiring the interaction of audition and production, such as verbal repetition.

Based on brain imaging studies, many have challenged the rigid disconnection model of conduction aphasia. For example, some advocate an expansion of the disconnection model to include any interruption in circuits linking language comprehension and speech production (Mendez & Benson, 1985). Others discount the disconnection

model based on metabolic studies of brain function (Metter et al. 1989).

The Bimodal Distribution Model

A variation on the disconnection model is found in the "bimodal distribution model" of conduction aphasia. This model suggests that conduction aphasia results from damage along a continuum extending from Wernicke's area to Broca's area (Kempler et al., 1988; Kertesz et al., 1977). Researchers have reported variability in the degree of fluency with the less fluent patients exhibiting more anterior lesions; those with higher fluency scores had more posterior lesions (Kertesz et al. 1977). Perhaps the clinical picture in conduction aphasia might shift toward that of Broca's aphasia or that of Wernicke's aphasia depending on the lesion locus.

The "Two" Conduction Aphasias

Most recent conceptions of conduction aphasia suggest that the label has actually been applied to two disorders with distinct pathophysiologic mechanisms (Gandour et al., 1991; Nadeau, 2001). One form, called *repetition conduction aphasia*, refers to a deficit in auditory short-term memory and is characterized by a disturbance only of verbal repetition tasks. The other form of conduction aphasia, labeled *reproduction conduction aphasia*, describes a more general language impairment affecting phonologic output processes. Individuals with reproduction conduction aphasia demonstrate deficits in word production across verbal tasks including conversation, naming, and oral reading, as well as repetition (Nadeau, 2001). Possibly the repetition and reproduction difficulties arise from lesions in functionally distinct but anatomically adjacent areas in the temporoparietal region (Gandour et al., 1991).

Nature and Differentiating Features

The definition of conduction aphasia ascribed to in this chapter conforms with descriptions of *reproduction conduction aphasia*. Thus, our definition of conduction aphasia denotes an individual who speaks with good intonation and generally understands what others say, but has trouble retrieving words. Paraphasic errors are produced (primarily phonemic paraphasias), which the individual recognizes and tries, though often abortively, to correct. Although the hesitations and correction efforts might mimic nonfluent disorders, the runs of fluency, preserved melody, and variety and complexity of syntactic structures found in the spontaneous speech of conduction aphasia distinguish it from Broca's aphasia and apraxia of speech. Also, the use of filler words with relatively few substantive words sometimes distinguishes these patients from those with Broca's aphasia (Benson et al. 1973). Relative preservation of auditory comprehension assists in distinguishing this disorder from Wernicke's aphasia, and the marked repetition deficit is a cardinal feature differentiating conduction aphasia from transcortical problems. Reading and writing problems appear to vary from patient to patient.

The primary criteria for diagnosis of conduction aphasia have been delineated as follows:

1. Fluent, paraphasic conversational speech
2. No significant difficulty in comprehension of normal conversation
3. Significant verbal repetition disturbance
4. A preponderance of phonemic paraphasias

Further Description of Salient Characteristics

FLUENCY

The term *fluent aphasia* has been used to describe easy, plentiful output (100 to 200 words per minute), good articulation, normal phrase length (averaging five to eight words per phrase), and normal melody, with particular difficulty on the "content" words, and, in some cases, paraphasic errors (Benson, 1993). Although conduction aphasia is considered one of the fluent aphasias, hesitations and self-correction attempts interrupt the flow of otherwise fluent speech. Thus, the output is best described as fluent but not quite as fluent as that of Wernicke's aphasia.

WORD FINDING

Difficulty in word retrieval is considered a prevalent aspect of the disorder with problems primarily on content words. Word-finding failures result in paraphasic substitutions, hesitations to access words, circumlocution, or empty speech in which content words are deleted. Interestingly, Kertesz (1979) has reported that some individuals with conduction aphasia do quite well on naming tests, suggesting variability across patients.

PARAPHASIAS

Phonemic paraphasias predominate in conduction aphasia. In fact, Kohn (1992) considers the production of phonemic paraphasias across verbal tasks to be the cardinal feature of conduction aphasia. Semantic paraphasias or neologisms occur less frequently in the speech of conduction aphasia than among the other fluent aphasias (Nadeau, 2001). Conduction aphasic speakers tend to produce more paraphasic errors and self-correction attempts on "target-oriented" tasks (those requiring a forced choice of specific target words) than in open-ended tasks or conversation (Ardila & Rosselli, 1993).

Because speech sound errors are a prevalent characteristic of conduction aphasia,

Broca's aphasia, and apraxia of speech, the nature of the errors has been studied to aid in differential diagnosis and to clarify underlying mechanisms contributing to errors. Although controversy continues, evidence suggests that the errors in conduction aphasia are a product of phonologic or linguistic deficit, whereas the errors in apraxia of speech and Broca's aphasia are related to faulty programming of articulatory movement (Clark & Robin, 1998; Nadeau, 2001; Seddoh et al. 1996). That is, errors in conduction aphasia seem to be attributable primarily to a linguistic or phonologic processing deficit, whereas Broca's aphasic patients evidence phonologic and phonetic deficits (see Nadeau, 2001, pp. 529–544, for a review of phonologic errors in aphasia).

Various models have been proposed to explain aphasic deficits. Nadeau (2001) has described a parallel distributed processing (PDP) model to explain errors in conduction aphasia. Also, single- and dual-stage psycholinguistic models of phonologic processing in aphasia have been advanced (Buckingham, 1992; Wilshire, 2002). For example, Wilshire (2002) explains a one-stage model as follows: "When a word is chosen for production, activation is transmitted to the representations of its phonemes, which in turn become activated themselves" (p. 191). In aphasia, faulty activation of these phonemic representations results in incorrect phoneme selection, hence phonologic errors. In two-stage models, phonologic errors might be attributed to a breakdown during retrieval of phonologic information from the lexicon, or during subsequent postlexical processing or reorganization of that information (Kohn & Smith, 1994).

These models provide theoretical distinctions between errors typical of conduction aphasia and errors typical of anterior aphasias (e.g., Broca's). For example, Kohn (1992) attributed errors in conduction aphasia to a disruption that occurs between the storage of phonologic representations in Wernicke's area and the coding of articulatory motor commands or programs in the frontal lobe. Thus, she distinguished the paraphasic errors in conduction aphasia from the articulatory errors of the anterior patients.

Distinctions between phonetic errors in apraxia of speech/Broca's aphasia and phonologic errors in conduction aphasia have been further supported by acoustic and physiologic studies that differentiate apraxic errors as a breakdown in specific aspects of motor control (Clark & Robin, 1998; Nadeau, 2001; Seddoh et al. 1996). Although the phonetic versus phonologic debate might appear to be excessive, the distinction bears considerable relevance to the focus and design of treatment programs. For example, use of linguistic cues versus articulatory cues might be differentially effective depending on the nature of the errors.

ERROR RECOGNITION

Kohn (1984) studied the *"conduite d'approche"* or sequences of self-correction attempts of individuals with aphasia. She found that people with conduction aphasia appear to recognize their errors much more frequently, but are no more successful than individuals with Wernicke's or Broca's in actually correcting the errors. Others suggest self-correction sequences are more successful in conversation than on repetition tasks in conduction aphasia (Buckingham, 1992). Although self-correction in conduction aphasia results in hesitations and what might appear to be nonfluent episodes in the context of otherwise fluent speech, the behavior appears qualitatively different from the struggle, articulatory posturing, and groping behavior of speakers with apraxia of speech.

REPETITION

A discriminating feature of conduction aphasia is the significant impairment in verbal repetition. Because several aphasia types show repetition difficulty, affixing the label of conduction aphasia based solely on faulty repetition would result in many mistaken diagnoses. For this reason, definitions of conduction aphasia invariably include reference to repetition as a "disproportionate" impairment. That is, there is a discrepancy between repetition and spontaneous speech production in conduction aphasia. Conversely, repetition is equivalent to performance on other verbal tasks in apraxia of speech, Broca's aphasia, and Wernicke's aphasia.

Repetition difficulty is most likely to appear on repetition of phrases, short sentences, polysyllabic words, and unfamiliar phrases. Errors tend to increase as the length and unfamiliarity of the material increases. Phonemic paraphasias are most evident on verbal repetition tasks. Errors in repetition are often paraphasic, or a rewording or paraphrase of the target. Interestingly, number repetition might be preserved in conduction aphasia or, if impaired, take the form of word substitutions rather than phonemic paraphasia (Goodglass et al., 2001).

The source of the repetition deficit has been a matter of intense debate. Researchers have postulated a variety of linguistic processing models that identify the "source" of repetition failure in conduction aphasia (Nadeau, 2001). Others have attributed the repetition deficit to an impairment of memory rather than to a more general language deficit (Saffrin & Martin, 1975). In fact, it is likely that the "disproportionate" repetition difficulty represents either an associated problem or different underlying sources in different patients, hence the distinction between pure repetition conduction disorders due to memory deficits and reproduction conduction aphasia associated with linguistic deficit.

Auditory Comprehension

By definition, the comprehension of the individual with conduction aphasia is characterized as near normal. However, clinical experience suggests that patients frequently fail to fit into our neat definitions; thus, it is not unusual to find individuals with conduction aphasia who exhibit impairment in the auditory modality. Such is the case as "jargon aphasia" or Wernicke's aphasia begins to improve in the direction of conduction aphasia. Also, it has been suggested that some individuals with conduction aphasia display

selective difficulty understanding syntax (Heilman & Scholes, 1976).

Reading

There has been controversy as to the exact nature of the reading deficit in conduction aphasia. Although some report good reading comprehension but paraphasic oral reading, others find oral reading to be minimally impaired (Benson et al. 1973; Green & Howes, 1977; Sullivan et al., 1986). Possibly the degree of oral reading and comprehension deficit correlates more with the site and extent of the lesion producing conduction aphasia than with the label of conduction aphasia per se.

Associated Problems

Frequently reported associated problems include oral and limb apraxia, ideomotor apraxia, parietal lobe signs, and right sensory impairment (Benson et al. 1973; Goodglass et al. 2001; Poncet et al., 1987).

Prognosis

Kertesz (1979) reported a favorable spontaneous recovery pattern associated with conduction aphasia. It is probable that patients presenting with conduction aphasia immediately postonset might show significant or even complete recovery (Benson et al. 1973). Other conduction aphasia patients appear to "evolve" from classifications such as "jargon aphasia" or Wernicke's aphasia. The evolved conduction aphasias might be expected to exhibit more residual language deficit.

Barring serious complications, even the patient with residual conduction aphasia frequently becomes a functional communicator. Because of the relatively good auditory comprehension, fairly copious verbal output, and an ability to supplement speech with nonverbal information, these patients tend to function well in situations that do not require single-word accuracy or specific responses. Furthermore, treatment that is appropriately designed and delivered should improve the outcome in such patients.

Evaluation

There are several potential goals of evaluation in conduction aphasia: (1) classification of conduction aphasia, (2) identification of cognitive/linguistic processing deficits, (3) description of communication strengths and weaknesses, (4) discovery of the "life consequences" of aphasia as perceived by those affected, and (5) assistance with intervention planning.

Evaluation of specialized areas can help distinguish conduction aphasia from other aphasia syndromes. Measurement of auditory comprehension, verbal repetition, confrontation naming, and spontaneous speech are considered key areas needed to classify conduction aphasia. Most of the formal aphasia batteries provide data to help identify conduction aphasia. However, supplemental measures are frequently used to gather additional information in these domains. In addition, since symptoms vary across individuals with conduction aphasia (Kohler et al., 1998), evaluation of individual performance helps appropriately plan intervention. For example, treatment might differ for individuals presenting primarily with a phonologic impairment versus individuals presenting with significant semantic level deficits. Neuropsychological processing deficits can be identified with tools designed specifically for this level of assessment such as the Psycholinguistic Assessments of Language Processing in Aphasia (PALPA), a test that is based on a cognitive neuropsychological model of language processing (Kay et al., 1992). Finally, measures that capture functional communication (Frattali et al., 1995), social participation (Simmons-Mackie & Damico, 2001), and quality of life (Holland & Thompson, 1998) provide information on the consequences of the disorder for those affected.

Auditory Comprehension

Because classic conduction aphasia is characterized by relatively good auditory comprehension, additional testing is often required to isolate subtle problems. For example, for-mal tests rarely evaluate syntactic comprehension, yet research suggests the potential for problems in this area (Heilman & Scholes, 1976). Available tests such as the Token Tests (McNeil & Prescott, 1978) and the syntax processing subtest of the Boston Diagnostic Aphasia Examination (BDAE) (Goodglass et al., 2001) or PALPA (Kay et al., 1992) might be useful in this regard. Finally, in cases of mild to moderate aphasia, asking the client to describe problems can be remarkably helpful.

Repetition

Typically, single-word repetition does not provide insight into the repetition deficit in conduction aphasia. Repetition testing should target multisyllable words and sentence length material such as items found on the repetition subtests of the BDAE (Goodglass et al., 2001). In addition, the influence of cues or prompts on repetition performance should be studied to aid in planning treatment. Finally, repetition testing of both words and nonwords provides information about the phonologic system, and might help the clinician tease out the level of deficit (see, for example, Best et al., 2002).

Word Finding

When focusing on word retrieval, the source of paraphasic errors and word-retrieval failures should be considered. As Best and colleagues (2002) noted, "On any model of word production . . . the minimum components necessary for successful word retrieval are semantic and phonologic representations and the links between these" (p. 158). Although conduction aphasia is most often associated with phonologic output problems, it is possible that semantic-level deficits exist also. Knowledge of the level of breakdown can help target treatment appropriately.

The most prevalent form of word-retrieval testing is confrontation naming. Aspects of word finding such as the severity of the deficit, types of words affected, types of errors, strategies used for repair, and potential word-retrieval facilitators should be noted. The Boston Naming Test (Kaplan et al., 2001) provides data on error types and the influence of word frequency and phonemic cues on naming. In addition, spontaneous speech samples might be analyzed for the following word-retrieval behaviors: (1) use of filled or unfilled pause or delay, (2) use of semantically related words or semantic paraphasia, (3) phonemic or literal paraphasia, (4) circumlocution or describing something about the intended words, and (5) using a general or empty word, such as "thing" in place of a target words.

Spontaneous Speech

Sampling spontaneous speech is critical in the evaluation of the individual with conduction aphasia. Spontaneous speech serves as the medium for assessing fluency and as the standard against which to contrast repetition. More importantly observation of natural communication without the constraints imposed in controlled situations allows the clinician to determine the patient's use of strategies and compare communication success to language accuracy. Moreover, sampling various types of connected speech is important in light of research that suggests that these patients perform differently in "open-ended" tasks as opposed to "target oriented" or structured situations. Information can be derived from partially structured tasks, such as picture descriptions, question–answer formats, barrier activities (i.e., describing a picture or object not visible to the listener), narratives (i.e., describing an event), or role playing. In addition, samples of genuine social communication provide data on the types and success of communication strategies used, methods of repair, effects of context, ability to initiate and terminate conversation, and strategies for maintaining the flow of social interaction.

Suitable methods of quantifying the spontaneous speech of individuals with conduction aphasia are numerous. Subjective rating scales such as the Profile of Speech Characteristics from the BDAE, or the fluency and information content scales used on the Western

Aphasia Battery (Kertesz, 1982) can be used independent of the formal test. Ratings of the degree of success in communicating an idea can be used instead of traditional measures of response accuracy. More objective measures might consist of actual frequency counts of specific error types, measures of response speed, or counts of "information units." For example, Nicholas and Brookshire (1993) have devised procedures for quantifying informativeness and efficiency of connected speech and completeness of main concepts.

More comprehensive analysis of connected speech might include analysis of phonemic paraphasias to identify error patterns, or discourse analysis as a means of identifying problems and strengths in spoken or written expression that are not apparent at the sentence level of analysis. Discourse analysis might focus on features such as organization, amount, complexity, efficiency, or cohesiveness of information conveyed. Qualitative methods such as the Conversation Analysis Profile for People with Aphasia (CAPPA) provide tools for analyzing the natural conversation of people with aphasia and their communication partners (Whitworth et al., 1997).

Assessment of natural communication should also focus on the level of enjoyment of communicative exchanges. In other words, clinicians must determine if communication is meeting the social goal of a satisfying human interaction in addition to the communicative goal of exchanging information. For example, clinicians can determine if the communication impairment is getting in the way of participation in society and quality of life from the perspective of the client and his/her significant others (LPAA, 2001). Observations of clients in natural situations allow the clinician to determine potential barriers to communication, and interviews with clients and family members provide insight into their perceptions of life with aphasia (Simmons-Mackie & Damico, 2001).

Treatment

The treatment of conduction aphasia shares the general goals common to the treatment of all individuals with aphasia. Treatment can be designed to (1) stimulate disrupted processes to promote recovery of function and functional reorganization, (2) teach the use of compensatory strategies to communicate in the face of residual deficits, (3) provide education and counseling to assist in living with aphasia, (4) foster self-confidence and positive attitude to promote successful communication and life participation, and (5) build a supportive communication environment.

In meeting one or more of the above goals, three general orientations can be used: (1) restorative approaches, (2) compensatory approaches, and (3) social model approaches to the management of aphasia. Restorative approaches include dynamic, organized treatment programs designed to facilitate restitution, recovery or reorganization of linguistic, and cognitive function. Restoration incorporates the concept of treating underlying processes to restore function toward premorbid levels. Approaches such as stimulation therapy (Duffy & Coelho, 2001) and cognitive neuropsychological therapy (Hillis, 2001) are examples of restorative treatments. Compensatory treatment approaches involve reinforcing or teaching alternative ways of communicating in the face of residual deficits. For example, restorative treatment might be directed at improving the word-retrieval process, whereas a compensatory approach might focus on teaching effective circumlocution to compensate when word retrieval fails. Often a particular treatment task incorporates both restorative and compensatory approaches such as teaching the use of a symbolic gesture to facilitate spoken word retrieval and simultaneously project a meaning in the place of the spoken word. Ultimately the goal of all treatment is to obtain more functional communication and achieve participation in life. Thus, the third orientation, social model approaches, focuses intervention toward achieving satisfying social participation in personally relevant life situations and improved quality of life with aphasia (LPAA, 2001; Simmons-Mackie, 2000, 2001). Social model approaches might include working on relevant aspects of

natural communication (e.g., conversation), removing social and environmental barriers to participating in communicative events, providing supported communication opportunities, and enhancing communicative confidence. In addition, ongoing education, counseling, and dialogue will improve understanding of aphasia by those affected, and increase the clinician's insight into the particular life consequences of aphasia.

Specific Treatment Targets

Verbal Repetition

Unlike the treatment of other aphasia types, therapy for conduction aphasia does not include verbal imitation as a powerful technique in deblocking access to spoken words. Because repetition is a primary deficit, it becomes a target of treatment rather than an approach to treatment. As verbal repetition improves, other behaviors (such as successful self-correction and word retrieval) follow suit.

Focusing therapy on verbal imitation involves (1) determining the level at which repetition begins to deteriorate; (2) determining the influences of such variables as word length, frequency of occurrence, phonemic complexity, and part of speech; and (3) determining what facilitates the client's verbal repetition. For instance, in spite of problems in reading aloud, repetition is frequently facilitated when the written words are provided. Difficulty is altered by varying the length and complexity of words, speaking in unison with the patient, "priming" the system by using the stimulus in other tasks prior to repetition work, enforcing delays (and even "filled" delays) between the spoken word and the patient's response, and varying syntactic complexity. Kohn and colleagues (1990) used sentence repetition as a treatment approach for reducing excessive self-correction behavior during conversation in an individual with conduction aphasia. Sentences were introduced in gradually increasing levels of difficulty to tax the patient's verbal output, and focus attention away from production accuracy. This patient improved in the efficiency of picture description and in the accuracy of sentence repetition. Unfortunately, in some cases, the repetition deficit seems incredibly resistant to our best efforts; in these situations, attention is redirected to more functional areas.

WORD RETRIEVAL

When a semantic level deficit is suspected, activities that provide practice of word retrieval under conditions that facilitate semantic processing (e.g., using word association, high-imagery pictures, written cues, gesture cues) and systematically increase the demand for "independent" word finding should improve the process of retrieving words. That is, if we attribute the source of errors to limited access to the lexicon, then semantic cues might prove most powerful in eliciting target words. Chapter 5 of this volume provides an overview of relevant approaches to word retrieval.

When phonologic-level processing deficits are suspected, treatment focuses on this level. For example, Lesser (1989) advised presenting words in written form or asking patients to visualize written forms to help break the word into phonologically manageable units. Cubelli et al. (1988) focused on "controlling" phonemic production by orienting clients to the phonemic structure of words. Written stimuli were used to build attention to phonemic selection and seriation. For example, clients were asked to match an object to a correct written word in a field with three phonologically similar choices; the therapist then read the client's choice aloud to allow him/her to confirm the accuracy of the choice. The authors also recommended having clients form words from a sequence of written syllables (e.g., "au–then–tic"); then clients read the formed word aloud. This task was made more difficult by increasing the length and complexity of word targets and by including "distracter syllables."

The use of initial phoneme cues to facilitate word finding, a universally popular cuing strategy with aphasia, has mixed results. Initial phoneme cues appear to be more powerful for clients with conduction aphasia than for those with Wernicke's aphasia. However, these cues are usually less powerful for conduction aphasia than they are with the anterior aphasias (Li and Canter, 1987). In fact, phonetic, timing, and facial posture cues are probably more appropriate when errors are articulatory (e.g., apraxic errors) rather than linguistic in nature.

When specific cues prove successful in facilitating communication in treatment, the patient can often learn to use or elaborate on these facilitators as self-cuing strategies. For example, clients who recognize paraphasic errors and compound the errors on repeated self-correction attempts might redirect efforts to finding an associated word ("What do I do with this?") or producing a gestural self-cue. Because additional information is often communicated in the process, the self-cue also serves to augment communication when word retrieval fails. Another strategy suggested for word-retrieval difficulty is self-imposed delay accompanied by relaxation to reduce the "blocking effect" caused by trying too hard (Lesser, 1989).

Although most word-retrieval programs focus at the single-word level, it is important to recognize the need to "find" words within and communicate at the discourse level. Productive circumlocution is an approach to compensate for failure to retrieve specific words in conversation. The purpose is to maintain the flow of conversation while preserving the communicative content. The patient is taught to talk around the inaccessible word purposefully though efficiently, rather than dwell on trying to access it.

Another approach to treatment of word-finding deficits involves improving "divergent" word retrieval (Chapey, 2001). Most traditional word-retrieval programming emphasizes "convergent" naming, that is, accessing a preselected target word, such as naming a pictured object or filling in an incomplete sentence. Divergent tasks are designed to stimulate the ability to provide a variety of alternate words or concepts (e.g., "Name as many foods as possible"). Facilitators, such as visual imagery (e.g., "Imagine walking through the grocery store"), can be provided to expand the behavior. Practice in divergent retrieval assists clients in effectively substituting acceptable alternative words when the target is inaccessible. The concept of divergent processing was applied in response elaboration training (RET), a program designed to build more elaborate conversational content. RET was successful in improving the number of content words conveyed in verbal picture description with an individual with conduction aphasia (Kearns & Scher, 1988). Divergent tasks can also be broadened to approximate the creative requirements of natural communication by providing open-ended topics or questions (e.g., "What do you think about nonsmoking policies in restaurants?").

SENTENCE PRODUCTION

For some clients it is necessary to counter the tendency to talk too much. Sometimes in the barrage of fluent speech, the good gets lost in the bad. Thus, rather than encouraging elaboration, treatment might target production of specific responses such as verbalization of a specific sentence structure using whatever variables assist in production. For instance, the patient might read each word of a sentence, or form a sentence, with the goal of *controlling* fluency, reducing occurrences of nonproductive verbalizations, and avoiding unsuccessful self-corrections. Judicious use of pauses and slow rate inhibit the tendency to launch furiously into verbiage. Instead of using "stop strategies" requiring exclamations of "Slow down," "Think," or other annoying reminders, the clinician encourages pacing or gestural accompaniment as a form of stop strategy. Pointing to each word as it is spoken or using a pacing board to slow the rate allows processing pauses and focuses attention. When the patient successfully formulates structured sentences, the stop strategies can be incorporated into more extended verbalization, such as picture description, answering questions, and conversation. During these activities, awareness that vague responses are as noncommunicative as errors can be fostered; however, it is important that the individual is ready for this type of approach. It would be unwise to inhibit fluency and circumlocutory strategies without a foundation of retrieval potential.

READING AND WRITING

Treating the person with conduction aphasia covers all areas of deficit including reading and writing. These areas are treated within the structure of language therapy, and are also excellent choices for homework and independent computer practice. As in the verbal realm, these activities should focus on success and functionality, not simply accuracy. For example, progress might be measured in terms of the time it takes to comprehend a paragraph or write a note, or the frequency with which the individual performs such behaviors in daily life. Use of computer programs, word processing with spell-check, and electronic mail are excellent graphic tasks. For example, composing or reading e-mail messages provides independent practice in functional graphic skills.

Facilitory Channels

VERBAL CUES

There are numerous types of verbal prompts available to facilitate word retrieval with people with aphasia. For example, word association has been used in a variety of formats, such as phrase completions ("cup of ___"), opposites ("hot and ___"), and semantic association (giving a synonym). One client with conduction aphasia demonstrated improvement in spontaneous speech using semantic contrasts to facilitate sentence production (Roberts & Wertz, 1986). Hierarchical stages were presented beginning with auditory and graphic presentations of a sentence to "prime" the client, followed by verbal imitation of the sentence ("The door is open."), with subsequent production of a contrasted sentence ("The door is closed.").

VISUAL CUES

In spite of reading impairments, graphic cues often prove helpful in strengthening access to desired responses. Initially providing written cues during verbal language tasks, then slowly fading the written cues, seems to help. In fact, improved verbal repetition, fewer paraphasias, and slower rate of speech have been reported when oral reading was used in the treatment of conduction aphasia (Boyle, 1988; Cubelli et al., 1988; Sullivan et al., 1986).

GESTURAL CUES

Gesture has proven to be a useful channel with some conduction aphasia patients. Although these patients often exhibit limb apraxia and may not spontaneously use symbolic or creative gestures, this modality can be strengthened and incorporated into treatment to facilitate word production and augment verbal expression. Initial practice of gestures without encouraging simultaneous verbal responses often reduces useless or empty verbiage. When used to facilitate and augment verbal output, gestures seem to help direct the listener's and the speaker's attention to the specific idea to be communicated. The use of such modalities should be extended to communication partners as well; it is likely that when both parties in an exchange use gesture (or drawing, writing, etc.), then the stigma of such "compensations" is reduced, and the likelihood of generalization is increased.

RHYTHM AND SONG

Melodic intonation therapy or prosodic cuing have not proven particularly useful approaches in improving the verbal expression of the patient with conduction aphasia.

Functional Communication

Because the goal of treatment is to promote communication outside of the structure and support of therapy, attention should be directed at functional, "real-life" communication. Unfortunately, the phrase "functional treatment" is often limited to activities such as ordering in a restaurant, making a grocery list, or paying bills; such tasks fall short of capturing the most widely used form of "functional" communication—social conversation. Therefore, it is imperative that treatment programs seek to understand and remedy problems as they occur in social conversation and individually relevant communication activities. Ultimately, improvement must make a difference in the quality of life as perceived by those affected by aphasia.

Programming realistic activities into treatment can facilitate improved communication in various conditions. For example, clinicians can "coach" clients as they practice activities that are relevant to their own lives as in discussing a television show with a partner, making a phone request, writing a letter to a friend, role playing a problem situation, or relating a humorous incident. The approach called Promoting Aphasic's Communicative Effectiveness (PACE) (Davis & Wilcox, 1985) incorporates rules of natural communication into semistructured treatment and is another means of improving functional communication in conduction aphasia. Incorporating guided experience with social conversation through conversation therapy (Simmons-Mackie, 2000, 2001), group therapy (see Chapter 3), and supported conversation (Kagan, 1998; Kagan & Gailey, 1993) can help build confidence and competence in natural communicative interactions (Pound et al., 2000).

In addition, extending treatment into natural communication settings ensures that changes in communication are meaningful and relevant to the particular individual's life situations. Thus, intervention might include promoting improved communication in the individual with aphasia and ensuring a supportive communication environment, including reducing environmental barriers to participation (Lubinski, 2001), training communication partners (Lyon, 1998; Kagan & Gailey, 1993; Kagan et al., 2001), and providing communicative supports such as pictographic resources, drawings, or written information (Kagan et al. 1996; Lyon,

1994). An excellent example of meaningful social intervention was provided by Booth and Perkins (1999). They observed conversational interactions between a man with aphasia and his brother. They noted that the brother often corrected the client's phonemic paraphasias, even though the intent was clearly communicated. The effect was to halt the flow of conversation and change the interaction from a peer relationship to a "teacher–student" relationship. This type of discourse style not only disrupted the social interaction, but also could undermine communicative confidence. Therefore, intervention focused on building more effective repair strategies within the dyad and teaching the brother that communicating the intent is generally more important than "perfect" productions. Thus, intervention provided a meaningful change in daily communicative life for this dyad. Such approaches that focus on promoting efficient and enjoyable communication are particularly relevant for people with conduction aphasia who are often able to communicate successfully in spite of vague productions or paraphasic errors.

Conclusion

This chapter has identified characteristics of conduction aphasia and discussed the difficult but rewarding job of client management. However, no single chapter can possibly encapsulate every aspect of evaluation and treatment. In treating individuals with conduction aphasia, it becomes readily apparent that there are as many variations in approaches as there are people with conduction aphasia and clinicians. However, there are many things that are successful with other types of aphasia, such as extensive auditory work with Wernicke's aphasia or syntax production programs with Broca's aphasia, that seem less useful with conduction aphasia. This chapter simply narrowed the field of therapy choices a bit without providing the proverbial cookbook. Perhaps in aphasia treatment "knowledge is power"; the more we know about the disorder and

how others handle it, the less time we need to spend sifting through the ever-growing bag of aphasia therapy tricks. Thus, treatment that integrates a knowledge of prognostic variables, an understanding of aphasia treatment principles, a grasp of theory, and a familiarity with relevant research into a caring, sensitive, and creative mixture assures the person with conduction aphasia of getting the most out of treatment.

References

Anderson, J., Gilmore, R., Roper, S., Crosson, B., Bauer, M., Nadeau, S., et al. (1999). Conduction Aphasia and the Arcuate Fasciculus: A Reexamination of the Wernicke-Geschwind Model. *Brain and Language, 70,* 1–12.

Ardila, A. & Rosselli, M. (1993). Language Deviations in Aphasia: A Frequency Analysis. *Brain and Language, 44,* 165–180.

Axer, H., Keyserlingk A., Berks, G. & Keyseringk, D. (2001). Supra- and Infrasylvian Conduction Aphasia. *Brain and Language, 76,* 317–331.

Benson, F. (1993). Aphasia. In: K. Heilman & E. Valenstein (Eds.), *Clinical Neuropsychology* (3rd ed., pp. 17–47). New York: Oxford University Press.

Benson, F., Sheremata, W., Bouchard, R., Segarra, Price, D. & Geschwind, N. (1973). Conduction Aphasia: A Clinicopathological Study. *Archives of Neurology, 28,* 339–346.

Best, W., Herbert, R., Hickin, J., Osborne, F. & Howard, D. (2002). Phonological and Orthographic Facilitation of Word-Retrieval in Aphasia: Immediate and Delayed Effects. *Aphasiology, 16,* 151–168.

Booth, S. & Perkins, L. (1999). The Use of Conversation Analysis to Guide Individualized Advice to Carers and Evaluate Change in Aphasia: A Case Study. *Aphasiology, 13,* 283–303.

Boyle, M. (1988). Reducing Phonemic Paraphasias in the Connected Speech of a Conduction Aphasic Subject. In: T. Prescott (Ed.), *Clinical Aphasiology* (pp. 379–394). Boston: College-Hill.

Buckingham, H. (1992). Phonological Production Deficits in Conduction Aphasia. In: S. Kohn (Ed.), *Conduction Aphasia* (pp. 77–116). Hillsdale, NJ: Lawrence Erlbaum.

Chapey, R. (2001). Cognitive Stimulation: Stimulation of Recognition/Comprehension, Memory and Convergent, Divergent, and Evaluative Thinking. In: R. Chapey (Ed.), *Language Intervention Strategies in Aphasia and related Neurogenic Communication Disorders* (4th ed., pp. 397–434). Philadelphia: Lippincott Williams & Wilkins.

Clark, H. & Robin, R. (1998). Generalized Motor Programme and Parameterization Accuracy in Apraxia of Speech and Conduction Aphasia. *Aphasiology, 12,* 699–713.

Cubelli, R., Foresti, A. & Consolini, T. (1988). Reeducation Strategies in Conduction Aphasia. *Journal of Communication Disorders, 21,* 239–249.

Davis, G. & Wilcox, J. (1985). *Adult Aphasia Rehabilitation: Applied Pragmatics*. San Diego: College Hill.

deBleser, R., Cubelli, R. & Luzzatti, C. (1993). Conduction Aphasia, Misrepresentations, and Word Representations. *Brain and Language, 45*, 475–494.

Duffy, J. & Coelho, C. (2001). Schuell's Stimulation Approach to Rehabilitation. In: R. Chapey (Ed.), *Language Intervention Strategies in Aphasia and related Neurogenic Communication Disorders* (4th ed., pp. 341–382). Philadelphia: Lippincott Williams & Wilkins.

Frattali, C., Thompson, C., Holland, A., Wohl, C. & Ferketic, M. (1995). *The American Speech-Language-Hearing Association Functional Assessment of Communication Skills for Adults (ASHA FACS)*. Rockville, MD: American Speech-Language-Hearing Association.

Gandour, J., Marshall, R., Kim, S. & Neuberger, S. (1991). On the Nature of Conduction Aphasia: A Longitudinal Case Study. *Aphasiology, 5*, 291–306.

Geschwind, N. (1965). Disconnexion Syndromes in Animals and Man. *Brain, 88*, 585–644.

Goodglass, H., Kaplan, E. & Barresi, B. (2001). *The Assessment of Aphasia and Related Disorders* (3rd ed). Baltimore: Lippincott Williams & Wilkins.

Green, E. & Howes, D. (1977). The Nature of Conduction Aphasia: A Study of Anatomic and Clinical Features and Underlying Mechanisms. In: H. Whitaker & H. Whitaker (Eds.), *Studies in Neurolinguistics* (vol. 3, pp. 123–156). New York: Academic Press.

Heilman, K. & Scholes, R. (1976). The Nature of Comprehension Errors in Broca's, Conduction and Wernicke's Aphasics. *Cortex, 12*, 258–265.

Henderson, V. (1992). Early Concepts of Conduction Aphasia. S. Kohn (Ed.), *Conduction Aphasia* (pp. 22–38). Hillsdale, NJ: Lawrence Erlbaum.

Hillis, A. (2001). Cognitive Neuropsychological Approaches to Rehabilitation of Language Disorders. In: R. Chapey (Ed.), *Language Intervention Strategies in Aphasia and related Neurogenic Communication Disorders* (4th ed., pp. 513–523). Philadelphia: Lippincott Williams & Wilkins.

Holland, A. & Thompson, C. (1998). Outcomes Measurement in Aphasia. In: C. Frattali (Ed.), *Measuring Outcomes in Speech-Language Pathology* (pp. 245–266). New York: Thieme.

Kagan, A. (1998). Supported Conversation for Adults with Aphasia: Methods and Resources for Training Conversation Partners. *Aphasiology, 12*, 816–830.

Kagan, A., Black, S., Duchan, J., Simmons-Mackie, N. & Square, P. (2001). Training Volunteers as Conversation Partners Using "Supported Conversation for Adults with Aphasia" (SCA): A Controlled Trial. *Journal of Speech, Language and Hearing Research, 44*, 624–638.

Kagan, A. & Gailey, G. (1993). Functional Is Not Enough: Training Conversation Partners in Aphasia. In: A. Holland & M. Forbes (Eds.), *Aphasia Treatment: World Perspectives* (pp. 199–226). San Diego, CA: Singular.

Kagan, A., Winckel, J. & Shumway, E. (1996). *Pictographic Communication Resources*. North York, Canada: Pat Arato Aphasia Centre.

Kaplan, E., Goodglass, H. & Weintraub, S. (2001). *Boston Naming Test*. Baltimore: Lippincott Williams & Wilkins.

Kay, J., Lesser, R. & Coltheart, M. (1992). *Psycholinguistic Assessments of Language Processing in Aphasia (PALPA)*. London, UK: Psychology Press.

Kearns, K. & Scher, G. (1988). The Generalization of Response Elaboration Training. In: T. Prescott (Ed.), *Clinical Aphasiology Conference Proceedings* (vol. 18, pp. 223–246). Boston: College-Hill.

Kempler, D., Metter, J., Jackson, C., Hanson, W., Riege, W., Mazziotta, J., Phelps, M. (1988). Disconnection and Cerebral Metabolism: A Case of Conduction Aphasia. *Archives of Neurology, 45*, 275–279.

Kertesz, A. (1979). *Aphasia and Associated Disorders*. New York: Grune & Stratton.

Kertesz, A. (1982). *The Western Aphasia Battery*. New York: Grune & Stratton.

Kertesz, A., Lesk, D. & McCabe, P. (1977). Isotope Localization of Infarcts in Aphasia. *Archives of Neurology, 34*, 590–601.

Kohler, K., Bartels, C., Herrmann, M., Dittmann, J. & Wallesch, C. (1998). Conduction Aphasia—11 Classic Cases. *Aphasiology, 12*, 865–884.

Kohn, S. (1984). The Nature of Phonological Disorder in Conduction Aphasia. *Brain and Language, 23*, 97–115.

Kohn, S. (1992). Conclusions: Toward a Working Definition of Conduction Aphasia. In: S. Kohn (Ed.), *Conduction Aphasia* (pp. 151–156). Hillsdale, NJ: Lawrence Erlbaum.

Kohn, S. & Smith, K. (1994). Distinction Between Two Phonological Output Deficits. *Applied Psycholinguistics, 15*, 75–95.

Kohn, S., Smith, K. & Arsenault, J. (1990). The Remediation of Conduction Aphasia Via Sentence Repetition: A Case Study. *British Journal of Disorders of Communication, 25*, 45.

Lesser, R. (1989). Some Issues in Neuropsychological Rehabilitation of Anomia. In: X. Seron & G. DeLoche (Eds.), *Cognitive Approaches to Neuropsychological Rehabilitation* (pp. 65–104). Hillsdale, NJ: Lawrence Erlbaum.

Li, E. & Canter, G. (1987). An Investigation of Luria's Hypothesis on Prompting in Aphasic Naming Disturbances. *Journal of Communication Disorders, 20*, 469–475.

Lichtheim, L. (1885). On Aphasia. *Brain, 7*, 433–484.

LPAA Project Group. (2001). Life Participation Approach to Aphasia. In: R. Chapey (Ed.), *Language Intervention Strategies in Aphasia and Related Neurogenic Communication Disorders* (4th ed., pp. 235–245). Philadelphia: Lippincott Williams & Wilkins.

Lubinski, R. (2001). Environmental Systems Approach in Adult Aphasia. In: R. Chapey (Ed.), *Language Intervention Strategies in Aphasia and related Neurogenic Communication Disorders* (4th ed., pp. 269–296). Philadelphia: Lippincott Williams & Wilkins.

Lyon, J.G. (1994). Drawing: Its Value as a Communication Aid for Adults with Aphasia. *Aphasiology, 9*, 33–50.

Lyon, J.G. (1998). Treating Real-Life Functionality in a Couple Coping with Severe Aphasia. In: N. Helm-Estabrooks & A. Holland (Eds.), *Approaches to the Treatment of Aphasia* (pp. 203–239). San Diego: Singular.

McNeil, M. & Prescott, T. (1978). *The Revised Token Test*. Baltimore: University Park Press.

Mendez, M. & Benson, F. (1985). Atypical Conduction Aphasia: A Disconnection Syndrome. *Archives of Neurology, 42*, 886–891.

Metter, E., Kempler, D., Jackson, C., Hanson, W., Mazziotta, J. & Phelps, M. (1989). Cerebral Glucose Metabolism in Wernicke's, Broca's and Conduction Aphasia. *Archives of Neurology, 46*, 27–34.

Nadeau, S. (2001). Phonology: A Review and Proposals from a Connectionist Perspective. *Brain and Language, 79*, 511–579.

Nicholas, L. & Brookshire, R. (1993). A System for Quantifying the Informativeness and Efficiency of the Connected Speech of Adults with Aphasia. *Journal of Speech and Hearing Research, 36*, 338–350.

Palumbo, C., Alexander, M. & Naeser, M. (1992). CT Scan Lesion Sites Associated with Conduction Aphasia. In: S. Kohn (Ed.), *Conduction Aphasia* (pp. 51–75). Hillsdale, NJ: Lawrence Erlbaum.

Poncet, M., Habib, M. & Robillard, A. (1987). Deep Left Parietal Lobe Syndrome: Conduction Aphasia and Other Neurobehavioral Disorders Due to a Small Subcortical Lesion. *Journal of Neurology, Neurosurgery and Psychiatry, 50*, 709–713.

Pound, C., Parr, S., Lindsay, J. & Woolf, C. (2000). *Beyond Aphasia: Therapies for Living with Communication Disability.* Bicester, UK: Speechmark.

Roberts, J. & Wertz, R. (1986). A Contrastive Language Treatment for Aphasic Adults. In: R. Brookshire (Ed.), *Clinical Aphasiology Conference Proceedings* (pp. 207–212). Minneapolis: BRK.

Saffrin, E. & Martin, O. (1975). Immediate Memory for Word Lists and Sentences in a Patient with Deficient Auditory Short-Term Memory. *Brain and Language, 2*, 420–433.

Seddoh, S., Robin, D., Sim, H., Hageman, C., Moon, J. & Folkins, J. (1996). Speech Timing in Apraxia of Speech Versus Conduction Aphasia. *Journal of Speech and Hearing Research, 39*, 590–603.

Simmons-Mackie, N. (2000). Social Approaches to the Management of Aphasia. In: L. Worrall & C. Frattali (Eds.), *Neurogenic Communication Disorders: A Functional Approach.* New York: Thieme.

Simmons-Mackie, N. (2001). Social Approaches to Aphasia Intervention. In: R. Chapey (Ed.), *Language Intervention Strategies in Aphasia and related Neurogenic Communication Disorders* (pp. 246–268). Philadelphia: Lippincott Williams & Wilkins.

Simmons-Mackie, N. & Damico, J.S. (2001). Intervention Outcomes: Clinical Application of Qualitative Methods. *Topics in Language Disorders, 21*, 21–36.

Sullivan, M., Fisher, B. & Marshall, R. (1986). Treating the Repetition Deficit in Conduction Aphasia. In: R. Brookshire (Ed.), *Clinical Aphasiology Conference Proceedings* (pp. 172–180). Minneapolis: BRK.

Wernicke, C. (1977). The Aphasia Symptom Complex: A Psychological Study on an Anatomic Basis, 1874. In: G. Eggert (trans.), *Wernicke's Works on Aphasia: A Sourcebook and Review* (pp. 91–145). The Hague: Mouton.

Whitworth, A., Perkins, L. & Lesser, R. (1997). *Conversation Analysis Profile for People with Aphasia.* London: Whurr.

Wilshire, C. (2002). Where Do Aphasic Phonological Errors Come from? Evidence from Phoneme Movement Errors in Picture Naming. *Aphasiology, 16*, 169–197.

11

The Transcortical Aphasias

ANN MARIE CIMINO-KNIGHT,
AMBER L. HOLLINGSWORTH, AND
LESLIE J. GONZALEZ ROTHI

Wernicke (1874) proposed that thought and language are distinct functions represented in separate anatomic brain locations. In addition, Wernicke delineated two distinct language functions that he also suggested were supported by separate anatomic regions in the left hemisphere. Specifically, he identified an "auditivo-verbal" center located in the first temporal convolution of the left hemisphere that contained the "stored memory images of auditory sensations corresponding to the audition of spoken language," and a "verbo-motor" center in the third frontal convolution of the left hemisphere that contained the "stored memory images of the sensations of movement corresponding to the production of articulated language" (Lecours et al., 1983). Wernicke also suggested a connection between these two centers and suggested there were three aphasia syndromes that reflected damage to each of the centers or the fibers that connect the centers. Lichtheim (1885) was the first to comment that Wernicke's model of language processing in the brain did not account for aphasia in which repetition was spared. He postulated that aphasias with spared repetition resulted not from a destruction of language centers ("central aphasias") but from a disconnection of the language centers and concept centers ("peripheral commissural aphasias"). Wernicke (1908) coined the term *transcortical aphasia* to refer to apha-

sia with spared repetition, with *transcortical motor aphasia* referring to a dissociation of language and "motivation" and *transcortical sensory aphasia* referring to a dissociation of language and "concepts." Goldstein (1948) referred to mixed transcortical aphasia as "isolation of speech." Transcortical motor aphasia is characterized as a nonfluent aphasia with relatively spared comprehension and spared repetition, transcortical sensory aphasia as a fluent aphasia with impaired comprehension and relatively spared repetition, and mixed transcortical aphasia as a nonfluent aphasia with impaired comprehension and relatively spared repetition. Study of these transcortical syndromes reveals anatomically and possibly psychologically distinct clinical syndromes.

Pathophysiology

Transcortical Motor Aphasia

Transcortical motor aphasia can be explained as either incomplete destruction of the cortical speech center, which is enough to impair spontaneous speech but not enough to impair repetition because spontaneous speech and repetition require differing levels of cortical excitability (Bastian, 1897), or spared repetition in the context of aphasia that represents the contribution of the right hemisphere in cases of left hemisphere damage (Mayendorf, 1911, as reported by Rubens and Kertesz, 1983). This notion of right hemisphere support of spared repetition in the context of aphasia has been expanded to all forms of transcortical aphasia (Berthier et al., 1991, 1997).

In a study using single photon emission computed tomography (SPECT), Berthier et al. (1997) examined the left perisylvian language cortex in patients with transcortical aphasia with lesions that involved or spared this region of interest. These investigators found that "repetition of words and sentences was preserved in spite of significant decrements of perfusion in various anatomical components of the language network represented in left perisylvian cortex." This study and others provide evidence that the integrity of left perisylvian cortex is not crucial for repetition of words and phrases, and propose that homologous regions of the right hemisphere may contribute to the mediation of residual aspects of repetition in patients with transcortical aphasia (Botez, 1964; Grossi et al., 1991; Pulvermuller & Schonle, 1993; Trojano et al., 1988).

Goldstein (1948) referred to two syndromes that could be categorized as transcortical motor aphasia. One form is considered "a heightening of the threshold of the motor speech performances," resulting from damage to the motor speech area, and the other is described as "an impairment of the impulse to speak at all," resulting from damage to the frontal lobe. The second form is distinguished by a "lack of any other speech disturbance or mental defect," whereas the first is distinguished by "more or less defects in the motor act of speaking." Goldstein also recognized that both motor speech performance and impulse to speak could be compromised in combination in a single case.

Botez (1960, 1964), Botez and Barbeau (1971), and Botez et al. (1983) suggest that the supplementary motor area (SMA) of the left hemisphere, a portion of premotor cortex, provides the starting mechanism for speech, and destruction of this area yields a lack of speech initiation. Others have hypothesized that the SMA is involved in programming motor subroutines prior to execution, implying that damage prohibits this preprogramming (Roland et al., 1980). For speech, this would mean that lack of speaking in left SMA–lesioned patients did not result from a lack of impulse or intention, but instead from a lack of a motor plan or program to execute.

According to Goldberg (1985), there are two distinct premotor systems, the lateral premotor system in which action generation is linked to the "external context" provided by the sensory systems, and the medial premotor system, which is involved in the "intentional process" whereby internal context influences the elaboration of action. The SMA is included in the medial premotor system, and Goldberg summarizes the role of SMA as mediating limbic influences on primary motor cortex, specifically in regard to intention to act and in preprogramming action prior to its execution. In speech and language, this can be translated so that lesions of the SMA would be anticipated to produce deficits of the intention to speak combined with deficits of preprogramming and planning verbal utterances prior to the act of speaking.

Possibly tying together these seemingly disparate perspectives on the mechanism of transcortical motor aphasia, Stuss and Benson (1986) discuss a continuum of syndrome manifestations that might be related to lesion localization within the left frontal lobe. With respect to transcortical motor aphasia, the structures of interest include medial and dorsal premotor cortex around or including the SMA (Naeser & Hayward, 1978; Rubens, 1975). The potential for variations in the anatomy of frontal lobe involvement and the behavioral variations of transcortical motor aphasia (Freedman et al., 1984) becomes apparent when looking at the vascular system supplying the frontal lobes. Two vessels supplied by the internal carotid artery supply the frontal lobe exclusively. These are the anterior cerebral artery, which supplies the medial portions of the frontal lobe, and the middle cerebral artery, which supplies the dorsolateral convexity of the frontal lobe.

Thus, pathology that might impede blood flow through these vessels selectively would involve the SMA and the lateral convexity of the premotor cortex (Stuss & Benson, 1986). For example, if the frontal lobe lesion affects the middle cerebral artery territory, motor speech deficits become evident. In contrast, with frontal lobe lesions that affect the anterior cerebral artery territory, aspontaneous speech is apparent. Most typically, when lesions are produced by vascular pathology, individuals with transcortical motor aphasia have lesions representing the watershed region between the middle cerebral and anterior cerebral arteries. In addition, significant frontal pathology resulting in transcortical motor aphasia is reported to be seen commonly in trauma (Liu et al., 1991), tumor (Costello et al., 1989), herpetic encephalitis (Brazzelli et al., 1994), and progressive diseases (Kartsounis et al., 1991).

Transcortical Sensory Aphasia

Lichtheim (1885) suggested that verbal information processed by the "auditivo-verbal" center was subsequently processed by the "verbo-motor" center, and he wrote of the association cortices linked to these two centers. Lichtheim described this syndrome as resulting from a disruption of the link between association cortices and language centers. Sparing of the link between the two language centers enables the patient with transcortical sensory aphasia to be able to repeat. Lichtheim called this the sensory version of "peripheral commissural aphasia"; subsequently, it was renamed "transcortical sensory aphasia" by Wernicke (1908).

McCarthy and Warrington (1987) propose a two-route functional model for the repetition of sentences or words. The first system is phonologically based and subserves word repetition, and the second system is semantically based and subserves sentence repetition. In the first system, input is processed into segmental phonologic representations and then converted to the corresponding output representations, allowing for repetition of nonwords as well as words. This system is influenced by stimulus length and is in-

sensitive to part of speech and frequency of words. Repetition errors emanating from reliance on this system include phonologic aberrations of the target. In the second system, access to output phonology is achieved via semantic mediation, but this semantic system cannot process nonwords. This system is sensitive to concreteness and part of speech but not to stimulus length (Caramazza et al., 1983). Repetition errors emanating from reliance on this system include semantic paraphasias. In a third, lexically mediated repetition system, a direct association exists between phonologic representations of the input and output lexicons without semantic mediation (Coslett et al., 1987; Kremin, 1987; Martin & Saffran, 1990). The third system, proposed by Coslett and coworkers (1987), is compatible with the lexical system proposed in Patterson and Shewell's (1987) model. Access to the phonologic addresses of words in the input and output lexicons are linked directly without semantic mediation. This system is influenced by word frequency and is insensitive to word length or concreteness. Repetition errors emanating from reliance on this system include lexicalization of nonwords. Only the semantic route, by accessing the "cognitive" system, allows us to apply meaning to what we hear as well as to produce words meaningfully, and this is the system that appears to be impaired in transcortical sensory aphasia (involving deficits A or B in Figure 11–1). This three-route functional model of repetition is reviewed in Figure 11–1.

Subtypes of transcortical sensory aphasia are predicted by this model. Specifically, Coslett and coworkers (1987) and Berndt et al. (1987) describe cases of transcortical sensory aphasia in which the patients are unable to comprehend what is said via the semantic system but who repeat lexically. Caramazza et al. (1986) report a case of a patient who showed a selective deficit of the acoustic phonologic conversion system who could not repeat nonwords but could repeat words. Caramazza et al. (1983) describe a patient whose performance indicated impairment of the lexical system and sparing of semantic processing. Davis et al. (1978)

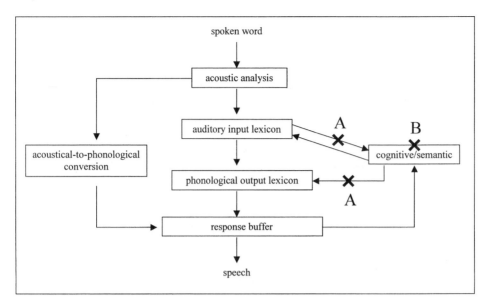

Figure 11–1. A cognitive-linguistic model of repetition.

found that during repetition tasks, patients with transcortical sensory aphasia were less able to recognize and correct semantic errors in the stimuli than were patients with transcortical motor aphasia. Berthier and coworkers (1991) found that within a group of nine patients with transcortical sensory aphasia, six patients corrected syntactic errors but did not correct semantic errors in a sentence repetition task, and all were able to repeat nonwords. In addition, Lesser (1989) as well as Coslett and coworkers (1987) describe transcortical sensory aphasia, in which repetition is accomplished via nonlexical phonologic analysis.

Regarding the anatomic substrate of transcortical sensory aphasia, Henschen (1920) described two associated etiologies: one involved with general cerebral atrophy, and the other with focal lesions. Freedman et al. (1991) have described a progressive disorder "of relatively focal but asymmetric biposterior dysfunction" that yields transcortical sensory aphasia. The mechanism of this disorder is unknown.

In addition, Poeck and Luzzati (1988) and Hodges et al. (1992) described a relatively circumscribed progressive fluent language disorder similar to that seen in transcortical sensory aphasia. Termed semantic dementia by Hodges et al. (1992), Patterson et al. (1993) report unilateral left or bitemporal lobe abnormalities with a "predilection for the temporal pole and the inferior middle, and superior gyri" (p. 65). This anatomy is agreed to by Breedin et al. (1994), but the pathologic mechanism of this disorder also remains unknown.

Kertesz et al. (1982), Hiltbrunner et al. (1987), and Rubens and Kertesz (1983) report that transcortical sensory aphasia from vascular causes is associated with focal lesions of the left inferior parietotemporo-occipital area. Furthermore, Boatman et al. (2000) induced transient transcortical sensory aphasia in six seizure patients by stimulating sites adjacent to Wernicke's area including the posterior superior and middle temporal gyri. The areas described as contributing to transcortical sensory aphasia (Boatman et al., 2000; Hiltbrunner et al., 1987; Kertesz et al., 1982; Rubens & Kertesz, 1983) are supplied by portions of the posterior and middle cerebral arteries or represent a watershed between the posterior cerebral and middle cerebral arteries. However, this localization remains controversial (Feinberg et al. 1986; Rothi & Feinberg, 1989).

Otsuki et al. (1998) and Maeshima et al. (1999) describe a total of three cases of transcortical sensory aphasia from frontal lobe lesions. In the two cases described by Otsuki and colleagues, the patients presented with infarctions of the left inferior frontal gyrus, middle frontal gyrus, and anterior inferior precentral gyrus. In the case described by Maeshima and colleagues, the patient presented with a hemorrhage that damaged the left superior, middle, and inferior frontal gyri but spared the precentral gyrus. Therefore, it seems that, like other types of transcortical aphasia, the symptom complex of transcortical sensory aphasia may occur with lesions in several different locations.

Mixed Transcortical Aphasia

Geschwind et al. (1968), studying a case of mixed transcortical aphasia resulting from carbon monoxide poisoning, anatomically confirm Goldstein's (1948) hypothesis that this syndrome resulted from lesions of association cortex that isolate but spare the left hemisphere perisylvian region, including Wernicke's area, Broca's area, and the connections between. Rubens and Kertesz (1983) report that mixed transcortical aphasia is typically associated with multifocal or diffuse damage to the aforementioned structures. Etiologies include hypoxia from such things as carbon monoxide poisoning, multiple infarctions involving vascular watershed zones, and dementing processes like Pick's disease. Others have reported the rare occurrence of mixed transcortical aphasia in association with cerebrovascular accidents (CVAs) involving the left internal carotid artery (Bogousslavsky et al., 1988), the left middle cerebral artery (Stengel, 1947), and the left anterior cerebral artery (Ross, 1980), although this has been refuted by Bogousslavsky et al. (1988) and Bougousslavsky and Regli (1990).

Rapcsak et al. (1990) reported a case of mixed transcortical aphasia from a left frontal lobe infarction, but SPECT showed "diminished blood flow over the left parietal convexity." Maeshima et al. (1996) reported a case of mixed transcortical aphasia from a left hemisphere lesion, and SPECT revealed "an area of low perfusion involving the entire left hemisphere except for the perisylvian speech areas." These studies along with another case reported by Maeshima et al. (2002), support the notion of "functional isolation" of the left posterior perisylvian language processing regions in mixed transcortical aphasia.

Interestingly, Bando et al. (1986) discuss a patient they labeled transcortical sensory aphasia but that they described as also disinclined to speak, a feature more compatible with mixed transcortical aphasia. In this study, the patient was given a Wada test (named for neurologist John A. Wada). This procedure consists of brief language and memory testing conducted following the injection of an anesthetic into the right or left carotid artery, which results in anesthesia of the corresponding brain hemisphere. This allows for isolated testing of the functions of the non-anesthetized hemisphere. When given a left-sided Wada test, the patient was able to repeat, but when given a right-sided Wada test, the patient could not repeat, suggesting to these authors that the repetition skill in their patient was being mediated by the right hemisphere. The same right hemisphere mechanism of repetition has also been proposed by Berthier and colleagues (1991, 1997) and Ohyama et al. (1996).

Nature and Differentiating Features

Transcortical Motor Aphasia

Transcortical motor aphasia is characterized by nonfluent verbal and written output in the context of spared repetition and comprehension. Verbal output is characterized by a reduction in the quantity, variety, and elaboration of output, a reduction in syntactic complexity, and a lack of motor precision in the execution of verbalizations. Any or all of these features may be present. With intense testing methods, some deficits of auditory comprehension of syntactically complex information may be noted (Rothi & Heilman, 1980); however, typically, auditory comprehension is considered to be spared.

Transcortical motor aphasia is most likely to be confused with Broca's aphasia or the other transcortical aphasias. In cases of transcortical motor aphasia, verbal productions during repetition tasks are far better than production skills during nonrepetition tasks, whereas in Broca's aphasia, this discrepancy is not typically noted. Unlike in transcortical sensory or mixed transcortical aphasia, comprehension skills in transcortical motor aphasia are relatively spared.

Many times in behavioral neurology differential diagnoses are made based on associated symptomatology. Therefore, it is important to know what behaviors are typically associated with transcortical motor aphasia. For patients with superior premotor involvement, associated signs may include transient urinary incontinence, contralateral grasp reflex, rigidity of the upper extremity, and a hemiparesis that involves the left leg more than the arm (Bogousslavsky & Regli, 1990). Initially, patients with supplementary motor area lesions may display mutism that quickly evolves into transcortical motor aphasia. Additionally, they may display bilateral ideomotor apraxia (Watson et al., 1986), akinesia (paucity of movement), or bradykinesia (slowness of movement).

Transcortical Sensory Aphasia

Lecours and Lhermitte (1983) describe transcortical sensory aphasia as including a normal flow of spoken output that is prosodically, phonetically, and phonemically relatively undisturbed but contains numerous verbal and syntactic paraphasias and discourse appears incoherent, circumlocutory, and typically contains a limited number of contentives and a significant number of stereotypic utterances. Naming is severely impaired and numerous word-finding pauses are noted during conversation. During naming failures, these patients are noted to repeat the correct label offered by the clinician without apparent recognition that it is the target. Written productions are qualitatively similar to verbal productions. It should be noted, however, that this deficit of verbal output

is not necessarily absolute. Heilman et al., (1981) describe a case of transcortical sensory aphasia that displayed relative sparing of verbal output in comparison with impaired auditory comprehension. Comprehension of spoken as well as written information is impaired in transcortical sensory aphasia. According to Albert et al. (1981), shifts in the context of verbal interactions make previously meaningful information difficult for the patients with transcortical sensory aphasia to comprehend. Reading aloud and repetition are significantly better than all other language skills, with these patients able to read or repeat long, complex information that they are unable to understand.

Neurologic impairments commonly associated with transcortical sensory aphasia include elements of the Gerstmann syndrome, alexia, constructional apraxia, and ideational apraxia (Albert et al., 1981). Albert et al. (1981) report that hemiparesis or hemisensory loss are rarely noted with transcortical sensory aphasia, whereas Mesulam (1985) reports that they are not uncommon in conjunction with a visual field defect.

Transcortical sensory aphasia is not uncommonly seen as the initial language disturbance of dementia of the Alzheimer's type (Albert et al., 1981; Cummings et al., 1985). This language disturbance evolves with Alzheimer's disease (AD), however, to a more severe language and cognitive disorder. In contrast, progressive transcortical sensory aphasia has been reported that is not associated with AD in which the language disorder (including alexia and agraphia) progresses over time while "other cognitive and behavioral abilities" remain stable (Chiacchio et al., 1993).

Recovery from transcortical sensory aphasia from other etiologies is reported to be quite good. Rubens and Kertesz (1983) report that transcortical sensory aphasia can occur as the result of trauma, but this posttraumatic syndrome is fleeting. Regarding focal ischemic lesions, several possible outcomes are described (Rubens & Kertesz, 1983). Lesions involving temporal cortex may initially result in Wernicke's aphasia that eventually evolves into chronic transcortical sensory aphasia (Kertesz et al., 1979). However, persistent difficulties with repetition in patients with aphasia have been noted to be associated with lesions involving damage to Wernicke's area (Selnes et al., 1985). What allows some but not all patients with Wernicke's aphasia with temporal lesions to evolve to transcortical sensory aphasia remains unclear, although the size of the lesion may be pertinent.

Another version begins with transcortical sensory aphasia with some patients evolving to anomia and possibly to full recovery, whereas others remain persistently aphasic. Kertesz and coworkers (1979) report that cases with this persistent form of transcortical sensory aphasia have parietal involvement. Alexander et al. (1989) noted transcortical sensory aphasia associated with left posterior cerebral artery distribution lesions involving "pathways in the posterior periventricular white matter adjacent to the temporal isthmus, pathways that are probably converging on the inferolateral temporooccipital cortex" (p. 885).

Mixed Transcortical Aphasia

Goldstein (1948) described the syndrome of mixed transcortical aphasia, characterized by severely diminished quantity of spontaneously generated verbal output, very poor auditory comprehension, and relative sparing of repetition, and called it "isolation of speech." In addition, echolalia is frequently associated with this syndrome, with automatic completion of unfinished sentences produced by the examiner (Stengel, 1947). Goldstein described two forms of this syndrome. In one form, the patient has an almost "compulsive" drive to repeat that which he hears when understanding word meaning and intention to repeat (considered to be "nonspeech mental processes") are not present. If these two factors are partially present, the mixed transcortical aphasia is characterized by "intentional repetition" (the second form). Goldstein proposed that the "compulsive repetition" form was probably

related to more extensive brain damage than the "intentional repetition" form. Although patients with mixed transcortical aphasia are noted to correct syntactically incorrect sentences during repetition tasks (Raymer et al., 2002), they are not noted to correct semantically incorrect sentences during repetition (Pirozzolo et al., 1981).

Although these patients are typically able to produce only a limited amount of verbal output and are especially unable to name objects, Heilman et al. (1976) and Nagaratnam and Nagaratnam (2000) report two remarkable cases of mixed transcortical aphasia in which the patients demonstrated all of the typical features of mixed transcortical aphasia but were able to name objects. Although very unusual and not typical of this syndrome, these cases confirm that it is possible to be able to produce object names while not comprehending their meaning. This evidence supports the hypothesis that different neural mechanisms underlie language comprehension and object recognition, and lends additional support to the conclusion of others (Berthier et al., 1991; Ohyama et al., 1996) that intact naming, like repetition, may be mediated by the contralateral hemisphere (Nagaratnam & Nagaratnam, 2000).

This form of transcortical aphasia has been reported to occur from nonfocal (Mehler, 1988; Whitaker, 1976) or multifocal (Bougousslavsky et al., 1988) brain disease or focal pathology specific to the left frontoparietal perisylvian region (Ross, 1980; Speedie et al., 1984). Neurologic signs possibly associated with mixed transcortical aphasia include echopraxia and grasp and suck reflexes (Schneider, 1938; Stengel, 1947).

Evaluation

Transcortical Motor Aphasia

The task of differential diagnosis requires the identification of transcortical motor aphasia in contrast to other forms of aphasia, as stated above. The first task is to establish that there is a difference in performance between spontaneous speech generation and repetition tasks. Speech obtained during repetition should be strikingly better than speech obtained during spontaneous generation. Repetition tasks should compare repetition of stimulus sentences that increase in length from single words to sentences of increasing length and complexity. The words and sentences used for these repetition tasks should also compare words of common usage versus words of infrequent usage and open-class (i.e., articles, prepositions) versus closed-class (i.e., nouns, verbs) words. Patients with transcortical motor aphasia have greater difficulty repeating longer stimuli, especially sentences loaded with closed-class words and infrequent words. To maximize the difficulty with repetition, these linguistic features should be emphasized in the stimuli. Spontaneous speech samples should involve response to questions as well as picture description and procedural discourse (i.e., "Tell me how you make your favorite sandwich"). The clinician should also assess the patient's ability to generate sentence where the clinician provides word pair stimuli that control the number of possible sentences available to the patient. For example, patients with transcortical motor aphasia who are able to produce sentences will have greater difficulty constructing a sentence with stimuli such as "apple and rhythm" than with "bed and sleep." Compatible with this, questions that do not provide information to the patient, such as "What did you have to eat today?" may be answered less completely than questions that provide information to the patient, such as "What kind of sandwich did you have for lunch?" These procedures should be repeated, and the patient should write his/her response.

Relevant errors in verbal productions would include the presence of speech signal distortion (reflecting a motor speech disturbance), echolalia, perseveration, reduction of syntactic complexity, and a lack of verbal elaboration. When a differential in performance on repetition tasks versus spontaneous generation is identified, transcortical aphasia should be suspected. The next task is to differentiate transcortical motor from sensory or mixed aphasias. This is typically accomplished by testing auditory or orthographic comprehension.

Finally, verbal generativity or word fluency, where the patient is asked to name words beginning with a certain letter in 60 seconds, has been reported to be deficient in patients with left frontal damage (Milner, 1964; Thurstone & Thurstone, 1943). Newcombe (1969) suggests that tasks utilizing the generation of words belonging to semantic categories do not show a similar deficit in these patients. Therefore, it would be important to test the verbal generativity of words beginning with specific letters (Benton et al., 1983) if transcortical motor aphasia is suspected.

Transcortical Sensory Aphasia

Transcortical sensory aphasia can be confused with Wernicke's aphasia or multimodal agnosia. Like those with Wernicke's aphasia, patients with transcortical sensory aphasia have deficient auditory comprehension and produce fluent verbal output containing numerous verbal paraphasias. However, performance in patients with Wernicke's aphasia does not improve with repetition tasks, whereas patients with transcortical sensory aphasia have relatively preserved repetition. Like patients with transcortical sensory aphasia, patients with a syndrome combining multimodal associative agnosia (tactile and visual modalities) and anomia (resulting from the same lesion noted above for transcortical sensory aphasia) can repeat but cannot name objects when seen or felt, or point to objects when named. Unlike those with transcortical sensory aphasia, patients with multimodal agnosia utilize auditorily presented information significantly better than information presented via the visual or tactile modality.

As with transcortical motor or mixed aphasia, testing for the presence of transcortical sensory aphasia requires use of a standard language exam that allows comparisons of auditory comprehension, verbal output, and repetition, such as the Boston Diagnostic Aphasia Exam (BDAE) (Goodglass & Kaplan, 1976) or the Western Aphasia Battery (WAB) (Kertesz, 1982). Auditory comprehension testing using these measures allows us to examine the differential between comprehension of words versus comprehension of sentences. Further evaluation of lexical and semantic information about single words is necessary with transcortical sensory aphasia. Using word comprehension testing that is especially sensitive to semantic distinctions is discussed by Martin and Saffran (1990). They describe the Lexical Comprehension Test developed by Saffran and Schwartz in which the examiner says a word and the patient is asked to point to one of four pictures that matches the word. The four pictures are either all unrelated or are all semantically related. Patients with deficient semantic processing confuse semantically related alternatives. In addition, Martin and Saffran describe a second test of the patient's sensitivity to semantic information about words, called the Synonymy Test developed by Saffran and Schwartz. In this test, the examiner says two words that may or may not be synonymous, and the patient is asked to judge whether the two words mean the same thing. A comparison is made between errors on related pairs versus unrelated pairs, with poorer performance on related pairs indicating semantic difficulties.

It is important that we carefully select the stimuli we use on repetition tests to evaluate the integrity of each of the systems reviewed in the Patterson and Schewell model (1987). The mechanism of the patient's spared repetition is especially important to evaluate in transcortical sensory aphasia because performance on this task also allows us to assess the integrity of the lexical system in patients believed to have deficient semantic processing or at least deficient access to semantic information (as tested above). For example, repetition testing should begin with single consonant-vowel-consonant (CVC) words and increase to longer words and word

strings to look at the influence of stimulus length. Pronounceable nonwords compatible in length with other word stimuli should be included on repetition tasks. These factors, as mentioned previously, influence the phonologic conversion system, and sensitivity to these factors may imply reliance on that system. Comparisons should be made between repetition performance using frequent versus infrequent words (sensitivity to which implies reliance on the lexical system) and concrete versus abstract words (sensitivity to which implies reliance on the semantic system). The nature of the errors on all repetition tasks should be noted, the relevance of which has been discussed in the preceding section.

Mixed Transcortical Aphasia

The differential diagnosis of mixed transcortical aphasia requires distinguishing this syndrome from other forms of transcortical aphasia and also from global aphasia. Using either the WAB or the BDAE, the diagnosis of any transcortical aphasia requires establishing that repetition is relatively selectively spared. If this is confirmed, then global aphasia can be ruled out. Depressed verbal fluency ratings indicate that transcortical sensory aphasia can be excluded. Poor auditory comprehension performance excludes transcortical motor aphasia. The same assessment procedures described for lexical comprehension and repetition in transcortical sensory aphasia would provide interesting information about those same skills in mixed transcortical aphasia. In addition, the word fluency and verbal generation measures described for transcortical motor aphasia would also be applicable.

Treatment

Transcortical Motor Aphasia

The prognosis for recovery from transcortical motor aphasia is considered to be good (Alexander & Schmitt, 1980; Geschwind & Kaplan, 1962; Kertesz & McCabe, 1977).

However, much of the literature represents conclusions drawn on single case descriptions or from groups of limited number. In contrast, one study that did not distinguish right- from left-sided anterior watershed lesions [anterior cerebral artery/middle cerebral artery (ACA/MCA)] suggested that 82% of their 22 patients remained "moderately to severely" disabled at discharge (Bougsslavsky & Regli, 1990). The mean discharge date of the group was noted to be 22 days postonset, and this may have been too early to experience the significant recovery seen by other authors. However, most authors noting significant recovery also reported that this recovery occurred early in the postonset course. The prognosis for recovery from transcortical motor aphasia, therefore, remains unclear.

Despite limited information regarding treatment efficacy, several authors have suggested treatment methodologies for transcortical motor aphasia. Restitutive rehabilitative strategies attempt to restore impaired functions, in contrast to substitutive rehabilitation strategies, which attempt to circumvent impaired functions [see Rothi and Horner (1983) and Rothi (1982, 1995) for a review]. Several authors have suggested using restitutive strategies with transcortical motor aphasia. For example, Johnson's (1983) treatment program emphasized remediation of motor function deficits in general and verbal motor skill in particular, which he felt needed to precede "traditional language retraining" methods. Specifically, he targeted those processes that "affected the volitional initiation of motor responses, maintenance of a required motor act, and/or voluntary inhibition or termination of motor acts."

"Conventional speech therapy" procedures were reportedly used by Kools (1983). Self-cuing strategies for naming were specifically emphasized. Lentz et al. (1983) report their attempts to emphasize expansion of the restricted sentence structure in a case with transcortical motor aphasia by capitalizing on spared naming skills. Huntley and Rothi (1988) report their attempts to treat verbal generativity of semantic category membership and spontaneous generation of complete sentences in a case of chronic transcortical motor aphasia. Although the behaviors specifically targeted by each of these treatment studies, reported above, have all responded to the aforementioned intervention strategies at least temporarily, the pervasive communication deficit of verbal aspontaneity in these patients remained relatively uninfluenced.

Less has been attempted using substitutive strategies. Luria and Tsvetkova (1968) and Luria (1977) suggest using a reorganizing technique that allows externally mediated sequencing to assist in the initiation and maintenance of speaking. For example, these authors note that a patient with transcortical motor aphasia may be completely unable to generate a desired sentence on command. However, when objects (unrelated to the words in the target sentence) are placed in front of the patient, equivalent in number to the number of words in the target sentence, and the person is asked to touch each object while saying target words of the sentence, the patient is able to produce more words of the sentence than without the objects to touch (Lebrun, 1995). Alexander and Schmitt (1980) note that this method was unsuccessful in their two subjects, but no further information is provided about their methodology. They conclude that "external rhythmic stimulation," which appears to be a slightly different conception of the strategy described by Luria (1977) "remains a plausible approach" for treating transcortical motor aphasia.

Recently, a case study was reported by Raymer et al. (2002), which described an effective treatment for sentence generation in a patient with transcortical motor aphasia. They describe a treatment method in which they paired nonsymbolic limb movements with the production of sentences. They proposed that because patients with transcortical motor aphasia have nonfluent verbal expression that is related to an inability to initiate and elaborate verbal messages, it might be possible that movements performed with the left hand in left space may engage right frontal mechanisms to enhance verbal initiation (Crosson et al., 2000). Raymer et al. (2002) applied this hypothesis to their treatment design. Sentence generation accuracy for trained and untrained stimuli improved when nonsymbolic movement of the left hand was part of the treatment method. Following treatment, the patient also produced increased numbers of words and sentences in connected speech samples.

Pharmacotherapy has been reported by Albert et al. (1988), who treated a patient with chronic transcortical motor aphasia from a left frontal intracerebral hemorrhage. They gave the patient the drug bromocriptine, a postsynaptic dopamine agonist, and noted improvement in aphasia characterized by decreases in response latency, improved naming, and fewer paraphasias. These improvements were noted to abate when the drug was discontinued. Gupta and Mlcoch (1992) and Bachman and Morgan (1988) reported the positive result of the use of bromocriptine with two cases of transcortical motor aphasia, whereas Sabe et al. (1992) showed positive results in three such cases. In contrast, in two subsequent studies a total of 11 patients with chronic stable transcortical motor aphasia were given bromocriptine with no resulting change in their aphasia (Gupta et al., 1995; Ozeren et al., 1995; Sabe et al., 1995).

Transcortical Sensory Aphasia

Treatment for the communication handicap posed by transcortical sensory aphasia has received no attention in the rehabilitation literature. One problem that may contribute to this lack of studies is that anosognosia is common in this syndrome, and a basic appreciation of the deficit by the patient is a necessary prerequisite to any successful treatment program. In cases in which denial of deficit impedes progress, the focus of treatment might initially be better directed at the denial rather than the aphasia.

Good treatment planning begins with an appreciation and accommodation for the etiology inducing the syndrome. In the case of progressive dementing processes, case management is very different from that for transcortical sensory aphasia resulting from ischemic infarct, and treatment of dementia is not within the purview of this chapter. Regarding vascular etiologies, chronicity and syndrome evolution should be very influential in treatment planning (Rothi & Horner, 1983). For the person who presents initially with transcortical sensory aphasia, treatment planning should be designed to anticipate a probable evolution in which verbal output and auditory comprehension of major lexical items improves. For the patient who evolved to chronic transcortical sensory aphasia from a more severe form of aphasia, the clinician should anticipate persistent deficits, and treatment planning should be designed to compensate for these deficits.

Furthermore, Robinson and Grossman (1997) suggest that rehabilitation should be guided by cognitive models of the brain and that therapeutic strategies "must be connected with physiological processes that represent neural recovery and must capitalize on the biological mechanisms thought to underpin neural recovery." Based on cerebral blood flow during positron emission tomography (PET) in a patient with transcortical aphasia who demonstrated a semantically based lexical retrieval deficit, Robinson and Grossman suggest that "treatment studies should be developed which capitalize on preserved visual and perceptual processing components in order to increase naming ability in patients with semantic impairments." For example, it is suggested that developing treatment strategies that are dependent on visual imagery and the integration of visuoperceptual and semantic information is thought to maximize the participation of spared cerebral areas. It should be noted that these suggested treatment methodologies have not been tested.

Mixed Transcortical Aphasia

Kertesz and McCabe (1977) suggest that although the prognosis for recovery from mixed transcortical aphasia in general is good, mixed transcortical aphasia has a poorer prognosis than the motor or sensory forms. The patients of Geschwind and co-workers (1968) and Heilman and coworkers (1976) remained severely impaired, chronically. Whitaker's (1976) case, due to the nature of her disease ("presenile dementia"), did not recover either. Therefore, the etiologies responsible for mixed transcortical aphasia may contribute to the lack of syndrome evolution to milder forms of language impairment.

Pulvermuller and Schonle (1993) investigated behavioral changes associated with treatment of a chronic case of mixed transcortical aphasia. The treatment paradigm involved encouraging the patient to "perform speech acts by repetition." For example, the clinician would present a sentence/question with two alternative responses and the patient was instructed to select and repeat the alternative that best suited his communication intent. During the therapy, the patient's performance on speech production task improved and reaction time decreased. However, it is not known if improved performance generalized to untrained stimulus items or conversational speech because language testing and functional communication measures were not completed following treatment. Therefore, although this study provides some evidence that chronic patients with mixed transcortical aphasia may benefit from language treatment, further research is needed.

Specific Treatment Tasks

Two studies have outlined methods for treating lexical retrieval in aphasic patients (Greenwald et al., 1995; Wambaugh et al., 2001). In the semantic cuing treatments, naming was facilitated with semantic and visual information about the target picture using verbal descriptions of distinctive features (i.e., camel: "This animal has a hump and a long neck") (Greenwald et al., 1995) and semantically related sentence completion (i.e., duck: "He carved a wooden duck")

(Wambaugh et al., 2001). In the phonologic cuing treatment, naming was facilitated using phonologic models for the first few sounds in the target word (i.e., camel: "It starts with /kæ/") (Greenwald et al., 1995; Wambaugh et al., 2001) or by providing a verbal production of a nonword that rhymed with the target word (i.e., cake: "It rhymes with /zek/") (Wambaugh et al., 2001). All of the subjects studied experienced improved naming abilities as a result of the treatments. Although these strategies were tested in patients with anomic ($n = 3$), conduction ($n = 1$), and Wernicke's ($n = 1$) aphasia, they may be useful in treatment planning for patients with transcortical aphasia with phonologically or semantically based lexical retrieval deficits, as described earlier in this chapter.

Transcortical Motor Aphasia

Although a tested pathway is not yet available, it seems clear that behavioral treatments for transcortical motor aphasia need to emphasize further substitutive strategies, such as those suggested by Luria (1977; Luria & Tsvetkova, 1968). These strategies need to address the mechanisms proposed to account for this disorder. Regarding impairments in the intention to verbalize and in verbal preprogramming, treatment methods such as the externally mediated sequencing or external rhythmic stimulation techniques described above seem justified. Other external mediation strategies for verbal interaction might be considered, such as listing questions to be answered by the person during discourse. Further, if the disruption of verbal intention does result from disconnection of limbic influence on the verbo-motor system, utilization of right hemisphere mediation or emotionally intoned verbal stimuli for treatment tasks may be considered.

Transcortical Sensory Aphasia

At the present time, there has been no study of the efficacy of specific treatment tasks for transcortical sensory aphasia and, therefore, only speculation about treatment programming is possible. The overwhelming contribution to impaired communication in transcortical sensory aphasia is the inability to apply meaning to what is heard or what is said. Rothi and Feinberg (1989) suggest that if lesions A and B of Figure 11–1 truly represent the deficit that accounts for the patient's inability to link meaning to words in transcortical sensory aphasia, treatment programs should address the mechanisms of the deficit. For example, if a particular patient presents a disconnection between the cognitive system and the input plus output lexicons (A in Figure 11–1), treatment should emphasize pairing auditory input with another input modality or verbal output with another output mode. Although reading and writing are typically noted to be impaired in patients with transcortical sensory aphasia, even slight assistance from these and other modalities/modes would be helpful. In contrast, if the patient has a dysfunction of the cognitive system itself (B in Figure 11–1), emphasis should be placed on reconstruction of semantic relationships. The third possibility is that a patient with transcortical sensory aphasia is able to repeat via the sublexical phonologic conversion system but unable to utilize lexical or semantic information. These patients may represent the chronic form resulting from evolution from Wernicke's aphasia. Treatments applicable to Wernicke's aphasia, as reviewed in Chapter 9, might be more applicable in these cases.

Mixed Transcortical Aphasia

In our experience, the occurrence of the syndrome of mixed transcortical aphasia in its most complete and severe form is rare, but milder versions are not uncommon. In those milder cases, the treatment for the verbal deficits described above under transcortical motor aphasia and the treatments for the receptive deficits described above for transcortical sensory aphasia might be relevant. Finally, we pass along a word of caution originally suggested by Alexander and Schmitt (1980) regarding treatment of any person with transcortical aphasia. Treatment programs relying heavily on repetition skill do not produce significant therapeutic result because "they address a function that is preserved and performed almost automatically in these patients." However, those treatment programs that possibly begin with repetition but in which the focus is to move slowly away from the more automatic to the less automatic or intentional may be more likely to address the deficit of transcortical aphasia.

Conclusion

The topic of transcortical aphasias resulting from thalamic/subcortical infarction has not been discussed in this chapter (the interested reader is referred to Crosson, 1992). However, recognition of the occurrence of these syndromes underscores the point of Goldberg (1985) that subcortical and cortical structures are not only structurally but also functionally interconnected, forming systems that are dependent on all the component parts for the functional integrity of the whole. Therefore, lesions of subcortical structures may induce syndromes that in many ways resemble but do not necessarily exactly mimic (Lazzarino et al., 1991; Nagaratnam & Gilhotra, 1998) the cortically induced syndromes. However, it is not just the subcortical/cortical connections that explain the relationship between these syndrome variants. Intracortical connections can possibly explain the relationship within and among syndromes, and in this particular instance the relationships among the major categories of transcortical aphasia.

Pandya (1988; Pandya & Yeterian, 1990), in discussions of the cellular architectonic and connectional organization of the human frontal cortex, reviews the notion that "in the course of evolution, the adaptation of organisms to increasingly complex conditions is reflected in concomitant morphological features of the brain" (Pandya & Yeterian, 1990). From evidence across species and within primates specifically, Pandya and Yeterian review the hypothesis that all cortical regions have evolved from two sources, which they call moieties. Therefore, cortical regions that are widely distributed anatomically may have evolved from a common source. The authors ask two important questions: "Is there some organizational principle that accounts for and interrelates different cytoarchitectonic regions in the frontal lobe?" and "Is there some organizational principle that accounts for and interrelates anatomically distributed portions within cytoarchitectonic regions?" Pandya and Yeterian suggest that from one of these moieties (paleocortical) those cortical systems evolved that process sensory information, whereas from the other moiety (archicortical) those cortical systems evolved that process spatial information. It is the archicortical moiety that is most relevant to the transcortical aphasias as the frontal structures evolving from this moiety include dorsolateral prefrontal cortex, implicated in transcortical motor aphasia. Pandya (1988) points out that this system of connectivity projects back to the medial and central occipitotemporal region, among other structures. This is the same region related to transcortical sensory aphasia and provides a structural suggestion that transcortical sensory and motor aphasias are related by more than symptom similarity.

Heilman (personal communication, 1991) suggests that both syndromes, by virtue of the connectivity of the neural structures involved, may represent differing levels of deficit in the same functional system—activation of the semantic field. Individuals with transcortical sensory aphasia may be those in whom activation of the semantic field is possible only by internally generated stimulation. For patients with transcortical motor aphasia, activation of the semantic field may be possible only by externally generated stimulation (a notion supported by a case of transcortical motor aphasia reported by Gold et al., 1997). The result would yield symptoms characteristic of each of these syndromes.

The transcortical aphasias present both clinical and theoretical challenges. Continued insight will help us meet those challenges.

Acknowledgments

This material is based on work supported by the Veterans Administration (VA) Office of Academic Affairs and the VA Rehabilitation Research and Development Service, Department of Veterans Affairs. This work was also supported by the Department of Communication Sciences and Disorders in the College of Liberal Arts and Sciences, University of Florida.

References

Albert, M.L., Bachman, D., Morgan, A. & Helm-Estabrooks, N. (1988). Pharmacotherapy for Aphasia. *Neurology, 38,* 877–879.

Albert, M.L., Goodglass, H., Helm, N.A., Rubens, A.B. & Alexander, M.P. (1981). *Clinical Aspects of Dysphasia.* New York: Springer-Verlag.

Alexander, M.P., Hiltbrunner, B., Fischer, R.S. (1989). Distributed Anatomy of Transcortical Sensory Aphasia. *Archives of Neurology, 46,* 885–892.

Alexander, M.P. & Schmitt, M.A. (1980). The Aphasia Syndrome of Stroke in the Left Anterior Cerebral Artery Territory. *Archives of Neurology, 37,* 97–100.

Bachman, D.L. & Morgan, A. (1988). The Role of Pharmacotherapy in the Treatment of Aphasia: Preliminary Results. *Aphasiology, 2,* 225–228.

Bando, M., Ugawa, Y. & Sugishita, M. (1986). Mechanism of Repetition in Transcortical Sensory Aphasia. *Journal of Neurological and Neurosurgical Psychiatry, 49,* 200–202.

Bastian, H. (1897). Some Problems in Connection with Aphasia and Other Speech Defects. *Lancet, 1,* 933–942, 1005–1017, 1131–1137, 1187–1194.

Benton, A.L., Hamsher, K., Varney, N.R., Spreen, O. (1983). *Contributions to Neuropsychological Assessment: A Clinical Manual.* New York: Oxford University Press.

Berndt, R.S., Basili, A., Caramazza, A. (1987). Dissociation of Functions in a Case of Transcortical Sensory Aphasia. *Cognitive Neuropsychology, 4,* 79–107.

Berthier, M.L., Posada, A., Puentes, C. & Hinojosa, J. (1997). Brain SPECT Imaging in Transcortical Aphasia: The Functional Status of Left Perisylvian Language Cortex. *European Journal of Neurology, 4,* 551–560.

Berthier, M.L., Starkstein, S.E., Leiguarda, R., Ruiz, A., Mayberg, H.S., Wagner, H., Price, T.R. & Robinson, R.C. (1991). Transcortical Aphasia: Importance of the Nonspeech Dominant Hemisphere in Language Repetition. *Brain, 114,* 1409–1427.

Boatman, D., Gordon, B., Hart, J., Selnes, O., Miglioretti, D. & Lenz, F. (2000). Transcortical Sensory Aphasia: Revised and Revisited. *Brain, 123,* 1634–1642.

Bogousslavsky, J. & Regli, F. (1990) Anterior Cerebral Artery Territory Infarction in the Lausanne Stroke Registry. *Archives of Neurology, 47,* 144–150.

Bogousslavsky, J., Regli, F. & Assal, G. (1988). Acute Transcortical Mixed Aphasia: A Carotid Occlusion Syndrome with Pial and Watershed Infarcts. *Brain, 111,* 631–641.

Botez, M.I. (1960). Clinical Contributions of the Tumoral Frontal Syndrome. *Psychiatria et Neurologia, 140,* 351.

Botez, M.I. (1964). The Starting Mechanism of Speech. *Ldegyogyasati, 1,* 13.

Botez, M.I. & Barbeau, A. (1971). Role of Subcortical Structures and Particularly of the Thalamus, in the Mechanisms of Speech and Language. *International Journal of Neurology, 8,* 300–320.

Botez, M.I., Lecours, A.R. & Berube, L. (1983). Speech and Language in the Frontal Syndrome. In: A.R. Lecours, F. Lhermitte & B. Bryan (Eds.), *Aphasiology* (pp. 124–140). London: Bailliere Tindall.

Brazzelli, M., Colombo, N., Della Sala, S. & Spinnler, H. (1994). Spared and Impaired Cognitive Abilities After Bilateral Frontal Damage. *Cortex, 30,* 27–51.

Breedin, S.D., Saffran, E.M. & Coslett, H.B. (1994). Reversal of the Concreteness Effect in a Patient with Semantic Dementia. *Cognitive Neuropsychology, 11,* 617–660.

Caramazza, A., Berndt, R.S. & Basili, A. (1983). The Selective Impairment of Phonological Processing: A Case Study. *Brain and Language, 18,* 128–174.

Caramazza, A., Miceli, G. & Villa, G. (1986). The Role of the (Output) Phonological Buffer in Reading, Writing and Repetition. *Cognitive Neuropsychology, 3,* 37–76.

Chiacchio, L., Grossi, D., Stanzione, M. & Trojano, L. (1993). Slowly Progressive Aphasia Associated with Surface Dyslexia. *Cortex, 29,* 145–152.

Coslett, H.B., Roeltgen, D.P., Rothi, L.J.G. & Heilman, K.M. (1987). Transcortical Sensory Aphasia: Evidence for Subtypes. *Brain and Language, 32,* 362–378.

Crosson, B. (1992). *Subcortical Functions in Language and Memory.* New York: Guilford.

Crosson, B., Singletary, F., Richards, K.S., Koehler, S.M. & Rothi, L.J.G. (2000). *Use of Nonsymbolic Gestures of the Left Hand to Enhance Word Finding in Nonfluent Aphasia.* Paper presented at the Second National Department of Veterans Affairs Rehabilitation Research and Development Conference. Arlington, Virginia.

Cummings, J.L., Benson, D.F., Hill, M.A. & Reed, A. (1985). Aphasia in Dementia of the Alzheimer's Type. *Neurology, 35,* 394–397.

Davis, L., Foldi, N.S., Gardner, H. & Zurif, E. (1978). Repetition in the Transcortical Aphasias. *Brain and Language, 6,* 996–238.

de Lacy Costello, A. & Warrington, E.K. (1989). Dynamic Aphasia: The Selective Impairment of Verbal Planning. *Cortex, 25,* 103–114.

Feinberg, T.E., Rothi, L.J.G. & Heilman, K.M. (1986). Multimodal Agnosia After Unilateral Left Hemisphere Lesion. *Neurology, 36,* 864–867.

Freedman, L., Selchen, D.H., Black, S.E., Kaplan, R., Garnet, E.S. & Nahmias, C. (1991). Posterior Cortical Dementia with Alexia: Neurobehavioral, MRI, and PET Findings. *Journal of Neurology, Neurosurgery and Psychiatry, 54,* 443–448.

Freedman, M., Alexander, M.P. & Naeser, M.A. (1984). Anatomical Basis of Transcortical Motor Aphasia. *Neurology, 34,* 409–417.

Geschwind, N. & Kaplan, E. (1962). A Human Cerebral Deconnection Syndrome. *Neurology, 12,* 675–685.

Geschwind, N., Quadfasel, F. & Segarra, J. (1968). Isolation of the Speech Area. *Neuropsychologia, 6,* 327–340.

Gold, M., Nadeau, S.E., Jacobs, D.H., Adair, J.C., Rothi, L.J. & Heilman, K.M. (1997) Adynamic Aphasia: A Transcortical Motor Aphasia with Defective Semantic Strategy Formation. *Brain and Language, 57,* 374–393.

Goldberg, G. (1985). Supplementary Motor Area Structure and Function: Review and Hypotheses. *Behavioural Brain Sciences, 8,* 567–616.

Goldstein, K. (1948). *Language and Language Disturbances.* New York: Grune and Stratton.

Goodglass, H., Kaplan, E. (1976). *The Assessment of Aphasia and Related Disorders.* Philadelphia: Lea and Febiger.

Greenwald, M.L., Raymer, A.M., Richardson, M.E. & Rothi, L.J.G. (1995). Contrasting Treatments for Severe Impairments of Picture Naming. *Neuropsychological Rehabilitation, 5,* 17–49.

Grossi, D., Trojano, L., Chiacchio, L., Soricelli, A., Mansi, L., Postiglione, A. & Salvatore, M. (1991). Mixed Transcortical Aphasia: Clinical Feature and Neuroanatomical Correlates. *European Neurology, 31,* 204–211.

Gupta, S., Mlcoch, A.G., Scolaro, C. & Moritz, T. (1995). Bromocriptine Treatment of Nonfluent Aphasia. *Neurology, 45,* 2170–2173.

Gupta, S.R. & Mlcoch, A.G. (1992). Bromocriptine Treatment of Nonfluent Aphasia. *Archives of Physical Medicine and Rehabilitation, 73,* 373–376.

Heilman, K.M., Rothi, L., McFarling, D. & Rottman, A. (1981). Transcortical Sensory Aphasia with Relatively Spared Spontaneous Speech and Naming. *Archives of Neurology, 38,* 236–239.

Heilman, K.M., Tucker, D.M. & Valenstein, E. (1976). A Case of Mixed Transcortical Aphasia with Intact Naming. *Brain, 99,* 415–426.

Henschen, S.E. (1920–1922). *Klinische und Anatomische Beitrage zur Pathologie des Gehirns* (vols. 5–7). Stockholm: Nordiska Bokhandel'n.

Hiltbrunner, B., Alexander, M.P. & Fischer, R.S. (1987). *Transcortical Sensory Aphasia: CT Anatomy and Neuropsychology.* Presented at the annual meeting of the Academy of Aphasia, Phoenix.

Hodges, J.R., Patterson, K., Oxbury, S. & Funnell, E. (1992). Semantic Dementia: Progressive Fluent Aphasia with Temporal Lobe Atrophy. *Brain, 115,* 1783–1806.

Huntley, R.A. & Rothi, L.J.G. (1988). Treatment of Verbal Akinesia in a Case of Transcortical Motor Aphasia. *Aphasiology, 2,* 55–66.

Johnson, M. (1983). Treatment of Transcortical Motor Aphasia. In: W. Perkins (Ed.), *Current Therapy of Communication Disorders.* New York: Thieme-Stratton.

Kartsounis, L.D., Crellin, R.F., Crewes, H. & Toone, B.K. (1991). Primary Progressive Nonfluent Aphasia: A Case Study. *Cortex, 27,* 121–129.

Kertesz, A. (1982). *The Western Aphasia Battery.* New York: Grune and Stratton.

Kertesz, A., Harlock, W. & Coates, R. (1979). Computer Tomographic Localization, Lesion Size, and Prognosis in Aphasia and Nonverbal Impairment. *Brain and Language, 8,* 34–50.

Kertesz, A. & McCabe, P. (1977). Recovery Patterns and Prognosis in Stroke. *Brain, 100,* 1–18.

Kertesz, A., Sheppard, A. & MacKenzie, R. (1982). Localization in Transcortical Sensory Aphasia. *Archives of Neurology, 39,* 475–478.

Kools, J. (1983). Congenital Transcortical Motor Aphasia. In: R. Talbott & V. Larson (Eds.), *Communicative Disorders, 12,* 171–172.

Kremin, H. (1987). Is There More Than Ah-Oh-Oh? Alternative Strategies for Writing and Repeating Lexically. In: M. Coltheart, R. Job & G. Sartori (Eds.), *The Cognitize Neuropsychology of Language* (pp. 295–335). London: Lawrence Erlbaum.

Lazzarino, L.G., Nicolai, A., Valassi, F. & Biasizzo, E. (1991). Language Disturbances from Mesencephalothalamic Infarcts. Identification of Thalamic Nuclei by CT-Reconstructions. *Neuroradiology, 33,* 300–304.

Lebrun, Y. (1995). Luria's Notion of "(Frontal) Dynamic Aphasia." *Aphasiology, 9,* 171–180.

Lecours, A.R. & Lhermitte, F. (1983). Clinical Forms of Aphasia. In: A.R. Lecours, F. Lhermitte & B. Bryans (Eds.), *Aphasiology* (pp. 76–108). London: Bailliere Tindall.

Lecours, A.R., Poncet, M., Ponzio, J. & Ramade-Poncet, M. (1983). Classification of the Aphasias. In: F. Lecours, F. Lhermitte & B. Bryans (Eds.), *Aphasiology.* London: Bailliere Tindall.

Lentz, S., Shubitowski, Y. & Rosenbek, J, et al. (1983). *Treating Spontaneous Speech Production in Transcortical Motor Aphasia.* Presented at the annual meeting of the American Speech and Hearing Association, Cincinnati, OH.

Lesser, R. (1989). Selective Preservation of Oral Spelling without Semantics in a Case of Multi-Infarct Dementia. *Cortex, 25,* 239–250.

Lichtheim, L. (1885). On Aphasia. *Brain, 7,* 433–484.

Liu, G.T., Moore, M.R. & Goldman, H. (1991). Transcortical Motor Aphasia Due to a Subdural Hematoma. *American Journal of Emergency Medicine, 9,* 620–622.

Luria, A.R. (1977). *Neuropsychological Studies in Aphasia.* Amsterdam: Swets and Zeitlinger BV.

Luria, A.R. & Tsvetkova, L.S. (1968). The Mechanisms of Dynamic Aphasia. In: *Foundations of Language* (vol. 4). Amsterdam.

Maeshima, S., Kuwata, T., Masuo, O., Yamaga, H., Okita, R., Ozaki, F., Moriwaki, H. & Roger, P. (1999). Transcortical Sensory Aphasia Due to Left Frontal Subcortical Hemorrhage. *Brain Injury, 13,* 927–933.

Maeshima, S., Toshiro, H., Sekiguchi, E., Okita, R., Yamaga, H., Ozaki, F., Moriwaki, H., Matsumoto, T., Ueyoshi, A. & Roger, P. (2002). Transcortical Mixed Aphasia Due to Cerebral Infarction in the Left Inferior Frontal Lobe and Temporoparietal Lobe. *Neuroradiology, 44,* 133–137.

Maeshima, S., Uematsu, Y., Terada, T., Nakai, K., Itakura, T. & Komai, N. (1996). Transcortical Mixed Aphasia with Left Frontoparietal Lesions. *Neuroradiology, 38,* S78–S79.

Martin, N. & Saffran, E.M. (1990). Repetition and Verbal STM in Transcortical Sensory Aphasia. *Brain and Language, 39,* 254–288.

McCarthy, R.A. & Warrington, E.K. (1987). The Double Dissociation of Short-Term Memory for Lists and Sentences. *Brain, 110,* 1545–1563.

Mehler, M.F. (1988). Mixed Transcortical Aphasia in Non-familial Dysphasic Dementia. *Cortex, 24,* 545–554.

Mesulam, M.M. (1985) *Principles of Behavioral Neurology.* Philadelphia: F.A. Davis.

Milner, B. (1964). Some Effects of Frontal Lobectomy in Man. In: J.M. Warren & K. Akert (Eds.), *Frontal Granular Cortex and Behavior* (pp. 313–334). New York: McGraw-Hill.

Naeser, M.A. & Hayward, R.W. (1978). Lesion Localization in Aphasia with Cranial Computed Tomography and the Boston Diagnostic Aphasia Exam. *Neurology, 28,* 545–551.

Nagaratnam, N. & Gilhotra, J.S. (1998). Acute Mixed Transcortical Aphasia Following an Infarction in the Left Putamen. *Aphasiology, 12,* 489–493.

Nagaratnam, N. & Nagaratnam, K. (2000). Acute Mixed Transcortical Aphasia with Bihemispheric Neurological Deficits Following Diffuse Cerebral Dysfunction. *Aphasiology, 14,* 893–899.

Newcombe, F. (1969). *Missile Wounds of the Brain: A Study of Psychological Deficits.* New York: Oxford University Press.

Ohyama, M., Senda, M., Kitamura, S., Ishii, K., Mishina, M. & Terashi, A. (1996). Role of the Nondominant Hemisphere and Undamaged Area During Work Repetition in Poststroke Aphasics: A PET Activation Study. *Stroke, 27,* 897–903.

Otsuki, M., Soma, Y., Koyama, A., Yoshimura, N., Furukawa, H. & Tsuji, S. (1998). Transcortical Sensory Aphasia Following Left Frontal Infarction. *Journal of Neurology, 245,* 69–76.

Ozeren, A., Sarica, Y., Mavi, H. & Demirkiran, M. (1995). Bromocriptine Is Ineffective in the Treatment of Chronic Nonfluent Aphasia. *Acta Neurologica Belgica, 95,* 235–238.

Pandya, D.N. (1988). Frontal Lobe Architecture and Connections. Presented at the annual meeting of the International Neuropsychological Society, New Orleans, LA.

Pandya, D.N. & Yeterian, E.H. (1990). Architecture and Connections of Cerebral Cortex: Implications for Brain Evolution and Function. In: A.B. Scheibel & A.F. Wechsler (Eds.), *Neurobiology of Higher Cognitive Function* (pp. 53–84). New York: Guilford.

Patterson, K., Graham, N. & Hodges, J.R. (1993). The Impact of Semantic Memory Loss on Phonological Representations. *Journal of Cognitive Neuroscience, 6,* 57–69.

Patterson, L. & Shewell, C. (1987). Speak and Spell: Dissociations and Word-Class Effects. In: M. Coltheart, G. Sartori & R. Job (Eds.), *The Cognitive Neuropsychology of Language* (pp. 273–294). London: Lawrence Erlbaum.

Pirozzolo, F.J., Kerr, K.L., Obrzut, J.E., Morley, G.K., Haxby, J.V. & Lundgren, S. (1981). Neurolinguistic Analysis of the Language Abilities of a Patient with a "Double Disconnection Syndrome": A Case of Subangular Alexia in the Presence of Mixed Transcortical Aphasia. *Journal of Neurology, Neurosurgery, and Psychiatry, 44,* 152–155.

Poeck, K. & Luzzati, C. (1988). Slowly Progressive Aphasia in Three Patients. *Brain, 111,* 151–168.

Pulvermuller, F. & Schonle, P.W. (1993). Behavioral and Neuronal Changes During Treatment of Mixed Transcortical Aphasia: A Case Study. *Cognition, 48,* 139–161.

Rapcsak, S.Z., Krupp, L.B., Rubens, A.B. & Reim, J. (1990). Mixed Transcortical Aphasia Without

Anatomic Isolation of the Speech Area. *Stroke, 21,* 953–956.

Raymer, A.M., Rowland, L., Haley, M. & Crosson, B. (2002). Nonsymbolic Movement Training to Improve Sentence Generation in Transcortical Motor Aphasia: A Case Study. *Aphasiology, 16,* 493–506.

Robinson, K.M. & Grossman, M. (1997). Hypothesis Driven Treatment of Naming Deficits. *Topics in Stroke Rehabilitation, 4,* 1–14.

Roland, P.E., Larsen, B., Lassen, N.A. & Skinhoj, E. (1980). Supplementary Motor Area and Other Cortical Areas in Organization of Voluntary Movements in Man. *Journal of Neurophysiology, 43,* 118–136.

Ross, E.D. (1980). Left Medial Parietal Lobe and Receptive Language Functions: Mixed Transcortical Aphasia After Left Anterior Cerebral Artery Infarction. *Neurology, 30,* 144–151.

Rothi, L.J.G. (1982). Theory and Clinical Intervention: One Clinician's View. In: J.A. Cooper (Ed.), *Aphasia Treatment: Current Approaches and Research Opportunities* (NIDCD Monograph, 2:91–98). Washington, DC: U.S. Government Printing Office.

Rothi, L.J.G. (1995). Behavioral Compensation in Brain Injury. In: R.A. Dixon & L. Bachman (Eds.), *Psychological Compensation: Managing Losses and Promoting Gains* (pp. 219–230). East Sussex, UK: Lawrence Erlbaum.

Rothi, L.J.G. & Feinberg, T.E. (1989). Patient with Left Posterior Circulation CVA, Now with Anomic Dysphasia, Can You Help? In: N. Helm-Estabrooks & J. Aten (Eds.), *Difficult Diagnoses in Neurogenic Communication Disorders* (pp. 93–100). San Diego: College-Hill Press.

Rothi, L.J. & Heilman, K.M. (1980). Transcortical Motor Aphasia and Syntactic Comprehension. Presented at the annual meeting of the Academy of Aphasia, Bass River, MA.

Rothi, L.J.G. & Horner, J. (1983). Restitution and Substitution: Two Theories of Recovery with Application to Neurobehavioral Treatment. *Journal of Clinical Neuropsychology, 5,* 73–81.

Rubens, A.B. (1975). Aphasia with Infarction in the Territory of the Anterior Cerebral Artery. *Cortex, 11,* 239–250.

Rubens, A. & Kertesz, A. (1983). The Localization of Lesions in Transcortical Aphasias. In: A. Kertesz (Ed.), *Localization in Neuropsychology* (pp. 245–268). New York: Academic Press.

Sabe, L., Leiguarda, R. & Starkstein, S.E. (1992). An Open-Label Trial of Bromocriptine in Nonfluent Aphasia. *Neurology, 42,* 1637–1638.

Sabe, L., Salvarezza, F., Cuerva, A.G., Leiguarda, R. & Starkstein, S. (1995). A Randomized, Double-Blind, Placebo-Controlled Study of Bromocriptine in Nonfluent Aphasia. *Neurology, 45,* 2272–2274.

Schneider, D.R. (1938). The Clinical Syndromes of Echolalia, Echopraxia, Grasping and Sucking. *Journal of Nervous and Mental Disease, 88,* 18–35, 200–216.

Selnes, O.A., Knopman, D.S., Niccum, N. & Rubens, A.B. (1985). The Critical Role of Wernicke's Area in Sentence Repetition. *Annals of Neurology, 17,* 549–557.

Speedie, L.J., Coslett, H.B. & Heilman, K.M. (1984). Repetition of Affective Prosody in Mixed Transcortical Aphasia. *Archives of Neurology, 41,* 268–270.

Stengel, E. (1947). A Clinical and Psychological Study of Echoreactions. *Journal of Mental Sciences, 93,* 598–612.

Stuss, D.T. & Benson, D.F. (1986). *The Frontal Lobes.* New York: Raven Press.

Thurstone, L.L. & Thurstone, T. (1943). *The Chicago Tests of Primary Mental Abilities.* Chicago: Science Research Associates.

Trojano, L., Fragassi, N.A., Postiglione, A. & Grossi, D. (1988). Mixed Transcortical Aphasia: On Sparing of Phonological Store in a Case. *Neuropsychologia, 63,* 633–638.

Wambaugh, J.L., Linebaugh, C.W., Doyle, P.J., Martinez, A.L., Kalinyak-Fliszar, M. & Spencer, K.A. (2001). Effects of Two Cueing Treatments on Lexical Retrieval in Aphasic Speakers with Different Levels of Deficit. *Aphasiology, 15,* 933–950.

Watson, R.T., Fleet, S., Rothi, L.J.G. & Heilman, K. (1986). Apraxia and the Supplementary Motor Area. *Archives of Neurology, 43,* 787–792.

Wernicke, C. (1874). *Der Aphasische Symptomenkomplex.* Breslau: Cohn and Weigart.

Wernicke, C. (1908). The Symptom-Complex of Aphasia. In: A. Church (Ed.), *Modern Clinical Medical Diseases of the Nervous System.* New York: Appleton.

Whitaker, H. (1976). A Case of Isolation of the Language Function. In: H. Whitaker & H.A. Whitaker (Eds.), *Studies of Neurolinguistics* (vol. 1). New York: Academic Press.

Suggested Readings

Albert, M.L., Goodglass, H., Helm, N., et al. (1981). *Clinical Aspects of Dysphasia.* New York: Springer-Verlag.

Berthier, M.L. (1999). *Transcortical Aphasias.* East Sussex, UK: Psychology Press.

Chapey, R. (2001). *Language Intervention Strategies in Aphasia and Related Neurogenic Communication Disorders* (4th ed.). Philadelphia: Lippincott Williams & Wilkins.

Coltheart, M., Job, R. & Sartori, G. (1987). *The Cognitive Neuropsychology of Language.* London: Lawrence Erlbaum.

Kertesz, A. (1994). *Localization and Neuroimaging in Neuropsychology.* San Diego: Academic Press.

Nadeau, S.E., Gonzalez-Rothi, L.J. & Crosson, B. (2000). *Aphasia and Language: Theory to Practice.* New York: Guilford Press.

Sarno, M.T. (1998). *Acquired Aphasia* (3rd ed.). San Diego: Academic Press.

12

Global Aphasia

MICHAEL COLLINS

The second edition of this book was published in 1997. At that time, the future of treatment for severe aphasia appeared threatened. Programs such as Lingraphica, C-VIC, and technology-driven behavioral advances such as Language Care Center (LCC) treatment programs were not yet realities. We continued to care for our patients, but often did so with limited resources and few viable options. We had not yet felt the demoralizing impact of the therapy cap, which placed even greater demands on our resourcefulness. Fortunately, for us and our patients, inventive clinicians continued to explore, invent, adapt, and treat, and our clinical armamentarium has continued to grow. I believe the future for these endeavors should encourage us. This chapter demonstrates and reinforces that optimism.

Defining Global Aphasia

Goodglass and Kaplan (1983) described global aphasia in this way: "All aspects of language are so severely impaired that there is no longer a distinctive pattern of preserved versus impaired components." Additionally, they state, "Auditory comprehension of conversation concerning material of immediate personal relevance may appear fairly good in comparison to the tests. That is, the patient may indicate 'yes' or 'no' correctly and with assurance in response to questions about family members, current medical problems, or recent personal events in the hospital or at home. We have also found that many of these patients have a remarkably well-preserved ability to understand geographic place names and locate them" (p. 97). Others, particularly physicians, use the term *global aphasia* to label an aphasia with relatively equal parts receptive and expressive deficits, regardless of severity of deficit. The severity of the deficits is not arguable. Globally aphasic patients have severe, persisting deficits across all communicative modalities. These deficits do not yield easily to traditional forms of treatment. This resistance is frequently due to nonverbal problem-solving deficits, such as those measured by the Colored Progressive Matrices (Raven, 1962), or to what often appears to be a profound volitional performance deficit, which some might call a profound oral-verbal, gestural apraxia. Rubens (1984), for example, found that globally aphasic patients were most frequently apractic, and that lesion size and gestural impairment were significantly related. The following definition of global aphasia summarizes what we know about it: Global aphasia is a severe, acquired impairment of communicative ability across all language modalities. No single communicative modality is preserved. Visual nonverbal problem-solving abilities are often severely depressed as well and are usually compatible with language performance. Patients often have a profound volitional performance deficit as well. Global aphasia usually results from extensive damage to the language zones of the left hemisphere.

In general, the larger the lesion and the greater its proximity to the primary language zones, the more severe the aphasia and the poorer the prognosis. Prognosis is frequently predicated on variability of performance in the early stages of recovery. Higher degrees of variability of performance among subtests or tasks suggest a better prognosis, whereas limited variability suggests that a chronic global aphasia will emerge.

Evaluating Global Aphasia

The validity of any measure is limited to the skill and insight of the tester, and the alertness, willingness, and tolerance of the patient. Formal testing in the early stages of recovery may provide valid results of abilities *at that moment in time*, but be valueless for identifying enduring strengths and weaknesses, predicting recovery, or focusing treatment. In the acute stage, formal assessment of severely aphasic patients may be impossible, and some would say unnecessary (Holland & Fridriksson, 2001). Until formal testing *is* possible and desired, multiple, brief interventions to determine basic communication skills are appropriate. The clinicians, the family, and the staff need to know a patient's ability to follow simple, one-step commands; use a communication board; use and comprehend simple gestures; read simple, functional materials; answer simple yes-no questions for activities of daily living and for personal information; and write or draw simple, communicative symbols; as well as the patient's supralinguistic abilities (inflection, emphasis, attention). Interaction, or attempts to interact with, those in the patient's environment, may be more eloquent than any of the baselined material.

Choice of diagnostic instruments reflect a clinician's training, biases, and clinical setting. This chapter reflects mine, but I also consider other measures that I value and that other clinicians have found to be useful. With that caveat, I would encourage clinicians to consider several other measures that seem to strike a balance between efficiency and comprehensiveness. These include the

Table 12–1. Summary of Approximate Performance Variables in Global Aphasia

Porch Index of Communicative Ability (PICA)
    Overall score: 3.15–8.38
    Overall percentile: 1–25
    Total variability: 3300

Boston Diagnostic Aphasia Examination (BDAE)
    Aphasia severity: 1
    Auditory comprehension: 1st–25th

Reading Comprehension Battery for Aphasia
    Total score: 0–30
    Yes-no questions: 0–40%

Following directions
    Body: 0–50%
    Nonbody: 0–30%

Apraxia Battery
    Request: 0–4
    Imitation: 0–8

Western Aphasia Battery (WAB), the Boston Assessment of Severe Aphasia, and the Burns Brief Inventory of Communication and Cognition (1997). In my clinic, a complete assessment of severe aphasia includes the Porch Index of Communicative Ability, or at least the short version; the Reading Comprehension Battery for Aphasia; a measure of oral and limb apraxia, for example "Open your mouth" (on request and imitatively) and "Make a fist" or "Wave good-bye"; clinician constructed yes-no assessments; body and nonbody commands; the Communicative Activities in Daily Living; and Raven's Colored Progressive Matrices (Table 12–1).

When to Assess

Traditionally, assessment is done when the patient has stabilized. But determining stability can be a complicated process, dependent on spontaneous recovery, acute and chronic conditions, psychological considerations, and their interactions. Most traditional discussions of aphasia distinguish acute from chronic. The distinction is not trivial, because measurements taken in the acute period are very likely to differ from those taken in the chronic period and are influenced by spontaneous recovery. When does spontaneous recovery end? No one knows, but many authorities have felt that recovery has begun to stabilize by about 1 month postonset (Porch et al., 1980). Marshall (1997a) feels that spontaneous recovery reduces the need for formal testing early in a patient's hospital stay.

Holland and Fridriksson (2001) state, "Most formal testing should be postponed until a stable level of performance on simple language tasks has been maintained for at least 2–3 days." They suggest that instead of initiating a formal assessment in the early stages of recovery, "clinicians can substitute for it very careful observation and documentation of a patients' language strengths and weaknesses" (pp. 21–22). They recommend very simple and well-practiced tasks, with changes from the previous day becoming the focus of documentation (Golper, 1996). Brief (~15 minute) and multiple (several times daily) sessions are encouraged, because "documentation of functional change can be achieved by carefully building reiterative activities into conversational interchanges and using them simultaneously for assessment and treatment." These activities might include reading get well cards; asking about the relationship of the person who sent the card(s); having the patient follow a few commands; asking the patient to read and write a few items from the menu; and noting responses/reactions to personally salient information. For example, if the patient is a Green Bay Packer fan, ask questions about a recent trade, a recent game, or a missed tackle. This approach makes some clinicians uncomfortable, perhaps because they have difficulty with the quasi-conversational nature of it. Many clinicians have difficulty equating conversation with assessment, and many have difficulty interacting with patients on that level. Many clinicians find more comfort in their objective measures, despite the discomfort these measures may cause the patient. I have personally used Holland and Fridriksson's approach for many years, and found it to be more valuable than formal tests in many settings. The information it yields is measurable, and although it is derived subjectively, it can be used with a fair amount of objectivity.

Holland and Fridriksson (2001) propose that assessment should take place in the patient's room for several reasons: it eliminates the time wasted in getting the patient to the clinician's office; it reduces the patient's fatigue; it increases the likelihood that one can be a model for family members, if they are present in the patient's room; it facilitates scheduling for family members; it provides a more familiar environment for patients; and it helps the clinician "maximize the positive rather than focusing on the deficits" (p. 22). In this approach, clinicians are encouraged to employ a conversational approach, with an emphasis on combining assessment and treatment, and to use careful observation and documentation in the assessment, rather than formal measures. At least one author takes exception to this approach. Peach (2001) argues that this approach, based on limited data, probably is not appropriate when evaluated under "best practice" standards, and ignores data that support clinical validity in the early stages of recovery.

One of the many things Bruce Porch taught us about managing the challenge of aphasia was that it was more important to know patients' capabilities than their deficits. In his view, determining the type of aphasia was less important than highlighting those abilities that could be capitalized on and enhanced; deficits are diagnostic and positive performance is prognostic. Determining patients' abilities requires the collection of as much data as can reasonably be obtained. Because clinical time has become so precious, evaluation is often undervalued. It should not be. Although measures should be both comprehensive and efficient, these qualities are not necessarily incompatible. For example, the short form of the Porch Index of Communicative Ability (PICA) (DiSimoni et al., 1975) meets both criteria. Although not as comprehensive as the standard version, it samples the same abilities on two items over 17 subtests. It allows for a determination of overall severity; prediction of recovery level; and "potentials" among modalities. Deficits and abilities can be presented objectively, and the test serves as a stable baseline to plot recovery.

Functional Communication Assessment

Functional communication has traditionally been defined as the ability to express basic needs; respond to questions with basic information, such as name, address, and telephone number; answer the telephone and take messages; and describe routine daily occurrences. To contemplate a communicative realm limited to these functions may not be conceivable to many of us, but the reality must be devastating to most severely aphasic patients. These skills do not begin to reach the richness of language required to discuss a hobby, tell someone you love them, tell a joke, read a prescription, write a memo, or, in most cases, return to work. Nevertheless, these skills are considered superfluous by most insurers. Some third-party payers, such as Medicare, continue to provide benefits as long as significant progress can be demonstrated (at least currently, while the $1500 cap has been suspended). The reality is that for many aphasic patients, therapy benefits end before the progress ends or these goals are reached.

Assessment of functional communication may be formal or informal, and range from subjective to objective. Formal, objective measures include the Functional Communication Profile (CFP), Communicative Abilities in Daily Living (CAD), Communicative Competence Evaluation Instrument (CEC), and the American Speech-Language-Hearing Association (ASHA) Functional Assessment of Communication Skills for Adults (ASHA FACS).

The result of the collaborative effort of many contributors over several years, the ASHA FACS is a deceptively sophisticated and useful instrument. Its 44 test items assess social communication, communication of basic needs, daily planning, and lexical and reading/writing/number concepts. The five-point scale used to assess these functions is multidimensional, and the result is a valid,

reliable, and standardized measure. More subjective assessment includes informal, conversational assessment; questionnaires; family member ratings of communication; and in vivo assessment.

The assessment measures discussed here are representative of the measures available. They are not equally sensitive, and the selection of one or more measures will be influenced by the patient's severity and responsiveness, and by time constraints. They should, however, adequately describe deficits, permit a reasonably stable baseline, and guide us in predicting recovery and focusing treatment.

Predicting Recovery

The prognosis for recovery from aphasia is influenced by several factors, including severity of aphasia, relative involvement of modalities, duration of illness, general health, psychological health, lesion size, etiology, and interaction among these variables. In this prognostic variable approach, patient (performance) can be compared with profiles from normative samples of age, health, etiology, etc., which are believed to influence eventual recovery levels. Peach (2001) reports that formal testing in the early stage, or early stages of spontaneous recovery, should be done to improve the ability to predict eventual recovery. I don't think this early approach to predicting recovery results is accurate, simply because behavior is too variable and there are too many variables. For reasonably precise predictions of recovery, even 1 month postonset may be too early. Porch et al. (1980) analyzed PICA scores retrospectively to determine whether multifactorial analysis of these scores, at 1, 3, and 6 months postonset, could be used to accurately predict recovery levels at 6 months postonset. We found that the *least stable* prediction cohort was from 1 month to 12 months. The *most stable* cohort was 6 month to 12 months. This suggests that, at a very minimum, formal testing, and all of the implications that it carries for the tremendously important issues such as return to work, treatment focus, and eventual recovery level, probably should not be done until the patient has *stabilized neurologically* or has at least reached what is admittedly a somewhat arbitrary benchmark of 1 month postonset.

Decisions in the Treatment of Global Aphasia

The evidence for the effectiveness of aphasia treatment seems to be very clear, both during the acute and the chronic settings (Denes et al., 1996). Robey (1998) reports that the effect of acute treatment is nearly twice as large as the effect of spontaneous recovery. This effect is much more difficult to measure because of the contribution of spontaneous recovery. Treatment in the chronic period is easier to measure, but it results in a smaller effect. The overwhelming evidence, however, suggests that aphasia treatment is efficacious, regardless of when it is started or what form it takes. With that knowledge, and the knowledge that speech and language therapy is more likely to be reimbursed in the acute stage, we are left with the need to determine appropriate treatment focus to make our treatment more efficient. Treatment for severe aphasia can be efficacious as well, and these patients must not be relegated to the least cost-effective end of the spectrum. This belief is reinforced by Rosenbek et al. (1989): "Globally aphasic people deserve treatment, and that treatment can be worth everyone's time. Verbal expression may not be a realistic long-term goal for such persons, but short-term attempts to establish or expand it are a legitimate therapeutic activity for both acute and chronically globally aphasic people" (p. 231). Successful treatment should be designed so that its effects can be measured. It should be based on formal and informal tests, and should be relevant to a patient's needs, and the treatment tasks should be organized in a hierarchy of difficulty.

When to Begin Treatment

When to begin treatment may be somewhat easier to determine than when to begin formal testing. Some form of treatment should probably start as soon as the patient is able to participate. Others, for example Sarno and Levita (1981), argue that, for some patients, treatment should be delayed. Sarno and Levita found that many of their globally aphasic patients made more gains in the second 6 months of their recovery than in the first. It is possible that psychodynamic factors influenced recovery in these patients, but physiologic effects such as diaschisis (decreased responsiveness and dysfunction of intact neurons remote from the lesion) (Rubens, 1977) cannot be ignored. Nevertheless, the best, most recent evidence suggests that treatment produces positive results. That effect has been demonstrated: untreated patients who were globally aphasic at 1 month postonset were likely to remain so at 6 months or 1 year (Pashek & Holland, 1988). In the Denes et al. (1996) study, however, the pattern of global aphasia was favorably modified by treatment, "evolving towards a form of aphasia that allowed a better, even if far from normal, verbal communication."

How Much to Treat

Denes et al. (1996) support the clinical intuition that more is better. In their study, globally aphasic patients treated intensively (130 individualized sessions over a 6-month period) showed a tendency to evolve toward a more favorable type of aphasia, when compared with a group receiving regular treatment (60 sessions over a 6-month period).

How Long to Treat

Treatment of less than 3 months has been shown to have a limited effect on recovery (Basso, 1992) and should probably be continued for at least 6 months. Treatment at any time postonset seems to have a significant effect (Collins & Wertz, 1983; Denes et al., 1996).

What to Treat

The targets of treatment are somewhat more controversial. Holland and Fridriksson (2001) propose that, with the exception of those patients who are capable of, and demanding, impairment-centered treatment, many patients could benefit from a combined approach stressing conversation and counseling, an alternative to deficit- or impairment-based treatment. Marshall (1997a) also advocates a conversation approach to treatment in the early stages of recovery for similar reasons. With very few exceptions, patients have never been asked the kinds of questions they're going to be asked in a formal language evaluation. Not only are they suddenly asked to cope with a devastating emotional trauma, they're asked to demonstrate, to a stranger, their incompetence. No wonder they get depressed.

Holland and Fridriksson (2001) stress conversation for several reasons. It is relatively easy to incorporate ongoing assessment into conversation, and to use the assessment to provide upbeat, positive understanding of the spontaneous recovery process. Because conversation is natural and expected, it is likely to expose strengths as well as to provide authentic opportunities for patients to develop and use effective strategies for circumventing communication problems. Preliminary information gathering from the family is important too. Ideally, clinicians should build communication protocols on personally salient information: vocation, avocations, family members, special interests, communicativeness, and communication style. Skilled clinicians can use this information to gain further information, and let the patients participate in a conversation to the degree they can, aided by the clinician to the level necessary. This may mean that most of the burden is on the clinician; learning how much of the burden the patient can share is key.

Holland and Fridriksson's (2001) approach to early intervention is much less directive and more counseling oriented than traditional, impairment-focused intervention. According to Peach (2001), aphasia treatment in the acute phase must be based on assessment results obtained using standardized instruments that "have demonstrated validity and reliability and that meet the demands of practice in the current health care environment" (p. 33).

Establishing the Conditions for a Positive Communication Environment

Educating the Patient, Family, and Staff

Optimism is strongest in the early stages of recovery. Dulling that optimism with data and your previous experience is neither wise nor helpful. A calm, rational, general discussion of severity, characteristics, and recovery is usually welcomed by the family. I've found that families eventually reach their own level of understanding and acceptance. As these increase, trust increases to sustain clinician and patient and family through the usually inevitable harder times.

Early in recovery is usually a good time to introduce literature, Web sites, and information regarding support groups. It is also a good time to demonstrate and reinforce communication techniques, learning more about the patient's communication as you do so. These techniques should include increased use of yes/no questions; slowed rate of speech; and input augmented with gestures, pictures, writing, and other visual aids. For many patients this is a good time to introduce a communication notebook, a multimedia collection including functional communication messages, for example, using the Boardmaker CD program, Writing with Symbols 2000. This is a good way to introduce patient and family to treatment without being too intrusive.

This is also a good time to inform the primary and ancillary care staff, such as occupational therapists, physical therapists, and nurses, about the patient's particular communication needs. Guidelines for establishing communication should be left in the patient's room, and the staff should be encouraged to observe at least part of several therapy sessions so that they can help extend the therapy outside of the sessions. The goal here is to create a positive communicative environment.

Towey and Pettit's (1980) program helps establish these conditions. They emphasize communicative competence in nonlinguistic areas such as eye contact, head nods, facial expressions, reciprocity of affect, physical proximity, and posture. They suggest that the clinician train all staff members to identify those nonlinguistic but communicative behaviors that occur in communicative interactions. In one aspect of the program, staff members are videotaped interacting with the patient. The tapes are then reviewed by the staff members and the speech pathologist in an attempt to identify the staff's thoughts and feelings experienced through the interactions and to increase empathic communication skills. As a result of this program, the authors suggested that several globally aphasic patients made significant gains in communication, but not in linguistic, skills. The primary guidelines for communicating with the severely aphasic patient are as follows: (1) Simplify: handle one idea at a time, use short sentences, speak more slowly, and change topics slowly. (2) Cue: make sure you have the patient's attention, by using gestures, facial cues, and pointing, and use redundant phrasing, e.g., "Are you hungry enough to eat dinner?" Repeat and reword until you communicate. (3) Allow time: allow the patient additional time to understand and to respond. Be patient, unhurried, and accepting of communication attempts. (4) Guess: determine the subject by asking increasingly specific questions. (5) Confirm: make statements about what you think the patient means. After the patient responds, ask a question that should elicit a different response from the patient. If the patient's response does not change, then you know you are not communicating. (6) Be clear: say "I'm sorry. I don't understand you" when necessary. Do not leave abruptly when attempts to communicate fail. (7) Reduce extraneous variables: avoid communicating in a noisy environment; don't try to communicate with the patient if other activities are going on, such as if the patient is listening to the radio or watching television; avoid situations in which more than one person is talking to the patient at a time. (8) Respect the patient: understand that the patient is an intelligent adult who is quite aware of his surroundings, even though language function is impaired. Include him in the conversation. Do not treat him as though he is not there, is deaf, or is mentally retarded.

Goals in the Treatment of Global Aphasia

The need to communicate, the desire to communicate, and the dependence on communication vary among patients. Clinicians should recognize this and respect it. Even many of the most resistant patients eventually accept therapy, at least grudgingly. Often, initial resistance can be overcome by more nondirect, covert therapy, including counseling and conversation. Several goals are reasonable and attainable for severely aphasic patients:

1. Improving auditory comprehension, supplemented with contextual cues, to permit consistent comprehension of one-step commands in well-controlled situations.
2. Improving production of "yes" and "no" as consistent, unequivocal responses in controlled situations.
3. Improving the ability to spontaneously produce several written responses, or approximations, of functional or salient words of daily living.
4. Improving production of several simple, unequivocal gestures.
5. Improving drawing so that several simple, unequivocal messages can be conveyed.
6. Ensuring that a small, basic core of communicative intentions can be conveyed in one or a combination of modalities.
7. Eliciting production of a few spoke words.

Specific Treatments for Global Aphasia

The selection of the specific techniques to reach these goals should be tailored to the patient. The techniques described in the following sections are demonstrably valid and efficacious but not all are appropriate for all patients. Appropriate techniques are determined by several factors, including time constraints, patient and family imperatives, resources, and relative patient strengths.

Treating the Equivocal Response

Establishing an unequivocal "yes" and "no" response can be frustrating for the clinician, but will yield important dividends, and may be the most important element in establishing communicative interaction. Responses may be equivocal not because the patient did not understand the questions, but because the response demands exceed the patient's capabilities, unless the input is very clear and the response channel is focused. This strategy seems to be effective with many patients, and it is one that can be employed by speech pathology assistants and family.

Shaping the Response

1. Make it very clear to the patient what is required. You might begin by saying "We need to work on 'yes' and 'no.' I'm going to say the word, and I want you to watch and listen while I say each word." Begin with "yes" and "no" printed on two cards. Present one card, point to it, and very clearly say the word accompanied by the gesture. Pause 5 seconds, and repeat the word and gesture. Repeat five times. Then present the other card and repeat the procedure.
2. Physically assist the patient with five repetitions of one response, and then the other response.
3. Present four, then three, then two "yes-no" stimuli while saying the word. Pause 5 seconds between responses. Always correct the response, and don't move on until a correct response has been produced.
4. Request gestured "yes" responses to two simple unambiguous questions while assisting with the gestures and saying the word. Do the same for "no" responses.

5. Request five repetitions of gestured "yes," then "no." Facilitate with physical or verbal cues, if necessary.
6. Alternate the requests for "yes" and "no" at 5-second intervals, facilitating if required.

Stabilizing the Response

1. Request gestured responses to simple questions, facilitating if necessary.
2. Permit only "yes" or "no" responses (verbal or gestural) while playing the card game "21."
3. Establish a performance baseline, then begin using personal, environmental, and informational questions.

Gestural Communication

Gestural communication is frequently as impaired, or nearly so, as other modalities. Some globally aphasic patients, however, may benefit from pantomimed instruction and combined pantomime and verbal instructions. We try to incorporate gestural training in our treatment program early in recovery. We assess spontaneous gestural ability informally and formally, and a part of each session is devoted to training these gestures.

We begin with one simple gesture, saying the word as we gesture. That gesture is treated until it is established or, after a fair trial and failure, abandoned. We add gestures as success is achieved in earlier gestures, making sure that the gestures are very different, and capitalizing on those gestures that seem to come easier. Once the patient has learned a few distinct gestures, uses them in response to questions, and recognizes the need for them, they are incorporated into a program of total communication.

Strengthening the Gestural Response

1. Clinician simultaneously gestures and says the word.
2. Clinician says word, and clinician and client gesture simultaneously (clinician assistance may be required).

3. Patient imitates gesture.
4. Patient imitates gesture after enforced delay.
5. Patient gestures in response to auditory stimulus.
6. Patient gestures as in 5, following delay.
7. Patient gestures to written stimulus.
8. Patient gestures as in 7, following delay.
9. Patient writes word in response to gesture with spoken word.
10. Patient gestures in response to appropriate stimuli.

Writing

Haskin's approach to writing has been used with some globally aphasic patients:

1. Clinician points to letters of the alphabet as the sound is produced, and increases the number of letters in sequence as success is achieved.
2. Clinician points to printed words after synthesizing the sounds of the words into a whole (e.g., "G-o," "c-a-t"), beginning with two sounds and gradually increasing the length of words.
3. Patient points to the letter after the clinician names it, or patient traces the letter after it is named.
4. Patient points to printed words after the clinician spells them, beginning with short, unrelated words that have varied spellings, and gradually increasing the complexity by selecting words with similar spellings.
5. Patient points to printed words after the clinician names them, beginning with four short, common words and increasing the display to 10 more abstract words as the patient improves.
6. Patient copies letters of the alphabet, beginning with printed capital letters, then small printed letters, and eventually transcribes these to cursive letters if improvement permits.
7. Patient writes letters of the alphabet to dictation, beginning with the alphabet in serial order, then in random order.

8. Patient writes words to dictation. These words should be words that have been practiced in previous sequences by tracing, pointing, etc.

Visual Action Therapy

Helm and Benson's program for global aphasia is called visual action therapy (VAT). The patient is trained to associate ideographic forms with particular objects and actions, and to carry out a series of tasks in association with these drawings. No verbalization is permitted during the training. Helm-Estabrooks et al. (1982) used VAT to treat eight globally aphasic patients who had not responded to traditional therapeutic interventions. When all training was completed, the authors grouped pre- and post-treatment PICA scores for 10 subtests: two pantomime tasks and two auditory comprehension tasks, which they labeled group one and predicted would improve; two reading subtests (group two), which they predicted might improve; and four verbal subtests (group three), which they predicted would not improve. They reported a significant, positive effect from the treatment for group one, with a significantly larger effect for the gestural subtests than for the auditory subtests, and no significant effect for groups two and three.

Although the primary purpose of VAT is to train globally aphasic patients to produce representational gestures for visually absent stimuli through the manipulation of real objects, this gestural focus seemed to generalize to other modalities. The authors suggest that their findings might be explained on the basis of these hypotheses:

1. Patients may use internal verbal monitoring during the training program.
2. VAT may improve general attentional skills.
3. VAT may improve visual spatial and visual search skills.
4. VAT may reintegrate some conceptual systems necessary for linguistic performance.

The authors feel that this program may help make the patient a better candidate for traditional treatment.

Speech

Some speech is probably attainable for many globally aphasic patients. Programs with the best chance of succeeding are those that employ a shaping/repetition model, such as the following:

1. Clinician produces the target.
2. Clinician produces the target utterance, shaping patient's response simultaneously.
3. Patient repeats target while clinician mimes the utterance.
4. Clinician produces the target utterance and patient repeats it.
5. Patient reads the target utterance, supported and augmented by clinician.
6. Clinician produces the target, and asks patient to respond after 5 seconds.
7. Patient responds with target to appropriate question.

Intersystemic Reorganization

Intersystemic reorganization involves the use of one communicative modality to facilitate use of another. In a program developed by Rosenbek et al. (1976), vision and gesture were combined with speech. In this program, we first attempted to teach gestures for simple verbs, such as "eat," "want," and "see." The four basic steps in this program are as follows:

1. Explain the rationale and procedure to the patient.
2. Teach several gestures.
3. Pair gestures with speech.
4. Fade gestures as speech becomes more functional.

Recently, an intriguing series of experiments has provided some evidence suggesting that *restriction* of gesture during speech might actually enhance speech in chronically aphasic patients. These authors demonstrated significant improvement in the speech of several chronically aphasic patients when gesturing with the intact limb was *constrained* (Pulvermuller et al., 2001). However, I alternated constrained and nonconstrained treatment with a severely aphasic patient recently and found no significant differences in speech.

Communication Boards

Communication boards are often the first thing other health professionals think of when they discover that a patient is unable to speak or gesture meaningfully. But not all patients can use a communication board effectively, no matter how simple it is. We've found that with great patience and the right materials, aphasic patients can communicate *if the conditions are optimized and the subject is important or salient.* Patients can make very effective use of a communication board or a communication book, which is a kind of "survival kit" for aphasic patients. Examples of what might be included in a small binder for a communication book are a small map, for example, a Rand-McNally 4-inch by 6-inch vacation atlas; an "aphasia card" from the National Aphasia Association; a small calendar; family pictures; pages for writing and drawing; and sections with indexes for people, things the patient needs, feelings (including a pain scale), food, beverages, places, clothing, and time. A good way to begin with more severe patients is to think of including some component of all of the above, but reduced to one page covered with acetate.

Successful use of a communication board or book requires training. Most clinicians begin training by some variation of pointing to a command, first with no foils and then gradually increasing the number of foils as the patient achieves a fairly high level of success, generally 80 or 90%. Many clinicians initially include divergent items on a page of no more than eight items (e.g., "bath," "cold," "eat," "sleep"), and as success is demonstrated combining them in separate "topic" pages (e.g., one containing family material, one containing familiar and personal objects, etc.).

Probably the most important attributes of communication boards are saliency and familiarity. Advertising icons are particularly communicative and recognizable, and can be used to construct a very effective communication board. Others, however, have demonstrated successful acquisition of novel lexicons. Johanssen-Horbach et al. (1985), for example, trained four globally aphasic patients to use blissymbols, and found that two of them were able to use these symbols to communicate with relatives. Steele et al. (1987) computerized a manual, visually representative, alternative communication system (C-VIC) for severely aphasic patients. Using this system, on two tasks (selecting an item from a field of objects and speaking the names of objects), C-VIC was found to be superior to natural language performance.

Other Innovative Programs

One of the most innovative programs in aphasia treatment is the Language Care Center (LCC) treatment programs using the Lingraphica system. This system utilizes a detailed patient care algorithm for directing treatment, a proprietary treatment technology called the Lingraphic system, and an extensive collection of prepared clinical exercises. These community-based programs are reported by the authors to be very successful. Most pertinent to this discussion is their report that of the nine aphasic patients classified as global by the WAB, four had been reassigned by the WAB after treatment to the diagnostic category of Broca's aphasia, with an average aphasia quotient (AQ) improvement of 8.6.

Group Treatment for Global Aphasia

Elman and Bernstein-Ellis (1999) have developed a very insightful and imaginative group communication treatment for adults with chronic aphasia. Much of their work is summarized in Chapter 3 of this book. A complete therapy program should include, if possible, significant time devoted to structured and unrehearsed group activity. The efficacy data for this treatment are compelling, and it should at least be considered as an adjunct to individual therapy. Vickers (1999) is an inspiring source of ideas for group treatment activities for adults.

Residential Treatment

Most residential treatment programs involve intensive treatment, often involving plans based on specific impairments and broader, functional limitations. Treatment programs can be geared to the individual or to groups, and many involve computer use. There are several of these programs now operating in the United States, for example the Pittsburgh Aphasia Treatment Research and Education Center, and the Residential Aphasia Program (RAP) at the University of Michigan. The typical program runs for 1 to 4 weeks. RAP is a very successful program that provides 15 hours of individual treatment, 5 hours of group treatment, and 3 hours of computer-assisted treatment 5 days a week for a 6-week period. This program can be modified in length and intensity. Given what we know about recovery from severe aphasia, I suggest that these patients not enroll in intensive, residential programs until approximately 6 months postonset. Also, these programs may not be appropriate for severely aphasic patients.

Programs employ a variety of treatment mixes. Medicare will usually pay for 1 hour of treatment daily, provided the patient meets treatment criteria and is improving. But most of what these programs do is not reimbursed, and so they entail using volunteers and graduate student clinicians, and they offer group sessions and counseling rather than individual sessions and therapy. This is not a mix that works well in the private sector and seems to work best as a not-for-profit enterprise, but some programs have made it work with a sliding scale or extended fee payment schedule.

There is a fairly abundant literature describing the efficacy of intensive treatment (Denes et al., 1996; Hinckley and Craig, 1998; McKenzie, 1991), and there are data on predicting which patients would benefit from intensive speech therapy (Legh-Smith et al., 1987), but apparently only anecdotal data for intensive residential treatment.

Computer-Assisted Treatment

There are several compelling reasons for considering computer-assisted treatment for severely aphasic patients, particularly to improve receptive skills. Less clear is the practical applicability of computers as an assistive device (Helm-Estabrooks and Walsh, 1982), although others (Beukelman et al.; Steele et al.) have found it to be effective. Most severely aphasic patients are capable of using this equipment, although modifications may be required and the equipment may have to be tailored to the patient. The majority of severely aphasic patients are capable of learning to use a full keyboard. Treatment programs may be customized to each patient's individual needs and skills. Independence in the use of the equipment gives the patient a sense of responsibility and control not possible in more traditional therapeutic encounters. Patients may be able to use equipment during "off hours," and be monitored and modified by the clinician at another time. Routine aspects of aphasia therapy, which are unavoidable in treating severe aphasia, are highly compatible with computer-assisted treatment. Cost-benefit ratios are high, and they greatly extend the treatment's range.

Promoting Aphasic's Communicative Effectiveness (PACE)

Promoting Aphasic's Communicative Effectiveness (PACE) (Davis & Wilcox, 1985) is a program of augmented communication that structures natural conversational interaction. It recognizes that not all communication channels are open to globally aphasic persons, but that they may communicate successfully when given free choice of responses. PACE is based on four principles: (1) The clinician and patient participate equally as senders and receivers of messages. (2) There is an exchange of new information between the clinician and patient. (3) The patient has free choice as to which communicate channels to use. (4). Feedback is provided by the clinician. The emphasis is not on communicative "accuracy" but on effectively conveying messages. The globally aphasic patient and those around him need to capitalize on these communicative strengths—facial expression, inflection, pointing, gestural recognition skills, intact memory for pictures, brands and faces, and ability to perform simple learned tasks, such as playing cards, particularly the game "21" and simple forms of poker; alternatively, the clinician can ask the patient to teach him a card game, and then can assist the patient in doing so.

Communication Partners

Jon Lyon's innovative work is the only program I'm aware of that pairs trained communicative volunteer partners with aphasic patients. These partners are trained to communicate with the patient and assist the patient in communication. Trained by the clinician to capitalize on a patient's most intact communication skills, the partners serve as respite for the patient's families and as communication lifelines for the patient. Although not practical for all patients, with the right patient and partner it can be remarkably effective.

When Treatment Should End

There is probably no logical conclusion to treatment. If we've done our job, the family will continue to serve as therapists, often with better skills than ours. If speech has not appeared in any consistent form, its position in the treatment hierarchy should be downgraded, and alternative and augmentative programs encouraged. Communication will never be easy or natural, but it may be spontaneous and should always be rewarded. When the patient and his family and friends have accepted the need for multimodal communication, and use it routinely, we should slowly and quietly step away.

A Few Caveats

This chapter concludes with a few caveats. First, we believe that treatment is effective, but evidence suggests that treatment is less effective for severely aphasic patients (Marshall, 1997a). We know that we need to manage our resources more effectively, and managed care and other financial pressures may require us to select our treatment candidates more carefully, perhaps rationing treatment to the best candidates, and limiting treatment with the less promising ones. One problem is that we still don't know how to do that and we can't ignore the best evidence we have: treatment works, even for the most severe patient, and that group data hide some of the most robust treatment effects. Wertz (1997) concurs: "Doubt is not a good reason to do anything, but it is a bad reason to do nothing." We have made remarkable progress in treating global aphasia in the past 5 years, and the future is bright.

References

Basso, A. (1992). Prognostic Factors in Aphasia. *Aphasiology, 6*, 337–348.

Code, C. (2001). Multifactorial Processing in Recovery from Aphasia: Developing the Foundations for a Multileveled Framework. *Brain and Language, 77*,25–44.

Collins, M. & Wertz, R. (1983). *Coping with Success: The Maintenance of Therapeutic Effect in Aphasia.* In: R. Brookshire (Ed.), Proceedings of the Conference on Clinical Aphasiology. Minneapolis: BRK.

Denes, G., Perazzolo, C., Piani, A. & Piccione, F. (1996). Intensive Versus Regular Speech Therapy in Global Aphasia: A Controlled Study. *Aphasiology, 10*, 385–394.

DiSimoni, F., Keith, R. & Darley, F. (1980). Prediction of PICA Overall Score by Short Versions of the Test. *Journal of Speech and Hearing Research, 23*, 511–516.

Elman, R. & Bernstein-Ellis, E. (1999). The Efficacy of Group Communication Treatment in Adults with Chronic Aphasia. *Journal of Speech, Language and Hearing Research, 42*, 411–419.

Golper, L. (1996) Language Assessment. In: G.L. Wallace (Ed.), *Adult Aphasia Rehabilitation* (pp. 78–68). Boston: Butterworth-Heinemann.

Goodglass, H. & Kaplan, E. (1983). *The Assessment of Aphasia and Related Disorders.* Philadelphia: Lea and Febiger.

Harris, V., Aftonomos, L. & Steele R. (1999). Improved Outcomes for Persons with Aphasia with advanced Treatment Programs. *Advance for Speech Pathologists,* October 18.

Helm-Estabrooks, N., Fitzpatrick, P. & Barresi, B. (1982) Visual Action Therapy for Global Aphasia. *Journal of Speech and Hearing Disorders, 47*, 385–389.

Hinckley, J. & Craig, H. (1998). Influence of Rate of Treatment on the Naming Abilities of Adults with Chronic Aphasia. *Aphasiology, 12*, 989–1006.

Holland, A. (1982). Observing Functional Communication of Aphasic Adults. *Journal of Speech and Hearing Disorders, 47*, 50–56.

Holland, A. & Fridriksson, J. (2001). Aphasia Management During the Early Phases of Recovery Following Stroke. *American Journal of Speech-Language Pathology, 10*, 19–28.

Holland, A., Fromm, D., DeRuyter, F. & Stein, M. (1996). Treatment Efficacy: Aphasia. *Journal of Speech and Hearing Research, 39*, 27–39.

Legh-Smith, J., Denis, R., Enderby, P. & Langton-Hewer, R. (1987). Selection of Aphasic Stroke Patients for Intensive Speech Therapy. *Journal of Neurology, Neurosurgery, and Psychiatry, 50*, 1488–1492.

Lingraphica System and Language Care Center Programs. *http://www.aphasia.com.*

Marshall, R. (1997a). Aphasia Treatment in the Early Post-Onset Period: Managing Our Resources Effectively. *American Journal of Speech-Language Pathology, 6*, 5–11.

Marshall, R. (1997b). Comments on "Comments." *American Journal of Speech-Language Pathology, 6*, 19–21.

McKenzie, C. (1991). Four Weeks of Intensive Aphasia Treatment and Four Weeks of No Treatment. *Aphasiology, 5*, 435–437.

Peach, R. (2001). Further Thoughts Regarding Management of Acute Aphasia Following Stroke. *American Journal of Speech-Language Pathology, 10*, 29–36.

Porch, B., Collins, M., Wertz, R. & Friden, T. (1980). Statistical Prediction of Change in Aphasia. *Journal of Speech and Hearing* Research, 23, 312–321.

Pulvermuller, F., Neininger, B., Elbert, T., Mohr, B., Rockstroh, B., Koebbel, P. & Taub E. (2001). *Stroke, 32*, 1621–1626.

Raven, J. (1962). *Coloured Progressive Matrices.* London: H.K. Lewis.

Robey, R. (1994). The Efficiency of Treatment for Aphasic Persons: A Meta-Analysis. *Brain and Language, 47*, 582–608.

Robey, R. (1998). A Meta-Analysis of Clinical Outcomes in the Treatment of Aphasia. *Journal of Speech and Hearing Research, 41*, 172–187.

Rosenbek, J., LaPointe, L. & Wertz, R. (1989). *Aphasia: A Clinical Approach.* Austin TX: Pro-Ed.

Rubens, A. (1977). The Role of Changes Within the Central Nervous System During Recovery from Aphasia. In: M. Sullivan & M. Kommers (Eds.), *Rationale for Adult Aphasia Therapy.* Lincoln, NE: University of Nebraska Medical Center.

Sarno, M. & Levita, E. (1981). Some Observations on the Nature of Recovery in Global Aphasia. *Brain and Language, 13*, 1–12.

Steele, R., Weinrich, M., Kleczewska, M., Wertz, R. & Carlson, S. (1987). Evaluating Performance of Severely Aphasic Patients on a Computer-Aided Visual Communication System. *Proceedings of the Conference on Clinical Aphasiology.* Minneapolis: BRK.

Towey, M. & Pettit, J. (1980). Improving Communicative Competence in Global Aphasia. In: R. Brookshire (Ed.), *Proceedings of the Conference on Clinical Aphasiology* (pp. 139–146). Minneapolis: BRK.

Vickers, C. (1999). *Communication Recovery: Group Conversation Activities for Adults.* San Antonio: Psychological Corporation.

Wertz, R. (1997). Comments on "Aphasia Treatment in the Early Post-Onset Period: Managing Our Resources Effectively." *American Journal of Speech-Language Pathology, 6*, 12–18.

13

Dementia

MICHELLE S. BOURGEOIS

The term *dementia*, defined as "being out of one's mind," has been around since the time of the Roman poet Lucretius (50 B.C.E.) (Berrios, 1987). Over the centuries, the term has evolved from one that described any change in intellect or judgment in the elderly, to a collection of cognitive and behavioral symptoms correlated with specific neuropathology. Currently, the aging process is thought to have three possible cognitive outcomes: (1) normal age-related decline, which is often described as normal and healthy aging; (2) age-associated memory impairment, which is not as severe and does not have all of the features of dementia; and (3) dementia, for which there are many types (Christensen & O'Brien, 2000). The *Diagnostic and Statistical Manual of Mental Disorders* (DSM-IV) (American Psychiatric Association, 1994) defines dementia as an impairment in short- and long-term memory with related changes in abstract thinking, judgment, other higher cortical functions, or personality that causes significant social and occupational impairments. Dementia is distinguished from disturbances of consciousness such as delirium, which is typically an acute and treatable physical condition, and other psychiatric morbidities such as depression and anxiety disorders for which there are pharmacologic remedies (Ballard, 2000). Evidence of an organic cause of the memory and intellectual impairments is also required for a DSM-IV diagnosis of dementia.

Dementia, therefore, is a clinical syndrome of chronic and progressive symptoms that result from acquired brain disease. As many as 70 different disorders may cause dementia or chronic cognitive impairment, including neurodegenerative diseases (e.g., Alzheimer's disease, Pick's disease, dementia with Lewy bodies), vascular diseases (e.g., multiinfarct dementia, Binswanger's disease), endocrine disorders (e.g., diabetes, thyroid disease), vitamin deficiencies (e.g., B_{12}, thiamine), systemic diseases (e.g., respiratory diseases, anemia), other neurologic disorders (e.g., normal pressure hydrocephalus, head injury, tumors, multiple sclerosis), and infections [e.g., syphilis, encephalitis, human immunodeficiency virus (HIV), Creutzfeldt-Jakob disease]. Approximately 13% of cases have a potentially reversible cause of dementia, such as drug toxicity, depression, thyroid disease, vitamin B_{12} deficiency, and normal pressure hydrocephalus (Eastley & Wilcock, 2000). A comprehensive, multidisciplinary clinical assessment of cognitive and noncognitive symptoms is crucial for accurate diagnosis. Clinicians have seen an increase in self-referrals for memory complaints due to the media coverage of the late former president Ronald Reagan's disclosure of his Alzheimer's diagnosis. Yet, memory impairment alone is not sufficient for diagnosis; in fact, subjective cognitive impairments, including poor concentration, thinking difficulties, and memory lapses, often signal depression.

Careful documentation of the presenting complaint and history of symptoms helps to identify areas of cognitive functioning (e.g., language impairment, orientation, initiation and execution of activities, visuospatial difficulties) and noncognitive functioning (e.g., change in personality, behavioral disturbance, and psychiatric symptoms). The gradual onset of symptoms over time may help to confirm a neurodegenerative condition, whereas a sudden, acute episode suggests a cerebrovascular infarct or stroke. Family members or significant others are often very helpful in supplementing patient information, particularly if they live with the person.

Review of the patient's medical conditions is important for determining if any existing medical condition could explain the symptoms. In particular, cardiovascular disease, diabetes, hypothyroidism, potentially anoxic or hypoxic conditions, liver and renal disease, and head trauma can all contribute to cognitive impairment. Follow-up blood screening is usually recommended to monitor known medical conditions, and to detect any previously undiagnosed ones.

Medication review is an increasingly vital component of the evaluation because of the incidence of polypharmacy in the elderly. Multiple medications for a range of physical illnesses can impact cognitive function and alter drug pharmacokinetics. Nonprescription drug use, such as cold and sleep remedies, and herbal products, such as Gingko Biloba, should also be documented for their potential contributions to impaired cognitive functioning and other side effects. Noncompliance with medication regimens often exacerbates known medical conditions and can be the result of forgetting to take the drugs as prescribed. The neurotoxic effects of drug and alcohol abuse, often overlooked in the elderly, can be reversed if detected and treated appropriately.

Physical and neurologic examinations are necessary for revealing any evidence of cardiovascular or respiratory impairment as indicated by measuring the pulse and blood pressure and listening to the heart, lungs, and abdomen. Cranial nerve examination looks for signs of facial weakness; abnormal eye movements; visual field defects; posture, gait, and movement disorders; grasp, sucking, and snout reflexes; and vibratory and proprioceptive sensation deficits that would signal specific medical or neurologic conditions. Assessment of the patient's mental status, language functioning, and mood help to differentiate focal impairments secondary to vascular lesions from psychotic symptoms related to psychiatric illness and the gradual deterioration of cognitive functioning in dementia. Clinical observations are usually correlated with radiologic evidence from computed tomography (CT) scans, magnetic resonance imaging (MRI), and single photon emission computed tomography (SPECT) scans, as well as electroencephalograph (EEG) studies.

Family and social history information includes documentation of relatives with dementia or other high-risk medical conditions, patient's education and occupation, social supports and resources, and living arrangements.

Pathophysiology

Changes in the brain are documented via radiologic procedures such as CT scans, MRI, positron emission tomography (PET), and SPECT scans. CT provides an x-ray image of intracranial structures to rule out brain tumors, cerebral lesions, cortical atrophy, and ventricular and white matter changes. CT is the scanning method of choice for cognitively impaired and agitated patients because it is faster and cheaper than MRI, but findings of cortical atrophy, ventricular enlargement, and reduced CT density may be similar to those seen with age-related changes and psychiatric disorders such as late-life depression and schizophrenia (Pearlson et al., 1991). Structural MRI uses electromagnetic forces to create a spatial representation of brain tissue, with improved resolution and superior soft tissue contrast of the images over CT scans. Because it does not use ionizing radiation, MRI can be used serially and for the study of normal controls (Barber & O'Brien, 2000).

MRI is helpful for differential diagnosis. In persons with suspected Alzheimer's disease (AD), MRI data reveal generalized atrophy of the whole brain and ventricles, wider cortical sulci, atrophy of the temporal lobes, hippocampi, and amygdala, with some of these changes evident before dementia symptoms occur. MRI evidence in persons diagnosed with dementia with Lewy bodies includes less medial temporal lobe atrophy than in AD and relative preservation of hippocampal volume. Frontotemporal dementia is characterized by bilateral and symmetrical prefrontal and anterior temporal lobe and basal ganglia atrophy in the absence of focal lesions. In vascular dementia a wide variety of focal cortical lesions; basal ganglia, thalamus, and white matter changes; generalized cerebral atrophy; and ventricular dilation are seen. MRI of persons with Huntington's disease reveals reduced basal ganglia volume, and widened frontal horns of the lateral ventricles. White matter and periventricular hyperintensities are seen in most dementias especially AD, vascular dementia (VaD), dementia with Lewy bodies (DLB), and multiple sclerosis (Barber & O'Brien, 2000).

Other types of imaging assess blood flow and biochemical changes for differential diagnosis. For example, functional MRI (fMRI) uses an intravenous injection of a contrast agent (gadolinium) to change the MRI signal as blood flows through the brain. Magnetic resonance spectroscopy (MRS) studies biochemical changes by measuring radiofrequencies (Frederick et al., 2000). SPECT uses gamma ray emitting substances to generate images that reflect the biochemical status of cells, including blood flow, synaptic density, and tumor metabolism. PET measures cerebral glucose metabolism by injecting radiolabeled glucose and recording the gamma rays produced when the isotope decays (Kennedy, 2000). The EEG technique for measuring the electrical activity of the brain often reveals increasing abnormalities with age, usually in temporal regions, and the progressive slowing of alpha activity and an increase in beta, theta, and delta activity in AD. EEG findings are more normal in VaD than in AD, except where there are focal changes and more severe intellectual decline (Erkinjuntti, 2000).

Due to the limitations of these radiologic assessment procedures, definitive diagnoses are still not possible until postmortem examination of the brain. The neurohistologic features of AD include senile or neuritic plaques (or lesions), neurofibrillary tangles (composed of cytoskeletal elements in the form of paired helical filaments and an abnormally phosphorylated isoform of tau, a glycoprotein), abnormal cytoplasmic structures called granulovacuoles, Hirano bodies, an estimated 36 to 46% decrease in neurons (particularly in the hippocampus), abnormal neurites, patterns of gliosis, vascular amyloid, and some white matter changes (leukoaraiosis) (Lantos & Cairns, 2000). The pathology of dementia with Lewy bodies is similar to that in AD and Parkinson's diseases, with the additional feature of Lewy bodies in both cortical and subcortical regions (e.g., substantia nigra as in Parkinson's disease), fewer neurofibrillary tangles, and minimal plaque (Ince et al., 2000). The histology of frontotemporal dementia (FTD) includes microvacuoles, Pick bodies, and motor neurone abnormalities (Brun et al., 1994). Creutzfeldt-Jakob disease, a virulent and rare dementia caused by a viral infection related to mad cow disease, is characterized by diffuse neuronal loss in the cortex, basal ganglia, thalamus, brainstem, and spinal cord.

Nature and Differentiating Features

Alzheimer's disease (AD), the most common form of dementia (60% of all cases), is reported to afflict ~6 to 10% of all individuals over the age of 65, up to 33% at age 90, and is expected to quadruple in the next 50 years (Ballard, 2000; Brookmeyer et al., 1998). The risk factors for AD include age, gender (women have higher incidence), family history of dementia (increases risk by 5% up to age 70, 16% up to age 80, and 33% up to age 90), less education, and history of head trauma with loss of consciousness (increases risk by 80%) (Jorm, 2000). Several genetic factors for AD have been discovered in recent years, including the mutation of the amyloid precursor protein gene on chromosome 21, presenilin genes on chromosomes 1 and 14, and the apolipoprotein E (Apo E) gene on chromosome 19. Of the 3 Apo E alleles (e2, e3, e4), the e4/e4 genotype was associated with 15 times the risk of AD compared with other genotypes. Studies suggest that anti-inflammatory medications and replacement estrogen for postmenopausal women may have protective effects (Jorm, 2000).

Memory loss is the hallmark symptom of AD. Most models describe memory as the encoding or registering of information, the storage of information, and the access to or retrieval of information (Baddeley, 1995). Sensory information is held temporarily in working memory or short-term storage before it is responded to or processed into long-term storage for later retrieval. These three subsystems are controlled by a central executive system, which is particularly vulnerable to the encoding and retrieval difficulties of persons with dementia. Although working memory remains intact in early AD, central executive function is impaired (Paulesu et al., 1993). Semantic memory loss may entail damage to memory stores or impaired retrieval (Hodges & Patterson, 1995). Remote, autobiographical memory gradually deteriorates over time (Greene et al., 1996). These memory changes affect language and communication behaviors as well. In the early stages, individuals have difficulty with word finding, comprehending abstract language, and following complex conversation. They are aware of their lapses in attention and concentration and have intact phonologic, syntactic, and pragmatic skills. As the disease progresses, there is a gradual worsening of semantic abilities, including increased word-finding deficits, increased use of indefinite pronouns, and difficulty comprehending complex instructions. Short-term memory losses are reflected in increased forgetting of recent events, difficulty maintaining a topic of conversation, and repetitive verbalization of anxious, delusional, and obsessive thoughts. Phonology and syntax remain intact, as well as oral reading, simple writing, and automatic, procedural memory tasks, such as playing the piano or getting dressed. In the late stages, verbal language becomes severely impaired in expression and comprehension, and ambiguous, echolalic, perseverative, and paraphasic utterances deteriorate to incoherent mumbling and eventual mutism. Individuals may respond to sensory stimuli, cues, and music with increased cooperation, smiling, and pleasant vocalizations (Bayles & Kaszniak, 1987; Lubinksi, 1991).

Behavioral symptoms prevalent in 90% of patients with AD include personality changes (disengagement, disinhibition, apathy); delusions (e.g., theft, persecution, one's house is not one's home, infidelity, abandonment, phantom boarder); hallucinations (visual, auditory, gustatory, olfactory, haptic); mood disorders (depression, mania, anxiety, anger); sleep, eating, and sexual disorders; and restlessness, pacing, wandering, and repetitive behaviors (Teri & Logsdon, 1994).

Vascular dementia (VaD) is differentiated from other forms of dementia due to arteriosclerotic changes in the blood supply to the brain and cerebrovascular disorders. VaD accounts for 10 to 50% of dementia cases and is considered the second most common cause of dementia. Other forms of VaD include multi-infarct dementia (MID) (large vessel or cortical disease) and Binswanger's disease (small vessel disease, lacunar infarcts). These conditions usually have an abrupt onset of cognitive symptoms and a stepwise, fluctuating, and progressive course. Early memory loss, executive dysfunction, personality changes, and increased incidence of depression are common clinical features. Language changes may be focal in nature and coexist with hemiparesis, facial weakness, visual field defects, and extrapyramidal signs (Erkinjuntti, 2000).

Frontotemporal dementias (FTD) include Pick's disease, progressive aphasia (left perisylvian frontotemporal lobes are affected), and semantic dementia (bilateral and selective atrophy of the anterior temporal neocortex) (Neary, 2000). It is estimated that 25% of dementia cases are FTD with a high familial incidence related to a specific gene mutation on chromosome 17. The onset of FTD is typically signaled by mood and personality changes such as depression, anxiety, and excessive sentimentality. Language changes are mostly expressive initially, with reduced output, increasing reliance on stereotypical remarks, perseverative and then echolalic responses, and eventual mutism. Comprehension, naming, reading, and written output are usually well preserved, as well as visual perception, spatial, and motor skills. Memory performance is variable; recall is enhanced with specific cues and direct and multiple-choice questions. There is more difficulty with sustained and selective attention and other executive function tasks. Behavioral symptoms include profound changes in personality and social conduct, including disinhibition, inappropriate jocularity, restricted verbal repertoire, impulsive, highly distractible, hyperorality, hypersexuality, stereotyped and ritualistic behavior, and repetitive behaviors (Mirea & Cummings, 2000).

Dementia with Lewy bodies (DLB) is characterized by attentional deficits and visuospatial deficits with relatively preserved memory early. There is a gradual increase of fluctuating cognition with recurrent visual hallucinations, delusions, and depression (McKeith et al., 1996). Symptoms of parkinsonism may eventually be exhibited in some patients, including tremor, rigidity, bradykinesia, gait abnormality, and postural change. On neuropsychological testing, persons with DLB are more impaired than those with AD on verbal fluency, psychomotor speed, executive function (problem solving, abstract reasoning), and visuospatial/constructional ability but are similarly impaired on episodic memory and language (Galasko et al., 1998).

Dementia affects approximately 10 to 15% of persons with Parkinson's disease, with prevalence increasing with age (Velakoulis & Lloyd, 2000). The extrapyramidal symptoms of tremor, hypokinesia, and rigidity precede global cognitive impairments and frontal dysfunction. Depression, anxiety, loss of self-esteem, suicidal thoughts, visual hallucinations, delusions, delirium, weight change, fatigue, and sleep disturbances may be related to treatment with dopaminergic drugs; dopamine agonists cause psychosis and nightmares (Liberman, 1998).

Dementia in Huntington's disease (HD), which is hereditary and progressive, includes motor, cognitive, and psychiatric symptoms. Involuntary and voluntary movement abnormalities range from chorea, dystonia, athetosis, and myoclonus to gait abnormalities, bradykinesia, and saccadic eye movements. Language is generally intact until the later stages when dysarthria and memory and attentional problems are prevalent. Personality alterations, mood disorders (depression), psychosis, aggressive behavior, apathy, irritability, emotional lability, disinhibition, impulsivity, and suicide are common in HD (Chua & Chiu, 2000).

Human immunodeficiency virus–associated dementia was first identified as a neuropsychiatric outcome of HIV disease in the past decade (Everall, 2000). Primarily a disorder of cognition, there are also associated problems with motor and psychological functioning. Early effects on speech are extrapyramidal, including slow, labored, and dysarthric speech; language, memory, and cognition worsen with disease progression. Mood changes range from depression to marked lability, irritability, and violent outbursts; in the late stages behavior deteriorates to mutism, immobility, and incontinence.

Evaluation

It is important to assess the specific cognitive, communicative, and functional strengths and impairments associated with dementia to manage disease symptoms appropriately. Brief standardized measures of cognition, or mental status, are useful for screening a broad range of cognitive abilities, including memory, language (e.g., naming, repetition, auditory comprehension, writing), spatial ability/praxis, set-shifting/calculation, orientation, personal knowledge, abstract thinking, construction, perception, concentration, and attention. Performance-based cognitive measures include the Mini-Mental Status Exam (MMSE) (Folstein et al., 1975), the Blessed Dementia Scale (BDS) (Blessed et al., 1968), the Cambridge Cognitive Examination (CAMCOG) (Blessed et al., 1991), and the Severe Impairment Battery (SIB) (Saxton et al., 1990). These measures are reliable, but the age, educational level, and cultural background of the person being assessed are known to influence performance and accuracy of identification of cognitive dysfunction (Mungas et al., 1996).

Mental status rating scales translate cognitive impairment into stages of disability, which can be useful for classifying patients and predicting relative treatment outcomes (Albert, 1994). Measures such as the Clinical Dementia Rating Scale (CDR) (Hughes et al., 1982) and the Global Deterioration Scale for Age-Related Cognitive Decline and Alzheimer's Disease (GDS) (Reisberg et al., 1982) involve a subjective evaluation of patients' cognitive skills (e.g., memory, orientation, judgment, problem solving, community affairs, home and hobbies, personal care, psychiatric symptoms, and performance on psychometric tests) by a skilled clinician who also may query family and other caregivers about behavioral functioning.

Comprehensive assessment batteries of cognitive and behavioral functioning include the Alzheimer's Disease Assessment Scale (ADAS) (Rosen et al., 1984), which evaluates cognitive (memory, language, and praxis) and noncognitive (mood and behavior) functioning, and the Consortium to Establish a Registry for Alzheimer's Disease (CERAD) (Welsh et al., 1994) battery, which includes subtests of fluency, naming, praxis, memory (free-recall and delayed recall), word recognition, and the MMSE. Subjective measures of clinician or caregiver impression of the patient's clinical change relative to screening, based on a brief interview with the patient, include the Clinician Interview-Based Impression (CIBI) and the Final Comprehensive Consensus Assessment (FCCA) (Knapp et al., 1994). Multicenter clinical drug trials use these measures to document treatment effects (Mohs, 1995).

The most pervasive symptom of dementia, memory impairment, has been assessed traditionally with the Revised Wechsler Memory Scale (WMS-R) (Russell, 1975). Bayles and Kaszniak (1987) reviewed other instruments that have been used to document the memory deficits of patients with dementia, including the Benton Revised Visual Retention Test (BVRT-R) (Benton, 1974) and the Fuld Object Memory Evaluation (Fuld, 1981). The increasing interest in memory, both from theoretical and applied perspectives, has led to the publication of measures of episodic or semantic memory (e.g., Pyramids and Palm Trees Test; Howard & Patterson, 1992), recognition memory (Recognition Span Test; Moss et al., 1986), retrograde amnesia (the Autobiographical Memory Interview, AMI; Kopelman et al., 1990), long-term memory (Doors and People; Baddeley et al., 1994), and everyday memory functioning (Rivermead Behavioral Memory Test, RBMT; Wilson et al., 1991), which assess a variety of performance-based tasks, such as lexical, semantic, and verbal priming, category fluency, and motor-skill learning tasks.

The language and communication disorders of persons with dementia have been assessed with a variety of comprehensive measures designed for patients with language impairments due to focal brain damage (e.g., Boston Diagnostic Aphasia Examination, Goodglass & Kaplan, 1983; Western Aphasia Battery, Kertesz, 1982). The Arizona Battery for Communication Disorders of Dementia (ABCD) (Bayles & Tomoeda, 1991) was designed specifically to measure the receptive and expressive oral and written language deficits of patients with dementia, and is therefore used extensively in diagnostic settings. Overall, comprehensive assessment tools are important in the differential diagnosis of language impairments due to brain damage because they sample a wide range of behaviors efficiently, although the administration of an entire comprehensive measure in one sitting may not be possible due to the attentional limitations of patients with dementia.

To document impairments in specific language domains, such as pragmatics, discourse, semantics, syntax, and phonology, many measures from the aphasia assessment literature are administered to patients with dementia. For an analysis of dementia patient performance on standardized language measures, such as the Peabody Picture Vocabulary Test (Dunn & Dunn, 1981), the Boston Naming Test (Kaplan et al., 1983), the FAS Word Fluency Measure (Borkowski et al., 1967), the Auditory Comprehension Test of Sentences (Shewan, 1979), and the Token Test (DeRenzi & Faglioni, 1978), see Bayles and Kaszniak (1987). Due to the many limitations on the use of these measures with patients with dementia, Bayles and colleagues developed their comprehensive assessment battery [the Arizona Battery for Communication Disorders of Dementia (the ABCD)] and standardized it with an extensive population of patients across the cognitive continuum. For other useful reviews of language and cognitive impairment measures, see Lubinski (1991) and Ripich (1991).

Assessment of the daily functional status of patients with dementia is necessary for determining patients' level of need for rehabilitative services. Disability in this population can be documented for a variety of functional behaviors such as language, daily living skills, and problem behaviors, and in a variety of settings (e.g., hospital, work, home, and nursing home). Frattali (1994) reviewed measures used to screen functional skills, such as the Functional Linguistic Communication Inventory (FLCI) (Bayles & Tomoeda, 1994) and the Communication Outcome Measure of Functional Independence (COMFI) (Santo Pietro & Boczko, 1997b), the Communicative Abilities in Daily Living (CADL) (Holland et al., 1999), and the Functional Assessment of Communication Skills for Adults (ASHA-FACS) (Frattali et al., 1995). The ASHA Task Force on Treatment Outcome and Cost Effectiveness has also developed the Functional Communication Measures (FCM) for rating (on a seven-point scale) 13 different communication disorders of any population. This tool was designed to measure change in FCM rating to demonstrate achievement of functional outcomes resulting from clinical intervention; studies to verify the reliability and validity of the measure are ongoing (Baum et al., 1997).

The rehabilitation potential of persons with dementia is also determined by assessing the status of their activities of daily living (ADL), including dressing, bathing, toileting, transfer, feeding, and mobility (for a review of measures see Kane & Kane, 2000) and instrumental activities of daily living (IADL), such as using the telephone, managing money, meal preparation, housework, and shopping (for a review of measures and critical analysis of disability assessment see Kovar & Lawton, 1994). Subtests of certain IADL measures may be relevant outcome measures for communication treatments because they include communication skills (using the telephone) and higher-order cognitive skills (money management, shopping).

The behavioral disturbances of patients with dementia also affect their everyday functional status. Teri and Logsdon (1994) review 28 measures of behavioral disturbance; some of the more popular rating scales include the Behavioral Pathology in Alzheimer's Disease Rating Scale (BEHAVE-AD) (Reisberg et al., 1987), the Cohen-Mansfield Agitation Inventory (Cohen-Mansfield & Billig, 1986), the Nursing Home Behavior Problem Scale (Ray et al., 1992), and the Multidimensional Observation Scale for Elderly Subjects (MOSES) (Helmes et al., 1987), which also measures cognitive and psychosocial functioning.

The degree to which dementia symptoms influence the quality of the lives of the afflicted and the persons in their environments has been the focus of much recent research. Quality of life (QL) is a broad concept that Lawton (1991) has proposed and includes measures of objective environment, self-perceived quality of life, psychological well-being, and behavioral competence (health, functional health, cognition, time use, and social behavior). Since Howard and Rockwood's (1995) review of the QL literature, several new measures have been developed including the Alzheimer Disease-Related Quality of Life (ADRQL) (Rabins et al., 1999) and the Quality of Life Assessment Schedule (QOLAS) (Selai et al., 2000). When QL is assessed using self-report questionnaires, the ability of persons with dementia, who may have memory and communication constraints, to reliably report their feelings, may be in question. Many researchers circumvent the reliability of self-report data with observational measures and caregiver-completed rating scales of behaviors believed to approximate QL indicators, such as affect, mood, depressive symptoms, and pleasant events. But proxy informants' ability to answer reliably for the person with dementia depends on the nature of the relationship, the amount of time spent with the person, the objectivity of the questions, and the severity of the person's cognitive and communicative deficits (Zimmerman & Magaziner, 1994). Observational measures have their own limitations. Schulz et al. (1994) reviewed tools for measuring the emotions, moods, and feeling states of the elderly; although most were self-report measures, the Philadelphia Geriatric Center Affect Rating Scale (Lawton et al., 1996) is completed by a clinician after a 10-minute observation period, during which the duration of affective states (pleasure, anger, anxiety/fear, sadness, interest, and contentment) are rated on a five-point scale. A measure of behaviors that have the potential to contribute to pleasant experiences of patients with dementia is the Pleasant Events Schedule-AD (PES-AD) (Teri & Logsdon, 1991). This caregiver-completed inventory of pleasant experiences rates each of 54 items on their frequency, availability, and enjoyability during the past month and has the potential to document change in patients' positive experiences.

The impact of dementia on caregivers cannot be overlooked. There is a burgeoning literature on the caregivers' role in maintaining the person in quality surroundings and the impact caregiving has on the care provider (Ory et al., 2000). Although caregiving for any disabled individual is burdensome, the range, frequency, and severity of cognitive deficits and problem behaviors associated with dementia can produce stresses that are physically demanding and unremitting. As level of patient dysfunction increases, caregiver outcomes such as perceived burden and depression have been found to increase (Schulz & Williamson, 1991). As a result, a plethora of caregiving interventions, ranging from information and resources, individual and family counseling, and support groups, to reducing caregiver stress and teaching skills to manage patient behaviors have appeared in the literature (Bourgeois et al., 2002; Kennet et al., 2000). Specific techniques to improve communication (i.e., the FOCUSED approach; Ripich et al., 1998) and cognition (Quayhagen et al., 1995) have utilized caregivers as trainers. Although it is too early for strong causal relationships to be seen, a working hypothesis of caregiver interventionists is that a happier, or less burdened, caregiver will make for a more contented patient and an overall improvement in the quality of life of all members of the patient's environment. In contrast, when caregivers are frustrated and burdened by caregiving challenges, patients are more likely to be institutionalized (Steele et al., 1990).

Treatment

The two approaches to treatment of dementia are pharmacologic and behavioral. In the past 20 years neuropathologic advances have led to a cholinergic hypothesis of geriatric memory dysfunction and the resultant development of a series of cholinesterase-inhibiting drugs that have produced statistically significant improvements in cognitive functioning in patients with dementia (Wilkinson, 2000). The first promising drug, tacrine (Cognex), showed significant improvements over placebo on cognitive testing, but serious liver function and gastrointestinal side effects prevented 70% of the patients from completing the 30-week study trial (Knapp et al., 1994). Subsequent variant compounds, donepezil (Aricept), rivastigmine (Exelon), and galantamine (Reminyl), have addressed many of the problems with side effects, dosing frequency, and tolerability and have shown increased efficacy on measures of cognitive functioning and activities of daily living. In addition, rivastigmine has been reported to improve noncognitive symptoms such as apathy, delusions, hallucinations, and agitation in patients with dementia with Lewy bodies. Unfortunately, the positive effects of these drugs are not maintained for longer than a couple of years, after which the degenerative nature of the disease continues its downward trajectory.

Many of the difficult behavioral symptoms of dementia, including mood disturbance, altered perception, agitation, aggression, anxiety, and sleep and appetite disturbances, are treated pharmacologically with a variety of antipsychotics, anxiolytics, sedatives, antidepressants, and other medications (Rosenquist et al., 2000). Because clinical trials and efficacy data for specific drugs and targeted behaviors are very limited, clinicians are advised to prescribe drugs only after nonpharmacologic approaches have been exhausted. Further recommendations are to start with low doses, to increase dose slowly, and to monitor target behaviors and signs of toxicity.

The nonpharmacologic, or behavioral, approaches to treating the challenging symptoms of dementia have seen an explosion in interest and publications in recent years. The old nihilistic attitude that nothing could be done for the patient so only focus on the caregiver has been replaced by a more holistic and humanistic approach intended to maintain function and prevent excess disability (Clark, 1995). Since ASHA's Committee on Communication Problems of the Aging published its mandate for speech-language pathologists to increase their involvement in the evaluation and management of patients with dementia, there has been an increase in the development of treatment programs designed to facilitate or maintain functional communication and to improve the quality of life of these individuals and their families (ASHA, 1988). Professionals in disciplines ranging from physical, occupational, music, and recreation therapy to psychology, psychiatry, and nursing have produced a plethora of therapeutic strategies and approaches, some with empirical support, others steeped in clinical lore (Bird, 2000).

Memory Treatment Strategies

Treatment of memory impairment is either internal or external in focus. Internal strategies involve some mental manipulation of the information to be remembered, such as mnemonic techniques and visual association strategies, and may be more useful for people experiencing normal memory changes due to aging. Even in the early stages of dementia, however, persons might not have the learning ability or motivation to use these techniques; instead, techniques that aim to reduce the demand on a person's memory and compensate for the impairment may be more effective (Camp et al., 2000). External memory strategies take advantage of cues in the environment to trigger recall. For example, written reminders, calendars, memo boards, notepads, sticky notes, and designated places for objects can help persons to remember to do a task, to keep an appointment, or to operate an appliance, such as the television remote control, especially if they are kept in close proximity to the relevant task or activity. Bourgeois (1990) explored the use of written and picture cues, in the form of Memory Wallets, to assist in the retrieval of personal information necessary to maintain conversations between persons with AD and their caregivers. Simple declarative sentences, one per page, and a relevant photograph or illustration were sufficient to cue the reading of that sentence, to elicit elaborated comments about the topic, and to reduce the frequency of ambiguous and repetitive verbalizations. Increased turn-taking and topic maintenance and reduced partner prompting and conversational dominance were found with the use of memory aids (Bourgeois, 1993; Hoerster et al., 2001). Subsequent studies demonstrated that persons with various degrees of cognitive impairment were able to improve their conversations using memory books that were modified to address their specific functional impairments (e.g., enlarging print size, making them wearable for wanderers) (Bourgeois, 1992). Specific problem behaviors, such as repetitive questions about a dead relative or the status of a tax return, were addressed by including a page in the memory book that answered the question (e.g., "Mary died in 1994 and is buried in Westlawn Cemetery"; "Your pension checks are deposited in the bank on Monday."). The repetitive verbalizations of patients with dementia were reduced by training spouses to use written cuing strategies (e.g., cue cards, memo boards, memory book pages) (Bourgeois et al., 1997). Institutional caregivers, nursing assistants, were trained to use portable, laminated memory books to increase comprehension and cooperation with care activities, such as bathing and grooming, by residents with dementia (Bourgeois et al., 2001).

A memory training procedure, spaced retrieval, involves the retention of and ability to recall information for long time periods by recalling information over successively longer intervals (Brush & Camp, 1998). Based on the principles of classical conditioning and repetition priming, spaced retrieval takes advantage of the relatively preserved skills of reading, motor learning, and procedural memory to help patients remember specific facts (e.g., family members' names, their room number) and functional strategies (e.g., use of a memo board or scheduled activities card, safe swallowing steps). Camp et al. (1996) programmatically evaluated the spaced-retrieval method of learning and retraining information to train tasks such as face-name association, object-location associations, and calendar use.

Environmental Strategies

Lindsley (1964) advocated the use of prosthetic environments, or more supportive physical and social environments, to overcome the declining competencies of old age. Dementia-specific environments, such as

special care units in the nursing home, use physical design and culture of care changes to effect a minimally challenging environment for patients that maximizes their quality of life (Cohen, 1994). A variety of other treatment approaches that change the stimulus characteristics of the environment, or something in the environment, have led to promising outcomes (Table 13–1). Listening to pleasant "white noise" (waterfall and nature sounds) via headphones reduced the disruptive vocalizations of nursing home residents with dementia (Burgio et al., 1996). The delivery of verbal cues at regularly scheduled intervals is the basis of prompted voiding techniques for reducing incontinence due to forgetting (Schnelle, 1990). Visual barriers, in the form of stop signs, directional signs, grid lines on the floor, or nature posters, have been used to prevent exit seeking and to promote safe wandering (Namazi et al., 1989). Subjects in a "breakfast club" intervention demonstrated increases in cross-conversation, questioning, use of each other's name, eye contact, and topic maintenance when using a variety of verbal, visual, and tactile prompts (Santo Pietro & Boczko, 1997a). Lund et al. (1995) used video respite tapes to increase engagement in a group activity as measured by the duration of time patients remained seated, were paying attention, and were smiling, laughing, and making verbal comments in response to the tape. Similarly, Orsulic-Jeras et al. (2000) documented significantly more constructive engagement, less passive engagement, and more pleasure when residents with dementia participated in Montessori-based activities (Camp, 1999). Music was demonstrated to reduce agitation during meals (Goddaer & Abraham, 1994). Cognitive skills training and a multitude of activity-focused techniques from various disciplines have produced skill maintenance and problem behavior reduction in persons with dementia (Arkin, 1999; Eisner, 2001; Hellen, 1992; Lawton & Rubinstein, 2000; Tappen, 1997; Volicer & Bloom-Charette, 1999).

The past decade has seen vast advances in the diagnosis and treatment of dementia in its many forms. There is increasing hope

Table 13–1. Specific Treatment Tasks

When Memory Impairments Cause:	*Suggested Treatment Techniques Are:*
Impaired conversation (word finding problems, ambiguity, inaccuracy, repetition)	Memory wallets, books, cards, notebooks Caregiver training
Encoding, short-term memory problems (repetitive questions, forgetting the answers to the questions, losing or misplacing things)	Variety of stimulus modalities for encoding information Repetition and practice: spaced retrieval Establish routines and schedules
Comprehension deficits (lack of cooperation)	Written cues: cards, memo boards Use one-step verbal instructions
Information retrieval deficits	Written, auditory, tactile cues Use two-choice questions; use personal objects, pictures, music, smells to trigger memories
Confusion and agitation	Calming music and nature sounds, other sensory stimulation (tactile: stuffed animals, dolls; visual: interest albums)
Apathy, lack of interest	Activity programs: Montessori, music, therapeutic recreation, pet therapy
Swallowing problems	Written cues Spaced retrieval to use cue card Caregiver training

that the causes of dementia will soon be identified and effective cures will follow in due time. In the interim, creative and effective management strategies are lessening the daily challenges of these unremitting diseases.

References

Albert, M.S. (1994). Brief Assessments of Cognitive Function in the Elderly. In: M.P. Lawton & J.A. Teresi (Eds.), *Annual Review of Gerontology and Geriatrics Focus on Assessment Techniques* (vol. 4, pp. 93–106). New York: Springer.

American Psychiatric Association (1994). *Diagnostic and Statistical Manual of Mental Disorders (DSM-IV)* (4th ed.). Washington, DC: APA.

Arkin, S. (1999). Elder Rehab: A Student-Supervised Exercise Program for Alzheimer's Patients. *The Gerontologist, 39,* 729–735.

ASHA Committee on Communication Problems of the Aging. (1988). The Roles of Speech-Language Pathologists and Audiologists in Working with Older Persons. *ASHA, 30,* 80–84.

Baddeley A. (1995). The Psychology of Memory. In: A.D. Baddeley, B.A. Wilson & F.N. Watts (Eds.), *Handbook of Memory Disorders* (pp. 3–26). New York: John Wiley.

Baddeley, A., Emslie, H. & Nimmo-Smith, I. (1994). *Doors and People.* England: Thames Valley.

Ballard, C. (2000). Criteria for the Diagnosis of Dementia. In: J. O'Brien, D. Ames & A. Burns (Eds.), *Dementia* (2nd ed., pp. 29–40). London: Arnold.

Barber, R. & O'Brien, J. (2000). Structural and Functional Magnetic Resonance Imaging (MRI). In: J. O'Brien, D. Ames & A. Burns (Eds.), *Dementia* (2nd ed., pp. 115–130). London: Arnold.

Baum, H., Swigert, N. & Gallahger, T. (1997). Treatment Outcomes Data for Adults in Health Care Environments. *ASHA, 39,* 26–31.

Bayles, K.A. & Kaszniak, A.W. (1987). *Communication and Cognition in Normal Aging and Dementia.* Boston: College-Hill Press.

Bayles, K.A. & Tomoeda, C. (1991). *The Arizona Battery for Communication Disorders of Dementia.* Tuscon, AR: Canyonlands.

Bayles, K.A. & Tomoeda, C. (1994). *Functional Linguistic Communication Inventory.* Tuscon, AR: Canyonlands.

Benton, A.L. (1974). *Revised Visual Retention Test: Clinical and Experimental Application* (4th ed.). New York: Psychological Corporation.

Berrios, G.E. (1987). History of the Functional Psychoses. *British Medical Bulletin, 43,* 484–498.

Bird, M. (2000). Psychosocial Management of Behaviour Problems in Dementia. In: J. O'Brien, D. Ames & A. Burns (Eds.), *Dementia* (2nd ed., pp. 603–613). London: Arnold.

Blessed, G., Block, S., Butters, T. & Kay, D. (1991). The Diagnosis of Dementia in the Elderly: A Comparison of CAMCOG (the Cognitive Section of the CAMDEX), the AGE-CAT Program, DSM-II, the Mini-Mental State Examination and Some Short Rating Scales. *British Journal of Psychiatry, 159,* 193–198.

Blessed, G., Tomlinson, B.E. & Roth, M. (1968). The Association Between Quantitative Measures of Dementia and of Senile Changes in the Cerebral Grey Matter of Elderly Subjects. *Journal of Psychiatry, 114,* 797–811.

Borkowski, J.G., Benton, A.L. & Spreen, O. (1967). Word Fluency and Brain Damage. *Neuropsychologia, 5,* 135–140.

Bourgeois, M. (1990). Enhancing Conversation Skills in Alzheimer's Disease Using a Prosthetic Memory Aid. *Journal of Applied Behavior Analysis, 23,* 29–42.

Bourgeois, M. (1992). Evaluating Memory Wallets in Conversations with Patients with Dementia. *Journal of Speech and Hearing Research, 35,* 1344–1357.

Bourgeois, M. (1993). Effects of Memory Aids on the Dyadic Conversations of Individuals with Dementia. *Journal of Applied Behavior Analysis, 26,* 77–87.

Bourgeois, M., Burgio, L., Schulz, R., Beach, S. & Palmer, B. (1997). Modifying Repetitive Verbalization of Community Dwelling Patients with AD. *The Gerontologist, 37,* 30–39.

Bourgeois, M., Dijkstra, K., Burgio, L. & Allen-Burge, R. (2001). Memory Aids as an AAC Strategy for Nursing Home Residents with Dementia. *Augmentative and Alternative Communication, 17,* 196–210.

Bourgeois, M., Schulz, R., Burgio, L. & Beach, S. (2002). Skills Training for Spouses of Patients with Alzheimer's Disease: Outcomes of an Intervention Study. *Journal of Clinical Geropsychology, 8,* 53–73.

Brookmeyer, R., Gray, S. & Kawas, C. (1998). Projections of Alzheimer's Disease in the United States and the Public Health Impact of Delaying Disease Onset. *American Journal of Public Health, 88,* 1337–1342.

Brun, A., Englund, B., Gustafson, L., Passant, U., Mann, D., Neary, D. & Snowden, J. (1994). Consensus Statement. Clinical and Neuropathological Criteria for Fronto-Temporal Dementia. *Journal of Neurology, Neurosurgery and Psychiatry, 4,* 416–418.

Brush, J.A. & Camp, C.J. (1998). *A Therapy Technique for Improving Memory: Spaced Retrieval.* Beachwood, OH: Menorah Park Center for the Aging.

Burgio, L., Scilley, K., Hardin, J., Hsu, C. & Yancy, J. (1996). Environmental "White Noise": An Intervention for Verbally Agitated Nursing Home Resident. *Journals of Gerontology, 51,* P364–373.

Camp, C.J. (1999). *Montessori-Based Activities for Persons with Dementia* (vol 1). Beachwood, OH: Menorah Park Center for the Aging.

Camp, C., Bird, M. & Cherry, K. (2000). Retrieval Strategies as a Rehabilitation Aid for Cognitive Loss in Pathological Aging. In: R. Hill, L. Backman & A. Stiggsdotter-Neely (Eds.), *Cognitive Rehabilitation in Old Age* (pp. 224–248). Oxford: Oxford University Press.

Camp, C., Foss, J.W., Stevens, A.B. & O'Hanlon, A.M. (1996). Improving Prospective Memory Task Performance in Alzheimer's Disease. In: M.A. Brandimonte, G.O. Einstein, & M.A. McDaniel (Eds.), *Prospective Memory: Theory and Applications* (pp. 351–367). Mahwah, NJ: Lawrence Erlbaum & Assoc.

Christensen, H. & O'Brien, J. (2000). Age-Related Cognitive Decline and Its Relationship to Dementia. In: J. O'Brien, D. Ames & A. Burns (Eds.), *Dementia* (2nd ed., pp. 15–27). London: Arnold.

Chua, P. & Chiu, E. (2000). Huntington's Disease. In: J. O'Brien, D. Ames & A. Burns (Eds.), *Dementia* (2nd ed., pp. 827–843). London: Arnold.

Clark L. (1995). Interventions for Persons with Alzheimer's Disease: Strategies for Maintaining and Enhancing Communicative Success. *Topics in Language Disorders, 15,* 47–65.

Cohen, G. (1994). Foreword: Towards New Models of Dementia Care. *Alzheimer Disease and Associated Disorders, 8,* 2–4.

Cohen-Mansfield, J. & Billig, N. (1986). Agitated Behavior in the Elderly. 1. A Conceptual Review. *Journal of the American Geriatrics Society, 34,* 711–721.

DeRenzi, E. & Faglioni, P. (1978) Normative Data and Screening Power of a Shortened Version of the Token Test. *Cortex, 14,* 41–49.

Dunn, L.M. & Dunn, L.M. (1981). *Peabody Picture Vocabulary Test–Revised.* Circle Pines, MN: American Guidance Service.

Eastley, R. & Wilcock, G. (2000). Assessment and Differential Diagnosis of Dementia. In: J. O'Brien, D. Ames & A. Burns (Eds.), *Dementia* (2nd ed., pp. 41–47). London: Arnold.

Eisner, E. (2001). *Can Do Activities for Adults with Alzheimer's Disease.* Austin, TX: Pro-Ed.

Erkinjuntti, T. (2000). Vascular Dementia: An Overview. In: J. O'Brien, D. Ames & A. Burns (Eds.), *Dementia* (2nd ed., pp. 623–634). London: Arnold.

Everall, I. (2000). Human Immunodeficiency Virus Type 1 Associated Dementia: Pathology, Clinical Features and Treatment. In: J. O'Brien, D. Ames & A. Burns (Eds.), *Dementia* (2nd ed., pp. 877–896). London: Arnold.

Folstein, N.F., Folstein, S.E. & McHugh, P.R. (1975). Mini-Mental State: A Practical Method for Grading the Cognitive State of Patients for the Clinician. *Journal of Psychiatric Research, 12,* 189–198.

Frattali, C. (1994). Functional Assessment. In: R. Lubinski and C. Frattali (Eds.), *Professional Issues in Speech-Language Pathology and Audiology* (pg. 306–320). San Diego, CA: Singular.

Frattali, C., Thompson, C., Holland, A., Wohl, C. & Ferketic, M. (1995). The FACS of Life: ASHA FACS—A Functional Outcome Measure for Adults. *ASHA, 37,* 40–46.

Frederick, B., Moore, C. & Renshaw, P. (2000). Magnetic Resonance Spectroscopy in Dementia. In: J. O'Brien, D. Ames & A. Burns (Eds.), *Dementia* (2nd ed., pp. 131–149). London: Arnold.

Fuld, P.A. (1981). *The Fuld Object Memory Evaluation.* Chicago: Stoelting Instrument Company.

Galasko, D., Salmon, D.P., Lineweaver, T., Hansen, L. & Thal, L.J. (1998). Neuropsychological Measures Distinguish Patients with Lewy Body Variant from Those with Alzheimer's Disease. *Neurology, 50,* A181.

Goddaer, J. & Abraham, I.L. (1994). Effects of Relaxing Music on Agitation During Meals Among Nursing Home Residents with Severe Impairment. *Archives of Psychiatric Nursing, 8,* 150–158.

Goodglass H. & Kaplan, E. (1983). The Boston Diagnostic Aphasia Examination. In: H. Goodglass & E. Kaplan (Eds.), *The Assessment of Aphasia and Related Disorders* (rev. ed.). Philadelphia: Lea & Febiger.

Greene, J.D.W., Patterson, K., Xuereb, J. & Hodges, J.R. (1996). Alzheimer's Disease and Nonfluent Progressive Aphasia. *Archives of Neurology, 53,* 1072–1078.

Hellen, C.R. (1992). *Alzheimer's Disease: Activity-Focused Care*. Boston: Andover Medical Publishers.

Helmes, E., Csapo, K.G. & Short, J.A. (1987). Standardization and Validation of the Multidimensional Observation Scale for Elderly Subjects (MOSES). *Journal of Gerontology, 42*, 395–405.

Hodges, J.R. & Patterson, K. (1995). Is Semantic Memory Consistently Impaired Early in the Course of Alzheimer's Disease: Neuroanatomical and Diagnostic Implications. *Neuropsycholgia, 33*, 441–459.

Hoerster, L., Hickey, E. & Bourgeois, M. (2001). Effects of Memory Aids on Conversations Between Nursing Home Residents with Dementia and Nursing Assistants. *Neuropsychological Rehabilitation, 11*, 399–427.

Holland, A., Frattali, C. & Fromm, D. (1999). *Communicative Abilities in Daily Living—CADL 2*. Austin, TX: Pro-Ed.

Howard, D. & Patterson, K. (1992). *Pyramids and Palm Trees*. England: Thames Valley.

Howard, K. & Rockwood, K. (1995). Quality of Life in Alzheimer's Disease. *Dementia, 6*, 113–116.

Hughes, C.P., Berg, L., Danziger, W.L., Cohen, L.A. & Martin, R.L. (1982). A New Clinical Scale for the Staging of Dementia. *British Journal of Psychiatry, 140*, 566–572.

Ince, P., Perry, R. & Perry, E. (2000). Pathology of Dementia with Lewy Bodies. In: J. O'Brien, D. Ames & A. Burns (Eds.), *Dementia* (2nd ed., pp. 699–717). London: Arnold.

Jorm, A.F. (2000). Risk Factors for Alzheimer's Disease. In: J. O'Brien, D. Ames & A. Burns (Eds.), *Dementia* (2nd ed., pp. 383–390). London: Arnold.

Kane, R.A. & Kane, R.L. (Eds.) (2000). *Assessing Older Persons: Measures, Meaning, and Practical Applications*. New York: Oxford University Press.

Kaplan, E., Goodglass, H. & Weintraub, S. (1983). *Boston Naming Test*. Philadelphia: Lea & Febiger.

Kennedy, A. (2000). Positron Emission Tomography in Dementia. In: J. O'Brien, D. Ames & A. Burns (Eds.), *Dementia* (2nd ed., pp. 163–177). London: Arnold.

Kennet, J., Burgio, L. & Schulz, R. (2000). Interventions for In-Home Caregivers: A Review of Research 1990 to Present. In: R. Schulz (Ed.), *Handbook on Dementia Caregiving* (pp. 61–126). New York: Springer.

Kertesz A. (1982). *Western Aphasia Battery*. New York: Grune and Stratton.

Knapp, M.J., Knopman, D.S., Solomon, P.R., Pendlebury, W.W., Davis, C.S., Gracon, S.I. (1994). A 30-Week Randomized Controlled Trial of High-Dose Tacrine in Patients with Alzheimer's Disease. *Journal of the American Medical Association, 271*, 985–991.

Kopelman, M., Wilson, B. & Baddeley, A. (1990). *The Autobiographical Memory Interview*. England: Thames Valley.

Kovar, M.G. & Lawton, M.P. (1994). Functional Disability: Activities and Instrumental Activities of Daily Living. In: M.P. Lawton & J.A. Teresi (Eds.), *Annual Review of Gerontology and Geriatrics Focus on Assessment Techniques* (vol. 4, pp. 57–75). New York: Springer.

Lantos, P. & Cairns, N. (2000). The Neuropathology of Alzheimer's Disease. In: J. O'Brien, D. Ames & A. Burns (Eds.), *Dementia* (2nd ed., pp. 443–459). London: Arnold.

Lawton, M.P. (1991). A Multidimensional View of Quality of Life in Frail Elderly. In: J.E. Birren, J.E. Lubben, J.C. Rowe & D.E. Deutchman (Eds.), *The Concept and Measurement of Quality of Life in the Frail Elderly* (pp. 3–27). San Diego: Academic Press.

Lawton, M.P. & Rubinstein, R.L. (Eds.). (2000). *Interventions in Dementia Care: Toward Improving Quality of Life*. New York: Springer.

Lawton, M.P., Van Haitsma, K. & Klapper, J. (1996). Observed Affect in Nursing Home Residents with Alzheimer's Disease. *Journal of Gerontology: Psychological Sciences, 51B*, P3–P14.

Liberman, A. (1998). Managing the Neuropsychiatric Symptoms of Parkinson's Disease. *Neurology, 50*, S33–38.

Lindsley, O.R. (1964). Geriatric Behavioural Prosthetics. In: R. Kastenbaum (Ed.), *New Thoughts on Old Age*. New York: Springer.

Lubinski, R. (Ed.). (1991). *Dementia and Communication*. Philadelphia: B.C. Decker.

Lund, D.A., Hill, R.D., Caserta, M.S. & Wright, S.D. (1995). Video Respite: An Innovative Resource for Family, Professional Caregivers, and Persons with Dementia. *Gerontologist, 35*, 683–687.

McKeith, I.G., Fairbairn, A. & Harrison, R. (1996). Management of the Non-Cognitive Symptoms of Lewy Body Dementia. In: Perry, R.H., McKeith, I.G. & Perry, E.K. (Eds.), *Dementia with Lewy Bodies* (pp. 381–396). London: Cambridge University Press.

Mirea, A. & Cummings, J. (2000). Neuropsychiatric Aspects of Dementia. In: J. O'Brien, D. Ames & A. Burns (Eds.), *Dementia* (2nd ed., pp. 61–79). London: Arnold.

Mohs, R.C. (1995). Assessment of Cognition in Clinical Trials of Drugs for the Treatment of Dementia. In: M. Bergener & S.J. Finkel (Eds.), *Treating Alzheimer's and Other Dementias* (pp. 347–357). New York: Springer.

Moss, M.B., Albert, M.S., Butters, N. & Payne, M. (1986). Differential Patterns of Memory Loss Among Patients with Alzheimer's Disease, Huntington's Disease, and Alcoholic Korsakoff's Syndrome. *Archives of Neurology, 43*, 239–246.

Mungas, D., Marshall, S.C., Welson, M., Haan, M. & Reed, B.R. (1996). Age and Education Correction of Mini-Mental State Examination for English- and Spanish-Speaking Elderly. *Neurology, 46*, 700–706.

Namazi, K., Rosner, T. & Calkins, M. (1989). Visual Barriers to Prevent Ambulatory Alzheimer's Patients from Exiting Through an Emergency Door. *The Gerontologist, 29*, 699–702.

Neary, D. (2000). Frontotemporal Dementia. In: J. O'Brien, D. Ames & A. Burns (Eds.), *Dementia* (2nd ed., pp. 737–746). London: Arnold.

Orsulic-Jeras, S., Judge, K. & Camp, C.J. (2000). Montessori-Based Activities for Long-Term Care Residents with Advanced Dementia: Effects on Engagement and Affect. *The Gerontologist, 40*, 107–111.

Ory, M., Yee, J., Tennstedt, S. & Schulz, R. (2000). The Extent and Impact of Dementia Care: Unique Challenges Experienced by Family Caregivers. In: R. Schulz (ed.), *Handbook on Dementia Caregiving* (pp. 1–32). New York: Springer.

Paulesu, E., Frith, C.D. & Frackowiak, R.S.J. (1993). The Neural Correlates of the Verbal Components of Working Memory. *Nature, 362*, 342–345.

Pearlson, G.D., Rabins, P.V. & Burns, A. (1991). CT Changes in Centrum Semiovale White Matter in

Dementia of Depression. *Psychological Medicine, 21,* 321–328.

Quayhagen, M.P., Quayhagen, M., Corbeil, R.R., Roth, P.A. & Rodgers, J.A. (1995). A Dyadic Remediation Program for Care Recipients with Dementia. *Nursing Research, 44,* 153–159.

Rabins, P.V., Kasper, J.D., Kleinman, L., Black, B. & Patrick, D.L. (1999). Concepts and Methods in the Development of the ADRQL: An Instrument for Assessing Health-Related Quality of Life in Persons with Alzheimer Disease. *Journal of Mental Health and Aging, 5,* 33–48.

Ray, W.A., Taylor, J.A., Lichtenstein, M.J. & Meador, K.G. (1992). The Nursing Home Behavior Problem Scale. *Journals of Gerontology: Medical Sciences, 47,* M9–M16.

Reisberg, B., Borenstein, J., Salob, S.P., Ferris, S.H., Franssen, E. & Georgotas, A. (1987). Behavioral Symptoms in Alzheimer's Disease: Phenomenology and Treatment. *Journal of Clinical Psychiatry, 48*(suppl.), 9–15.

Reisberg, B., Ferris, S., deLeon, M. & Crook, T. (1982). The Global Deterioration Scale for Assessment of Primary Degenerative Dementia. *American Journal of Psychiatry, 139,* 1136–1139.

Ripich, D. (1991). Language and Communication in Dementia. In: D. Ripich (Ed.), *Geriatric Communication Disorders* (pp. 255–292). Austin, TX: Pro-Ed.

Ripich, D., Ziol, E. & Lee, M.M. (1998). Longitudinal Effects of Communication Training on Caregivers of Persons with Alzheimer's Disease. *Clinical Gerontologist, 19,* 37–55.

Rosen, W.G., Mohs, R.C. & Davis, K.L. (1984). A New Rating Scale for Alzheimer's Disease. *American Journal of Psychiatry, 141,* 1356–1364.

Rosenquist, K., Tariot, P. & Loy, R. (2000). Treatments for Behavioral and Psychological Symptoms in Alzheimer's Disease and Other Dementias. In: J. O'Brien, D. Ames & A. Burns (Eds.), *Dementia* (2nd ed., pp. 571–601). London: Arnold.

Russell, E.W. (1975). A Multiple Scoring Method for the Assessment of Complex Memory Functions. *Journal of Consulting & Clinical Psychology, 43,* 800–809.

Santo Pietro, M.J. & Boczko, R. (1997a). The Breakfast Club and Related Programs. In: B. Shadden and M.A. Toner (Eds.), *Aging and Communication* (pp. 341–359). Austin, TX: Pro-Ed.

Santo Pietro, M.J. & Boczko, R. (1997b). *Communication Outcome Measure of Functional Independence (COMFI Scale).* Vero Beach, FL: Speech Bin.

Saxton, J., McGonigle-Gibson, K., Swihart, A., Miller, V. & Boller, F. (1990). Assessment of the Severely Impaired Patient: Description and Validation of a New Neuropsychological Test Battery. *Psychological Assessment, 12,* 298–303.

Schnelle, J.F. (1990). Treatment of Urinary Incontinence in Nursing Home Patients by Prompted Voiding. *Journal of the American Geriatrics Society, 38,* 356–360.

Schulz, R., O'Brien, A.T. & Tompkins, C. (1994). The Measurement of Affect in the Elderly. In: M.P. Lawton & J.A. Teresi (Eds.), *Annual Review of Gerontology and Geriatrics: Focus on Assessment Techniques* (pp. 210–233). New York: Springer.

Schulz, R. & Williamson, G.M. (1991). A 2-year Longitudinal Study of Depression Among Alzheimer's Caregivers. *Psychology and Aging, 6,* 569–578.

Selai, C.E., Trimble, M.R., Rossor, M.N. & Harvey, R.J. (2000). The Quality of Life Assessment Schedule (QOLAS)—A New Method for Assessing Quality of Life (QOL) in Dementia. In: S.M. Albert and R.G. Logsdon (Eds.), *Assessing Quality of Life in Alzheimer's Disease* (pp. 31–50). New York: Springer.

Shewan, C.M. (1979). *Auditory Comprehension Test for Sentences.* Chicago: Biolinguistics Clinical Institutes.

Steele, C., Rovner, B., Chase, G. & Folstein, M. (1990). Psychiatric Symptoms and Nursing Home Placement of Patients with Alzheimer's Disease. *American Journal of Psychiatry, 147,* 1049–1051.

Tappen, R.M. (1997). *Interventions for Alzheimer's Disease: A Caregiver's Complete Reference.* Baltimore, MD: Health Professions Press.

Teri, L. & Logsdon, R.G. (1991). Identifying Pleasant Activities for Alzheimer's Disease Patients: The Pleasant Events Schedule-AD. *The Gerontologist, 31,* 124–127.

Teri, L. & Logsdon, R.G. (1994). Assessment of Behavioral Disturbance in Older Adults. In: M.P. Lawton & J.A. Teresi (Eds.), *Annual Review of Gerontology and Geriatrics: Focus on Assessment Techniques* (pp. 107–124). New York: Springer.

Velakoulis, D. & Lloyd, J. (2000). Parkinson's Disease and Dementia: Prevalence and Incidence. In: J. O'Brien, D. Ames & A. Burns (Eds.), *Dementia* (2nd ed., pp. 845–852). London: Arnold.

Volicer, L. & Bloom-Charette, L. (Eds.). (1999). *Enhancing the Quality of Life in Advanced Dementia.* Philadelphia: Brunner/Mazel.

Welsh, K.A., Butters, N., Mohs, R.C., Beekly, D., Edland, S., Fillenbaum, G. & Heyman, A. (1994). The Consortium to Establish a Registry for Alzheimer's Disease (CERAD). Part V. A Normative Study of the Neuropsychological Battery. *Neurology, 44,* 609–614.

Wilkinson, D. (2000). How Effective are Cholinergic Therapies in Improving Cognition in Alzheimer's Disease. In: J. O'Brien, D. Ames & A. Burns (Eds.), *Dementia* (2nd ed., pp. 549–558). London: Arnold.

Wilson, B., Cockburn, J. & Baddeley, A. (1991). *The Rivermead Behavioral Memory Test* (rev. 2nd ed.). England: Thames Valley.

Zimmerman, S. & Magaziner, J. (1994). Methodological Issues in Measuring the Functional Status of Cognitively Impaired Nursing Home Residents: The Use of Proxies and Performance-Based Measures. *Alzheimer Disease and Associated Disorders, 8,* S281–S290.

14

Right Hemisphere Syndrome

MARGARET LEHMAN BLAKE

The notion that the right cerebral hemisphere adds important contributions to language processing was first considered by Hughlings Jackson in the 1870s (Jackson, 1874/1958). However, only during the past quarter century have we realized how important this "nondominant" side of the brain is for efficient communication processes. These discoveries were made in the 1970s when aphasiologists using adults with right hemisphere brain damage (RHD) as "control" subjects noticed that these individuals did not perform as well as non-brain-damaged adults on language tasks (Gardner, 1994). Much of the research that grew out of these observations was largely descriptive, as is necessary upon initial consideration of a disorder. The past 10 years have seen an increase in carefully controlled experimental studies designed to go beyond description of the problems to identifying underlying deficits and at what stages of processing breakdowns may occur. The eventual goal of this research is to improve the techniques used for evaluation and treatment of individuals with RHD. As our understanding of the deficits improves, so will our ideas on how best to approach them in a clinical setting.

This chapter discusses our current knowledge about the disorders associated with RHD, and our best existing assessment and treatment methods. Despite the increased interest and research in this area, we currently do not have a standard or well-accepted term for the deficits associated with RHD.

Common labels include right hemisphere syndrome, right hemisphere cognitive-communicative deficits, and right hemisphere cognitive-linguistic deficits. The words *communication* or *linguistic* often are used in clinical settings to ensure payment of services by third-party payers. The lack of an accepted label creates difficulties in communicating about the disorders with our patients, their families, and other medical professionals.

Pathophysiology

Damage to the right hemisphere is caused by the same mechanisms that cause damage to the left hemisphere: stroke, tumors, head injury, or disease processes. Despite the similarity in etiologies, there are striking differences in our understanding of localization within the left and right hemispheres. Unlike our study of the left hemisphere, we have not found any obvious localization of language or communication processes within the right hemisphere. Difficulties establishing localization of function within the right hemisphere could be partially due to the fact that many studies to date have used only a gross classification of lesion location, simply anterior versus posterior to the central sulcus. This division may be too imprecise to identify specific localizations. Another factor is that the right hemisphere has more white matter and less gray matter than the left side of the brain, suggesting more intrahemispheric connections between neurons within the right hemisphere (Gur et al., 1980). Thus, specific abilities may be the result of processing by large networks instead of relatively restricted areas dedicated to specific functions. For example, attentional processes, which frequently are impaired after RHD, are posited to arise from a large network that involves several cortical and subcortical areas, including the frontal and parietal lobes as well as the cingulate gyrus, hypothalamus, and the reticular system (Cohen, 1993).

One could speculate that complex neuronal networks would be necessary for various communicative processes impacted by RHD. For example, discourse comprehension involves linking multiple sentences together to understand main ideas or themes, or integrating disparate clues to generate a single interpretation; interpretation of humor, affect, or sarcasm may require reinterpretation of a literal meaning based on contextual, situational, or prosodic cues. Disorders of these communicative processes could be due to damage to neuronal networks within the right hemisphere that integrate information from various sources, rather than damage to small localized areas.

Nature and Differentiating Features

One obstacle in diagnosing RHD deficits is that there are no clear boundaries between normal and abnormal behavior for many of the pragmatic and cognitive abilities affected by RHD, given the wide range of what is considered "normal" in the general population. Thus, it is critical to discuss a patient's behaviors with his/her family to determine which ones may be new, or abnormal, and which ones are consistent with the patient's pre-stroke behavior.

It is important to remember that not all individuals with RHD exhibit communication deficits. Estimates suggest that approximately half of a nonselect group of adults with RHD have verbal communication impairments (Joanette & Goulet, 1994),

whereas 95% of adults with RHD admitted to a rehabilitation unit may have some type of cognitive or communicative deficit (Blake et al., 2002). Additionally, the patterns of deficits and severity of those deficits may differ widely across individuals.

Adults with RHD may seem to be communicatively competent upon initial or superficial contact. Deficits usually appear with more in-depth conversational exchange and social interaction. After RHD, individuals may exhibit either hypo- or hyperresponsivity. A person with the typical hyporesponsive characteristics exhibits paucity of speech, producing short, curt answers to questions. Affective responsivity may be reduced, as expressed through facial expression, prosody, and/or lexical selection. Conversely, a person with typical hyperresponsive characteristics produces verbose responses that may be tangential. She may talk excessively without ever really answering a question or getting to the point; her responses may include various details that are related to the topic, but the main idea must be inferred by the listener. She may laugh easily, tell inappropriate jokes or otherwise display inappropriate humor, and appear hyperanimated. The limited data available indicate that hyporesponsivity is as common as hyperresponsivity (Blake et al., 2002).

Whether hypo- or hyperresponsive, an individual's responses may be tangential to the questions, and he often may not be aware of the listener's knowledge. He may not notice when communication breakdowns occur, but even if he does, he can't always fix them. He may not make appropriate eye contact. Often it is such pragmatic aspects of communication that are the most striking, and offer the first clue that something is not quite right. The patient may deny that he has any deficits, or report that he has been told that he has problems, without personally accepting those deficits (e.g., "The doctor says I have trouble seeing things").

Potential difficulties in the cognitive realm become apparent with more in-depth communicative exchange or observation of performance on nonverbal tasks. Sequencing, organizing, problem solving, and reasoning all may be inefficient. Deficits in attention and perception also frequently occur. Again, any or all of these deficits may be present after RHD, and all may vary in severity from patient to patient.

We are beginning to refine our understanding of right hemisphere syndrome, going beyond simply describing all of the problems that can occur to determining cause, prevalence, and patterns of co-occurrence. Blake and colleagues (2002) conducted a retrospective study of a large group of adults with RHD in an inpatient rehabilitation unit. The results indicate that the most commonly diagnosed deficits are disorders of attention, visuoperception, and learning/memory. Exploratory analyses suggest that deficits in attention and learning/memory tend to co-occur, whereas difficulties with calculation and basic linguistic skills are not closely related to the other deficits. Identifying these patterns is one step in determining the underlying impairment(s) that cause the behaviorally diagnosed deficits.

For current purposes, the myriad deficits associated with RHD are divided into three general categories: communication, attention/perception, and cognition. These categories are for expository purposes only; in a patient with RHD, deficits in one area impact deficits in another area, and in some cases they may be difficult to separate. Throughout the discussion of RHD deficits, two commonalities are apparent. First, problems often surface when multiple interpretations are possible, and the comprehender must select the most appropriate meaning. Second, deficits often appear with increased demands on cognitive resources. Thus, an individual with RHD may have little difficulty with an "easy" or straightforward task, but may break down when the task becomes more "difficult." Factors that increase difficulty level include adding time constraints, inferences, or metalinguistic/metacognitive demands, such as requiring consideration of another person's point of view.

Communication

Adults with RHD usually have little or no difficulty with basic comprehension and expression. Mild deficits in word finding, verbal fluency, or auditory comprehension may be present, although careful assessment is necessary to determine whether these problems are actually due to linguistic impairments, or to other factors, such as reduced attention (Myers, 1999b; Tompkins, 1995).

FIGURATIVE/NONLITERAL LANGUAGE

One of the most commonly described RHD deficits is the misinterpretation of nonliteral language. Adults with RHD often do not fully appreciate the abstract meaning of words and phrases (Kempler et al., 1999; Myers & Linebaugh, 1981). Early research suggested that their responses reflected a literal interpretation. For example, when presented with four pictures and asked to identify which one depicts the phrase "He's a chip off the old block," a patient may select a wooden block with a piece missing rather than a father and son. However, adults with RHD do recognize idioms in implicit tasks that do not require metalinguistic judgments, despite problems in explicitly explaining those same idioms (Tompkins et al., 1992). Careful examination of patients' responses indicates they usually are not completely concrete. For example, when asked to explain the proverb "Don't cry over spilled milk," one patient said, "Don't cry about something spilled or thrown out because you can get something to take its place that may be better." She included literal aspects of the phrase, but also some fragments of the abstract meaning.

Indirect requests, such as "Can you open the window?" also can be interpreted literally. An individual with RHD may respond with a verbal response ("yes") to that question, instead of performing the action that the speaker was indirectly suggesting (Weylman et al., 1989). However, such requests are more likely to be interpreted correctly if they are used in a natural context than when taken out of context, as in experimental conditions (Vanhalle et al., 2000).

Inferencing

Generation and interpretation of inferences also may be problematic after RHD. This may cause literal, often disjointed interpretations of discourse, and may account for the factual but disorganized verbal output, which can resemble a list of details or sentences rather than a coherent story (Beeman, 1993; Benowitz et al., 1990; Wapner et al., 1981). Inferencing in adults with RHD is not completely absent, but rather the likelihood of inferencing problems depends on the type of inferences required, whether inference revisions are needed, and the availability of cognitive resources (Brownell et al., 1986; Lehman & Tompkins, 2000; Myers & Brookshire, 1996; Tompkins et al., 1994).

Basic inferences necessary to link two sentences together create few or no problems for an adult with RHD. Elaborative inferences, those that add information to a passage but are not necessary for basic understanding (e.g., predictions and character emotions), are thought to require more cognitive resources and are more likely to be impaired after RHD (see Lehman & Tompkins, 2000, for a review). However, for some individuals, even these more difficult inferences can be facilitated by a context that strongly biases toward a specific interpretation or outcome (Lehman-Blake & Tompkins, 2001).

Problems in comprehension often occur when multiple interpretations are possible and the comprehender has to select the most appropriate meaning, or when an initial interpretation must be revised. For example, the sentence "Amy admired the historic farmhouse" leads most comprehenders to believe that Amy is a tourist. However, the addition of the second sentence "If she sold it, her commission would be especially large" changes Amy's role to a realtor. Tompkins's suppression deficit hypothesis suggests that adults with RHD are able to generate multiple interpretations, but have difficulty when they must decide which of the possible interpretations is most plausible (Tompkins & Lehman, 1998; Tompkins et al., 2000, 2001). Difficulties also may occur in the presence of metacognitive demands such as attributing emotions to a story character that are different from the comprehender's emotions. An adult with RHD may provide an interpretation that is possible, but not plausible for the specific context (Wapner et al., 1981). Such inferencing deficits also are present in story description tasks. These individuals often can adequately describe a straightforward picture (e.g., a picnic scene), but are less able to comprehend and/or express nuances of inferentially complex pictures, such as Norman Rockwell prints (Myers, 1999b; Myers & Brookshire, 1996).

Discourse Organization (Macrostructure)

Difficulties with the structure of discourse are similar to problems with inferencing. RHD frequently causes deficits in the ability to identify main ideas or themes in a discourse, and/or reduced cohesion of discourse production. Adults with RHD may have difficulty explicitly identifying main ideas from written or spoken texts (Brookshire & Nicholas, 1984; Hough, 1990), and may not efficiently use themes as clues to help organize sentences into coherent stories (Schneiderman et al., 1992; Wapner et al., 1981).

Discourse production, as suggested earlier, may be characterized as off-target, disjointed, and not very organized. However, not all adults with RHD exhibit discourse production deficits (Chantraine et al., 1998; Joanette et al., 1986). When problems are present, they can occur in self-generated stories, or descriptions of pictured scenes or videos (Cherney et al. 1997; Joanette et al., 1986; Urayse et al., 1991). When discourse is based on scripts—overlearned, routinized descriptions of common activities—deficits are not readily apparent (Lojek-Osiejuk, 1996; Roman et al., 1987).

Humor

After RHD, an individual may be drawn to physical, slapstick humor. He may not be sensitive to the situation or communication partner, and thus may tell inappropriate jokes. One prevailing theory of humor appreciation suggests that comprehension of humorous material requires a two-step process: (1) detection of an incongruity, and (2) reinterpretation of the incongruous information to create coherence between the punch line and the preceding text (Brownell & Gardner, 1989). Deficits in humor caused by RHD seem to impair the second stage of humor processing, the reinterpretation. This is similar to the difficulties in inference revision discussed above. An individual with RHD often can identify that something "doesn't fit," and knows that there needs to be an element of surprise in a humorous item, but may not be able to describe why a punch line is funny, or be able to pick out an appropriate punch line that provides an adequate (and funny) explanation of the incongruity (Brownell et al., 1983; Winner et al., 1998).

PRAGMATICS

Pragmatics involves the relationship between language and social contexts, including the intent of the communication exchange. It has been suggested by some to be the crux of RHD deficits (Joanette & Ansaldo, 1999; Myers, 2001). Careful examination of conversational structure and other pragmatic features is important given the wide range of "normal" pragmatic behaviors seen in the non-brain-damaged population and evidence that efficiency of communication declines in old age (Mackenzie et al., 1999). In studies of conversational behavior, adults with RHD take fewer turns, and talk more about themselves than healthy older adults. They also may attempt to prolong conversations instead of terminating them upon cues from their conversational partner (Kennedy, 2000; Kennedy et al., 1994). They produce both direct and indirect requests in conversation, although they may not provide a reason why they are making a specific request, which healthy older adults usually do (Brownell & Stringfellow, 1999).

In discourse comprehension, adults with RHD may have difficulty using context to interpret an indirect request or a literally false statement (sarcasm or a lie) produced by a conversation partner (Stemmer et al., 1994; Weylman et al., 1989; Winner et al., 1998). They may have problems detecting tangential statements that block the normal flow of conversation, and in fixing conversational breakdowns. Additionally, they can have trouble judging the overall appropriateness of a conversation (Rehak et al., 1992).

A disruption of theory of mind has been suggested as one explanation of the pragmatic disorders that occur after RHD (Brownell & Martino, 1998; Winner et al., 1998). Theory of mind is "the ability to attribute thoughts and feelings to self and others" (Happe et al., 1999; p. 211). It involves seeing another person's point of view, and understanding how much another person knows, particularly if it is different from what you know. Adults with RHD seem to interpret information based on their own viewpoint, not taking into account another person's perspective [see also Sabbagh's (1999) description of communicative intentions]. This can explain the overpersonalization seen in their conversation, and difficulties with accurately attributing emotions to characters in a story, among other deficits. It is not clear whether RHD pragmatic deficits are best explained in relation to theory of mind impairments, or if they could be associated with the problems dealing with multiple interpretations (e.g., the patient's point of view versus a partner's perspective).

PROSODY

Prosody provides the melody of speech, and can convey meaning beyond the literal interpretation of the words in a sentence. Fundamental frequency, intensity, and duration all are manipulated to create varying intonation patterns during normal speech production. These intonation patterns convey both linguistic and emotional information.

Adults with RHD may have difficulties with both comprehension and production of prosody, a disorder called aprosodia. Listening to someone with aprosodia, you hear flat, monotone speech that may sound fast, with a robotic quality. It can be difficult to determine the speaker's emotional state, and the listener may miss important information that is not marked with emphatic stress. In addition to deficits of production, individuals with aprosodia may not appropriately interpret meaning signaled by prosodic cues. As with previously described findings regarding inferencing and humor, prosodic comprehension deficits often are most pronounced when conflicting interpretations are present, such as with sarcasm, in which the semantics and the prosody convey opposite meanings (Bowers et al., 1987; Kaplan et al., 1990).

One proposal suggests that aprosodias can be divided into various types that mirror the aphasia types, both in terms of behavioral characteristics and localization (Gorelik & Ross, 1987; Ross, 1981). However, evidence for this correspondence is equivocal (Baum & Pell, 1999). During diagnosis, aprosodia should be differentiated from dysarthria, a motor speech disorder that also may be present after a right hemisphere stroke.

AFFECT

Reduced appreciation of emotional material and altered expression of emotion may occur after RHD (Borod, 1992; Brownell & Martino, 1998; Gardner, 1994). Nearly all of the research in this area has focused on hypoaffectivity, although some patients exhibit increased emotional expression (hyperaffectivity) (Blake et al., 2002; Gardner, 1994). Findings from affective studies suggest that adults with RHD frequently can comprehend emotion conveyed in words, but deficits often appear when inferences are necessary, such as to infer mood either from a situation or from personality characteristics. Comprehension of affect from stories or short texts is easier when the context strongly biases toward a specific emotion (Gardner, 1994; Tompkins, 1991). Adults with RHD also may be less effective at verbalizing emotion.

They may use less expressive words, and may have more difficulty telling a story about an emotional event than a nonemotional one (Bloom et al., 1990; Borod et al., 2000; Cimino et al., 1991). There is no clear evidence that RHD impairs negative emotions more than positive (as purported by the valence hypothesis), or vice versa (see Borod et al., 2000, for a review).

Attention and Perception

ATTENTION

Attention is the ability to focus on stimuli, both internal and external, and to filter out unwanted stimuli. Disorders of attention may be due to reduced attentional capacity, difficulties in assessing how much attention is needed for any given task, and/or problems with allocating the needed amount of attention. In any case, if more "mental energy" is needed to modulate attention, then there is less energy available for other cognitive or communicative processes. Deficits in attention may impact any of the specific disorders discussed in this chapter. For example, attention may affect comprehension (auditory and reading) if a patient is unable to sustain attention long enough to comprehend the incoming information, or if fluctuations in attention cause the patient to miss information. Attentional problems may help explain the tangential conversation seen in adults with RHD: An individual may be unable to maintain her attentional focus on a single topic, becoming distracted by her own thoughts. Attentional deficits have been proposed as one explanation for why adults with RHD often have problems with cognitively demanding tasks but not on relatively "easier" tasks (e.g., Tompkins et al., 1994).

NEGLECT

Neglect is an attentional disorder in which stimuli perceived by the sensory systems (e.g., vision, hearing) are not consciously processed by the brain (Heilman et al., 1985). Neglect typically affects the side of space contralateral to the brain lesion. Thus, an individual with neglect caused by RHD seems to ignore stimuli in the left side of space. The area that is neglected is not absolute (e.g., everything to the left of midline), but can shift depending on the specific position of a stimulus, the presence of other stimuli in the visual field, or the patient's attentional focus. Neglect has been reported in olfaction, audition, sensation, and vision (Myers, 1999b). Visual neglect is one of the most common types, and it frequently affects communication, particularly reading and writing, but also verbal communication when an item referred to in conversation or the conversational partner is located in the left visual field. Additionally, the disruption of attentional processes in neglect has consequences for communication abilities beyond simply not "seeing" objects (Myers, 1999b).

Estimates suggest that 30 to 60% of patients with RHD exhibit visuospatial neglect (Myers, 1999b). The wide range may be a result of which diagnostic tasks are used, as some are more sensitive than others, and several tasks may be necessary to accurately diagnose mild or moderate neglect (Karnath & Neimeier, 2002; Maeshima et al., 2001). Another factor is the time at which testing takes place, because neglect can resolve spontaneously during the acute stage. Individuals with large lesions that affect three or more cerebral lobes or subcortical areas are most likely to have persisting neglect (Maguire & Ogden, 2002).

Despite the fact that objects are not consciously processed by the brain, unconscious processing of neglected items can occur. In a classic study, Marshall and Halligan (1988) instructed adults with neglect to look at drawings of two houses, which were identical except that one had smoke coming out the left side. The patients reported that both houses were the same, but when asked which one they would rather live in, almost all picked the one without the smoke. A recent priming study reported evidence of semantic priming from words flashed in the left visual field (Kanne, 2002). Adults with RHD reported that they did not see the words, but nonetheless they were faster at

naming a subsequent target word when the target was related to the left-sided prime word than when the prime was unrelated to the target. Together these results indicate that items in the left visual field are processed by the brain, even when the subject is unaware of the stimuli.

Visuospatial neglect frequently affects reading (neglect dyslexia) and writing (neglect agraphia) (Heilman et al., 1985). Patients may not read words or letters placed in the left side of space, and oftentimes a patient will guess at what letters he does not see, to create a real word. While reading a paragraph, one patient read the word "thing" instead of "painting" (the word was printed on the left side of the page). He neglected the letters at the beginning of the word, then added an "h" to make a real word. During writing tasks, individuals with neglect frequently begin writing in the middle of the page instead of at the left margin.

Neglect also affects other language abilities. Individuals with an initial diagnosis of neglect, regardless of whether or not it resolved, have more difficulty with discourse-level language tasks than those who never had neglect (e.g., Myers & Brookshire, 1986; Tompkins et al., 1994). This may be because neglect is an attentional disorder, and the decreased attention impacts various communicative abilities.

ANOSOGNOSIA

Denial of illness, or anosognosia, may occur in up to 40% of individuals with RHD (Blake et al., 2002). It frequently occurs in conjunction with neglect. Patients with anosognosia do not always recognize their impairments, and are not fully aware of the limitations caused by the deficits. This reduced awareness can occur even with dramatic physical impairments such as dense hemiplegia. Some patients may express superficial awareness of deficits without really accepting them, saying, for example, that they've been told that they have problems seeing things on the left side; this response suggests that the patients do not really believe they have problems that everyone else seems to notice. The presence of anosognosia becomes particularly challenging in the clinical setting, because a patient is not likely to participate well in intensive therapy if she does not recognize her problems (Robertson & Murre, 1999).

VISUOPERCEPTION

Visuoperceptual deficits affect a person's interpretation of the world, and frequently occur after RHD. Blake and colleagues (2002) reported that perceptual deficits were diagnosed in over 60% of adults with RHD admitted to a rehabilitation unit. Such deficits cause difficulties in various communicative abilities, such as reading and writing, where problems include misperception of letters or words and disorganized writing. Performance on confrontation naming tasks also may be negatively affected by visuoperceptual deficits. Similarly, picture descriptions may include incorrect responses that are due to perceptual difficulties. In the Cookie Theft picture from the Boston Diagnostic Aphasia Examination (BDAE; Goodglass & Kaplan, 1983), for example, the water flowing over the sink may be perceived as a towel hanging below the sink. Careful examination of errors is necessary to determine whether errors are due to a language problem (anomia or paraphasia) or problems with interpreting or integrating visual cues, or are actually due to disturbed visual perception.

Cognition

Cognitive abilities such as organizing, sequencing, reasoning, and problem solving are impaired in approximately half of adults with RHD admitted to a rehabilitation unit (Blake et al., 2002). Cognitive deficits associated with RHD are not well explained, partly because of the wide range of cognitive abilities in the general population, but also because cognitive abilities are only imprecisely defined and the concepts are closely intertwined, making it difficult to isolate one problem from another.

Disruptions of cognition impact communication in various ways, and interact with other deficits previously described. Adults with RHD often have difficulties with relatively basic cognitive functions such as organization and sequencing. These may impact discourse production, causing a disorganized macrostructure that is difficult for listeners to follow. Relatively higher level skills, such as reasoning and problem solving (often referred to as executive functions), also may be inefficient (Tompkins, 1995). An individual with poor problem-solving ability may have difficulty determining how to repair conversational breakdowns, or figuring out the best way to convey her emotions if aprosodia limits her ability to use intonational contours.

Evaluation

Diagnosis of right hemisphere communicative and cognitive disorders should involve formal assessment as well as observation. Informal tools often also contribute to the overall picture of a patient's strengths and deficits, although conclusions drawn from nonstandardized measures must be made with caution. Formal measures of disorders associated with RHD can be used to provide a global assessment or to evaluate certain deficits in more detail. Reliability, validity, and standardization procedures vary widely across tests, and close scrutiny of the psychometric properties is important to guide the selection of a test that will provide valid and reliable results.

Observation of a patient's behaviors and interactions provides important information about pragmatic aspects of communication, awareness of deficits, and attention (e.g., distractibility) (e.g., Myers, 1999b). This information then can be integrated with the results from formal assessments to obtain a broad picture of a patient's deficits and how she deals with them in casual interactions. For adults with RHD, it is especially important to talk with their family or friends to get a sense of their pre-stroke level of functioning. Given the wide range of "normal" for pragmatic and cognitive abilities, it is important to isolate the aberrant behaviors that appeared subsequent to the brain injury, as these will become targets for treatment.

Treatment

Studies of treatment efficacy and outcomes are severely lacking in the realm of RHD. The only treatments that have been studied to any degree are those for attention and neglect. Specific treatments for other cognitive and communicative deficits are a mixture of tasks taken from other disorders (traumatic brain injury or aphasia), and clinician-generated tasks that have face validity. The treatments discussed here must be viewed in that light, and used with caution until carefully designed efficacy studies are conducted to evaluate their worth. Clinicians should be equally circumspect of computerized tasks and paper/pencil tasks, as limited efficacy data are available for any computer therapy program.

Treatment can be classified generally as either task-oriented or process-oriented (Myers, 1999a,b). Task-oriented treatment, as the name suggests, focuses on improving performance on a specific task or action. Working on writing accurate phone messages is one example. Task-oriented training is not expected to generalize to other tasks, and often is used to improve a specific skill that is necessary for daily functioning or increased independence. Process-specific treatments address deficits that are thought to underlie various behavioral disorders. Attention is one common example. Focusing treatment on remediation of attentional deficits is thought to strengthen the attentional processes that are needed for efficient and effective communication and cognitive abilities. Process oriented therapies can be categorized as facilitatory or compensatory (Myers, 1997; Robertson & Murre, 1999; Tompkins, 1995). Facilitatory treatment is treatment at the level of the impairment, such as one brain area "taking over" for the damaged area. Compensatory treatment

involves teaching the patient to accomplish a task in a way different from his usual (pre-stroke) approach (Robertson & Murre, 1999).

Calvanio and colleagues (1993) discuss some cautions of using compensatory strategies in cognitive rehabilitation. First, strategies or rules that are too specific may not generalize to similar tasks. Second, rules that are too general may be difficult to teach, and even more difficult for a patient to determine when and where they should be used. Third, individuals with brain damage may have deficits in abstract thinking and problem solving that are necessary for successful use of strategies. For example, many treatments designed to treat pragmatic deficits rely on metalinguistic or metacognitive skills that may or may not be intact in patients with brain damage (Penn, 1999). Fourth, patients may not be able to reliably use strategies when they are in attentionally demanding situations. Although a patient may show good visual scanning while completing a paper/pencil scanning task in a quiet treatment room, she may not be able to allocate attention to the scanning process when she is at home amidst various distractors.

Specific Treatment Tasks

Given the lack of efficacy or outcome data for specific treatments, the following discussion focuses on a small number of tasks that have either a theoretical basis or some data suggesting clinical usefulness for adults with RHD. Detailed descriptions of specific treatments and suggestions for a variety of communicative and cognitive deficits can be found in books by Myers (1999b) and Tompkins (1995).

The suppression deficit hypothesis (Tompkins & Lehman 1998; Tompkins et al., 2000, 2001) proposes that adults with RHD can, and do, generate multiple interpretations or inferences, but may have difficulty selecting the most appropriate interpretation. Thus, treatment for extralinguistic deficits involving nonliteral language, inferencing, or humor (or any situation in which more than one interpretation is possible), should involve determining which of several possible inferences is the most appropriate for a given situation or context (Tompkins & Baumgaertner, 1998). A variety of stimuli can be used, including pictured scenes, short vignettes, ambiguous newspaper headlines, jokes, cartoons, or videotapes of conversational interactions. The patient should participate in both (1) identifying the various interpretations and (2) explaining why one is more appropriate than another. Increasing difficulty may be accomplished by using longer or more inferentially complex stimuli, or providing similar situations in which many of the possible interpretations overlap, whereas the most probable inference differs. These suggestions, although theoretically motivated, have not been clinically tested.

Various treatments for neglect have been examined and several have been found to be effective in remediating leftward scanning, although generalization to new tasks is limited. Facilitation of visual scanning has been targeted using tasks such as cancellation, picture description, search tasks, and reading (see Myers, 1999b; Tompkins & Lehman, 1998; and Zoccolotti, 1999, for reviews). Treatment strategies have included verbal reminders ("Look to the left"), and visual or tactile cues at the left margin (a colored line, textured marker, or the patient's left arm). Other treatments emphasize voluntary movement of attention and exploration of space without external cues (Myers, 1997, 1999b). The most beneficial neglect treatments generally share several characteristics: First, the focus is clear yet narrow; second, there is a clear rationale for the goal and the tasks; third, treatment is intensive (5 hours/week for at least 4 weeks). In general, treatments that rely on external cues, such as the examiner repeating "Look to the left," are not highly successful, because performance deteriorates as soon as the cue is faded. Treatments in which the patient must actively participate are often more successful, although generalization is not assured (Calvanio et al., 1993; Myers, 1999b).

Conclusion

The right hemisphere plays an important role in effective communication, and RHD can cause devastating effects on interpersonal interactions. Our knowledge about the underlying mechanisms of RHD cognitive and communicative deficits is slowly expanding. There is a critical need for clinical research to apply these findings to treatments, and to evaluate the efficacy and outcomes of treatment for adults with RHD.

References

Baum, S.R. & Pell, M.D. (1999). The Neural Bases of Prosody: Insights from Lesion Studies and Neuroimaging. *Aphasiology, 13*, 581–608.

Beeman, M. (1993). Semantic Processing in the Right Hemisphere May Contribute to Drawing Inferences from Discourse. *Brain and Language, 44*, 80–120.

Benowitz, L.I., Moya, K.L. & Levine, D.N. (1990). Impaired Verbal Reasoning and Constructional Apraxia in Subjects with Right Hemisphere Damage. *Neuropsychologia, 28*, 231–241.

Blake, M., Duffy, J.R., Myers, P.S. & Tompkins, C.A. (2002). Prevalence and Patterns of Right Hemisphere Cognitive/Communicative Deficits: Retrospective Data from an Inpatient Rehabilitation Unit. *Aphasiology, 16*, 537–548.

Bloom, R.L., Borod, J.C., Obler, L.K. & Koff, E. (1990). A Preliminary Characterization of Lexical Emotional Expression in Right and Left Brain-Damaged Patients. *International Journal of Neuroscience, 55*, 71–80.

Borod, J.C. (1992). Interhemispheric and Intrahemispheric Control of Emotion: A Focus on Unilateral Brain Damage. *Journal of Consulting and Clinical Psychology, 60*, 339–348.

Borod, J.C., Pick, L.H., Andelman, F., Obler, L.K., Welkowitz, J., Rorie, K.D., Bloom, R.L., Campbell, A.L., Tweedy, J.R. & Sliwinski, M. (2000). Verbal Pragmatics Following Unilateral Stroke: Emotional Content and Valence. *Neuropsychology, 14*, 112–124.

Bowers, D., Coslett, H.B., Bauer, R.M., Speedie, L. & Heilman, K.M. (1987). Comprehension of Emotional Prosody Following Unilateral Hemispheric Lesions: Processing Defect Versus Distraction Defect. *Neuropsychologia, 25*, 317–328.

Brookshire, R.H. & Nicholas, L.E. (1984). Comprehension of Directly and Indirectly Stated Main Ideas and Details in Discourse by Brain-Damaged and Non-Brain-Damaged Listeners. *Brain and Language, 21*, 21–36.

Brownell, H. & Gardner, H. (1989). Neuropsychological Insights into Humor. In: J. Durant & J. Miller (Eds.), *Laughing Matters* (pp. 17–34). New York: Wiley.

Brownell, H. & Martino, G. (1998). Deficits in Inference and Social Cognition: The Effects of Right Hemisphere Brain Damage on Discourse. In: M. Beeman and C. Chiarello (Eds.), *Right Hemisphere Language Comprehension: Perspectives from Cognitive Neuroscience* (pp. 309–328). Mahwah, NJ: Lawrence Erlbaum.

Brownell, H.H., Michel, D., Powelson, J. & Gardner, H. (1983). Surprise But Not Coherence: Sensitivity to Verbal Humor in Right-Hemisphere Patients. *Brain and Language, 18,* 20–27.

Brownell, H.H., Potter, H.H., Bihrle, A.M. & Gardner, H. (1986). Inference Deficits in Right Brain-Damaged Patients. *Brain and Language, 27,* 310–321.

Brownell, H.H. & Stringfellow, A. (1999). Making Requests: Illustrations of How Right-Hemisphere Brain Damage Can Affect Discourse Production. *Brain and Language, 68,* 442–465.

Calvanio, R., Levine, D. & Petrone, P. (1993). Elements of Cognitive Rehabilitation After Right Hemisphere Stroke. *Behavioral Neurology, 11,* 25–57.

Chantraine, Y., Joanette, Y. & Ska, B. (1998). Conversational Abilities in Patients with Right Hemisphere Damage. *Journal of Neurolinguistics, 11,* 21–32.

Cherney, L.R., Drimmer, D.P. & Halper, A.S. (1997). Informational Content and Unilateral Neglect: A Longitudinal Investigation of Five Subjects with Right Hemisphere Damage. *Aphasiology, 11,* 351–364.

Cimino, C.R., Verfaellie, M., Bowers, D. & Heilman, K.M. (1991). Autobiographical Memory: Influence of Right Hemisphere Brain Damage on Emotionality and Specificity. *Brain and Cognition, 15,* 106–118.

Cohen, R.A. (1993). Attentional Control: Subcortical and Frontal Lobe Influences. In: R.A. Cohen (Ed.), *The Neuropsychology of Attention* (pp. 219–254). New York: Plenum Press.

Gardner, H. (1994). The Stories of the Right Hemisphere. Integrative Views of Motivation, Cognition and Emotion. *The Nebraska Symposium on Motivation, 41,* 57–69.

Goodglass, H. & Kaplan, E. (1983). *The Assessment of Aphasia and Related Disorders.* Philadelphia: Lea & Febiger.

Gorelik, P. & Ross, E. (1987). The Aprosodias: Further Functional-Anatomical Evidence for the Organization of Affective Language in the Right Hemisphere. *Journal of Neurology, Neurosurgery, and Psychiatry, 50,* 553–560.

Gur, R.C., Packer, I.K., Hungerbuhler, J.P., Reivich, M., Obrist, W.D., Amarnek, W.S. & Sackeim, H.A. (1980). Differences in the Distribution of Gray and White Matter in Human Cerebral Hemispheres. *Science, 207,* 1226–1228.

Happe, F., Brownell, H. & Winner, E. (1999). Acquired "Theory of Mind" Impairments Following Stroke. *Cognition, 70,* 211–240.

Heilman, K.M., Watson, R.T. & Valenstein, E. (1985). Neglect and Related Disorders. In: K.M. Heilman & E. Valenstein (Eds.), *Clinical Neuropsychology* (2nd ed., pp. 243–294). New York: Oxford University Press.

Hough, M.S. (1990). Narrative Comprehension in Adults with Right and Left Hemisphere Brain-Damage: Theme Organization. *Brain and Language, 38,* 253–277.

Jackson, J.H. (1958). On the Nature of the Duality of the Brain. In: J. Taylor (Ed.), *Selected Writings of John Hughlings Jackson* (vol. 2, pp. 129–145). New York: Basic Books. (Originally published 1874.)

Joanette, Y. & Ansaldo, A.I. (1999). Clinical Note: Acquired Pragmatic Impairments and Aphasia. *Brain and Language, 68,* 529–534.

Joanette, Y. & Goulet, P. (1994). Right Hemisphere and Verbal Communication: Conceptual, Methodological, and Clinical Issues. *Clinical Aphasiology, 22,* 1–23.

Joanette, Y., Goulet, P., Ska, B. & Nespoulous, J-L. (1986). Informative Content of Narrative Discourse in Right-Brain-Damaged Right-Handers. *Brain and Language, 29,* 81–105.

Kanne, S.M. (2002). The Role of Semantic, Orthographic, and Phonological Prime Information in Unilateral Visual Neglect. *Cognitive Neuropsychology, 19,* 245–261.

Kaplan, J.A., Brownell, H.H., Jacobs, J.R. & Gardner, H. (1990). The Effects of Right Hemisphere Damage on the Pragmatic Interpretation of Conversational Remarks. *Brain and Language, 38,* 315–333.

Karnath, H.-O. & Neimeier, M. (2002). Task-Dependent Differences in the Exploratory Behaviour of Patients with Spatial Neglect. *Neuropsychologia, 40,* 1577–1585.

Kempler, D., VanLancker, D., Marchman, V. & Bates, E. (1999). Idiom Comprehension in Children and Adults with Unilateral Brain Damage. *Developmental Neuropsychology, 15,* 327–349.

Kennedy, M.R.T. (2000). Topic Scenes in Conversations with Adults with Right-Hemisphere Brain Damage. *American Journal of Speech-Language Pathology, 9,* 72–86.

Kennedy, M., Strand, E., Burton, W. & Peterson, C. (1994). Analysis of First-Encounter Conversations of Right-Hemisphere Damaged Participants. *Clinical Aphasiology, 22,* 67–80.

Lehman, M.T. and Tompkins, C.A. (2000). Inferencing in Adults with Right Hemisphere Brain Damage: An Analysis of Conflicting Results. *Aphasiology, 14,* 485–499.

Lehman-Blake, M.T. & Tompkins, C.A. (2001). Predictive Inferencing in Adults with Right Hemisphere Brain Damage. *Journal of Speech, Language and Hearing Research, 44,* 639–654.

Lojek-Osiejuk, E. (1996). Knowledge of Scripts Reflected in Discourse of Aphasics and Right-Brain-Damaged Patients. *Brain and Language, 53,* 58–80.

Mackenzie, C., Begg, T., Lees, K.R. & Brady, M. (1999). The Communication Effects of Right Brain Damage on the Very Old and the Not So Old. *Journal of Neurolinguistics, 12,* 79–93.

Maeshmia, S., Truman, G., Smith, D.S., Dohi, N., Shigeno, K., Itakura, T. & Komai, N. (2001). Factor Analysis of the Components of 12 Standard Test Batteries, for Unilateral Spatial Neglect, Reveals that They Contain a Number of Discrete and Important Clinical Variables. *Brain Injury, 15,* 125–137.

Maguire, A.M. & Ogden, J.A. (2002). MRI Brain Scan Analyses and Neuropsychological Profiles of Nine Patients with Persisting Unilateral Neglect. *Neuropsychologia, 40,* 879–887.

Marshall, J.C. & Halligan, P.W. (1988). Blind-Sight and Insight in Visuo-Spatial Nelgect. *Nature, 336,* 766–767.

Myers, P.S. (1997). Right Hemisphere Syndrome. In: L.L. LaPointe (Ed.), *Aphasia and Related Neurogenic Language Disorders* (pp. 201–225). New York: Thieme.

Myers, P.S. (1999a). Process-Oriented Treatment of Right Hemisphere Communication Disorders. *Seminars in Speech and Language, 20,* 319–333.

Myers, P.S. (1999b). *Right Hemisphere Damage: Disorders of Communication and Cognition.* San Diego: Singular.

Myers, P.S. (2001). Toward a Definition of RHD Syndrome. *Aphasiology, 15,* 913–918.

Myers, P.S. & Brookshire, R.H. (1986). The Effect of Visual and Inferential Variables on Scene Descriptions of Right-Hemisphere-Damaged and Non-Brain-Damaged Adults. *Journal of Speech and Hearing Research, 39*, 870–880.

Myers, P.S. & Linebaugh, C.W. (1981). Comprehension of Idiomatic Expressions by Right-Hemisphere-Damaged Adults. In: R.H. Brookshire (Ed.), *Clinical Aphasiology* (vol. 11, pp. 254–261). Minneapolis: BRK.

Penn, C. (1999). Pragmatic Assessment and Therapy for Persons with Brain Damage: What Have Clinicians Gleaned in Two Decades? *Brain and Language, 68,* 535–552.

Rehak, A., Kaplan, J.A. & Gardner, H. (1992). Sensitivity to Conversational Deviance in Right-Hemisphere-Damaged Patients. *Brain and Language, 42,* 203–217.

Robertson, I.H. & Murre, J.M.J. (1999) Rehabilitation of Brain Damage: Brain Plasticity and Principles of Guided Recovery. *Psychological Bulletin, 125,* 544–575.

Roman, M., Brownell, H.H., Potter, H.H. & Seibold, M. (1987). Script Knowledge in Right Hemisphere-Damaged and Normal Elderly Adults. *Brain and Language, 31,* 151–170.

Ross, E. (1981). The Aprosodias: Functional-Anatomical Organization of the Affective Components of Language in the Right Hemisphere. *Archives of Neurology, 38,* 561–596.

Sabbagh, M.A. (1999). Communicative Intentions and Language: Evidence from Right-Hemisphere Damage and Autism. *Brain and Language, 70,* 29–69.

Schneiderman, E.I., Murasugi, K.G. & Saddy, J.D. (1992). Story Arrangement Ability in Right Brain-Damaged Patients. *Brain and Language, 43,* 107–120.

Stemmer, B., Giroux, F. & Joanette, Y. (1994). Production and Evaluation of Requests by Right Hemisphere Brain-Damaged Individuals. *Brain and Language, 47,* 1–31.

Tompkins, C.A. (1991). Redundancy Enhances Emotional Inferencing by Right- and Left-Hemisphere-Damaged Adults. *Journal of Speech and Hearing Research, 34,* 1142–1149.

Tompkins, C.A. (1995). *Right Hemisphere Communication Disorders: Theory and Management.* San Diego: Singular.

Tompkins, C.A. & Baumgaertner, A. (1998). Clinical Value of Online Measures for Adults with Right Hemisphere Brain Damage. *American Journal of Speech-Language Pathology, 7,* 68–74.

Tompkins, C.A., Baumgaertner, A., Lehman, M.T. & Fassbinder, W. (2000). Mechanisms of Discourse Comprehension Impairment After Right Hemisphere Brain Damage: Suppression and Enhancement in Lexical Ambiguity Resolution. *Journal of Speech, Language and Hearing Research, 43,* 62–78.

Tompkins, C.A., Bloise, C.G.R., Timko, M.L. & Baumgaertner, A. (1994). Working Memory and Inference Revision in Brain-Damaged and Normally Aging Adults. *Journal of Speech and Hearing Research, 37,* 896–912.

Tompkins, C.A., Boada, R. & McGarry, K. (1992). The Access and Processing of Familiar Idioms by Brain-Damaged and Normally Aging Adults. *Journal of Speech and Hearing Research, 35,* 626–637.

Tompkins, C.A. & Lehman, M.T. (1998). Interpreting Intended Meanings After Right Hemisphere Brain Damage: An Analysis of Evidence, Potential Accounts, and Clinical Implications. *Topics in Stroke Rehabilitation, 5,* 29–47.

Tompkins, C.A., Lehman-Blake, M.T., Baumgaertner, A. & Fassbinder, W. (2001). Mechanisms of Discourse Comprehension Impairment After Right Hemisphere Brain Damage: Suppression in Inferential Ambiguity Resolution. *Journal of Speech, Language and Hearing Research, 44,* 400–415.

Urayse, D., Duffy, R.J. & Liles, B.Z. (1991). Analysis and Description of Narrative Discourse in Right-Hemisphere-Damaged Adults: A Comparison with Neurologically Normal and Left-Hemisphere-Damaged Adults. *Clinical Aphasiology, 19,* 125–138.

Vanhalle, C., Lemieux, S., Joubert, S., Goulet, P., Ska, B. & Joanette, Y. (2000). Processing of Speech Acts by Right Hemisphere-Damaged Patients: An Ecological Approach. *Aphasiology, 14,* 1127–1142.

Wapner, W., Hamby, S. & Gardner, H. (1981). The Role of the Right Hemisphere in the Apprehension of Complex Linguistic Material. *Brain and Language, 14,* 15–32.

Weylman, S., Brownell, H.H., Roman, M. & Gardner, H. (1989). Appreciation of Indirect Requests by Left- and Right-Brain-Damaged Patients: The Effects of Verbal Context and Conventionality of Wording. *Brain and Language, 62,* 89–106.

Winner, E., Brownell, H., Happe, F., Blum, A. & Pincus, D. (1998). Distinguishing Lies from Jokes: Theory of Mind Deficits and Discourse Interpretation in Right Hemisphere Brain-Damaged Patients. *Brain and Language, 62,* 89–106.

Zoccolotti, P. (1999). Visual, Visuospatial and Attentional Disorders. In: G. Denes & L. Pizzamiglio (Eds.), *Handbook of Clinical and Experimental Neuropsychology* (pp. 875–885). Hove, East Sussex: Psychology Press.

Suggested Readings

Beeman, M. & Chiarello, C. (1998). *Right Hemisphere Language Comprehension: Perspectives from Cognitive Neuroscience.* Mahwah, NJ: Lawrence Erlbaum.

Myers, P.S. (1997). *Right Hemisphere Damage: Disorders of Communication and Cognition.* San Diego: Singular.

Tompkins, C.A. (1995). *Right Hemisphere Communication Disorders: Theory and Management.* San Diego: Singular.

Tompkins, C.A., Fassbinder, W., Lehman-Blake, M.T. & Baumgaertner, A. (2002). The Nature and Implications of Right Hemisphere Language Disorders: Issues in Search of Answers. In: A.E. Hillis (Ed.), *Handbook of Adult Language Disorders: Integrating Cognitive Neuropsychology, Neurology, and Rehabilitation* (pp. 429–448). Philadelphia: Psychology Press.

Tompkins, C.A. & Lehman, M.T. (1998). Outcomes Measurement in Cognitive Communication Disorders: Right-Hemisphere Brain Damage. In: C.M. Frattali (Ed.), *Measuring Outcomes in Speech-Language Pathology* (pp. 281–292). New York: Thieme.

15

Traumatic Brain Injury

BRENDA L.B. ADAMOVICH

Traumatic brain injury is the leading cause of death and long-term disability in the United States for children and adults age 40 and younger. Motor vehicle accidents are the main cause of injuries, with males age 15 to 24 having the greatest risk. There are 2,000,000 head injuries per year in the United States, with 500,000 requiring hospitalization. Approximately 200,000 to 300,000 patients acquire chronic cognitive disabilities (Winslade, 1998). The cost per year to society for these injuries, including medical treatment, rehabilitation, support services, and lost insurance, is $25 billion (Bigler, 1990). The survivors of traumatic brain insult experience permanent disabilities of varying degrees. Memory and other cognitive disturbances are typically the most long lasting and incapacitating sequelae of traumatic brain injury. The number of specialized programs for patients with traumatic brain injury has grown over the past 10 years from a handful of programs to almost 1,000 programs across the United States. The quality of care in general has improved from lifetime nursing home placements to interdisciplinary programs that focus on home and community reentry with emphasis on metacognitive skills, functional gains, and empowerment.

Pathophysiology

It is now generally acknowledged that acceleration-deceleration injuries are responsible for the predominant pathologic lesion in traumatic brain injury. More specifically, the head is accelerated and then suddenly stopped. The forces involved may be translational when movement is in a horizontal plane due to direct impact, or angular when there is a rotational or inertial component, with damage frequently occurring about the diencephalic-midbrain junction. It is generally accepted that the angular acceleration injury is most likely to produce the diffuse injury and the concussion associated with closed head injury.

Direct impact forces usually result in discrete focal lesions. Contusions may be found at the site of direct impact or, as the brain shifts in relation to the skull, contrecoup contusions may be found at sites remote from the point of direct impact. The distribution of these contusions relates to the rotational sources and to contact of the brain surface with certain bony prominences in the skull.

Focal cortical contusions are generally found in the frontal (frontopolar and orbitofrontal) and temporal (anterior temporal, but not necessarily medial temporal) lobes. Diffuse axonal injury of the white matter is associated with high acceleration injuries. The severity of diffuse axonal injury correlates with the severity of the posttraumatic coma and is associated with focal lesions in the corpus callosum and the dorsolateral quadrants of the midbrain.

Nature and Differentiating Features

Two classes of neurobehavioral sequelae occur following traumatic brain injury as a result of discrete, focal, or widespread diffuse brain lesions. Speech, language, voice, hearing, fluency, and/or swallowing deficits may occur secondary to the focal lesions most typical of those that occur following cerebrovascular accidents. Specific language problems may be confused with problems due to more general disruptions of attention, information processing, and/or cognition. For example, comprehension deficits may be due to memory disturbances rather than to linguistic disturbances.

Widespread, diffuse brain damage, which most typically occurs following closed head injury, generally results in communication disorders created by impaired attention, information processing, and cognition. To communicate effectively, an individual must possess attentional skills that allow the manipulation of the focus of attention in three basic ways: initiating and sustaining attention; shifting the focus of attention when appropriate; and inhibiting the inappropriate shifting of attention.

Information processing refers to the analysis and synthesis of information in sequential steps. *Cognition* is a complicated and misunderstood term around which an entire subscience in psychology has been formed. Generally, it refers to the knowledge base necessary to comprehend or use specific information. Cognitive processes include perception, discrimination, organization, recall, and problem solving, all of which may be integrated with and difficult to separate from language.

Assessment

Clinicians working with closed-head injured individuals must identify focal lesion disorders as well as attention, information processing, and cognitive deficits. Thus, diagnostic batteries should provide for at least a screening of the person's speech, fluency, voice, swallowing ability, visual processing (neglect, discrimination, and organization), hearing, and language. Specific deficits are often difficult to identify as they can be masked by severe cognitive deficits.

The Scales of Cognitive Ability for Traumatic Brain Injury (SCATBI) is a diagnostic test for adolescents and adults designed to assess cognitive-linguistic status after closed-head injury (CHI) and to describe the extent of changes during and following rehabilitation (Adamovich & Henderson, 1992). This test was constructed to measure performance on five scales, each representing a general area of cognitive ability that may be impaired after CHI and is ultimately necessary to function in day-to-day living. The five scales are perception; discrimination; orientation; organization; and recall and reasoning. In general, individual items within each scale were designed to progress in difficulty from easier to more difficult. Other diagnostic test batteries designed to measure cognitive processes include the Detroit Test of Learning Aptitude (Baker & Leland, 1935); the Neurobehavioral Rating Scale (Levin, 1987); the Orientation Group Monitoring System (Jackson et al., 1989); the Ross Test of Higher Cognitive Processes (Ross & Ross, 1976); and the Wechsler Adult Intelligence Scale (Wechsler, 1981).

Functional Outcome Measures

The functional independence measure (FIM) (Granger et al., 1986) is the most widely used outcome measure in medical rehabilitation programs in the United States. The FIM evaluates 18 functional activities on a seven-point/level scale. The functional assessment measure (FAM) (Hall et al., 1993) consists of 12 additional test items that can be added to the FIM to better assess communication, cognition, and behavior disturbances, which are the predominant disturbances following CHI. A study of 965 CHI patients from 11 brain injury rehabilitation programs revealed high internal reliability on the physical and cognitive components measured by the FIM and the FAM (Hawley et al., 1999). Other outcome measurement tools utilized with brain-injured patients include the Mayo-Portland Adaptability Inventory (Malec et al., 1993) and the Craig Handicap Assessment and Reporting Tool (Whiteneck et al., 1992).

Boake et al. (2001) defined productive outcome if the patient was competitively employed or enrolled full time in school. They evaluated whether early traditional neuropsychological testing was useful in predicting a productive outcome in 293 CHI adults. The greatest predictive indicator was normal range scores on 10 of the 15 neuropsychological tests administered. Sherer et al. (2002) found that of 388 adults with CHI, those scoring at the 75th percentile on neuropsychological tests of cognitive status had approximately two times greater odds of being productive 12 months postinjury. These studies support the occurrence of a ceiling effect whereby patients with CHI achieve normal scores on most traditional neuropsychological tests due to the lack of sensitivity to higher level cognitive deficits after CHI.

Treatment

Traditional methods of treatment, as outlined in other chapters in this text, are utilized to treat resulting focal lesion deficits, such as speech, language, voice, fluency, and swallowing, provided that attention and recall abilities allow the individual to actively participate in therapy. Nonvocal communication devices should be considered for head-injured patients who are unable to communicate verbally if patients possess the cognitive and physical abilities necessary to utilize these devices.

Schiff et al. (2002) advocate that fluctuating capacities of memory, attention, intention, and awareness in patients with severe-moderate brain injury provides clinical evidence that their limited functional capacities may not represent entirely irreversible damage. They further suggest that mechanisms of plasticity and dynamic reorganization are available to the brain and could be harnessed for therapeutic advantage. According to Robertson (1999), evidence for experience-dependent plasticity of the brain, including cell regeneration, means that rehabilitation should focus on restituting impaired cognitive function, as well as on training compensatory strategies for lost function. It is suggested that restitution-oriented rehabilitation approaches are feasible in the case of lesions that spare a proportion of connections in a lesioned circuit. Facilitatory and inhibitory stimulation of cognitive systems may potentially rescue circuits that would otherwise disintegrate. For the most part, memory rehabilitation has not resulted in direct and lasting improvement through restitution-oriented therapies. Therefore, compensatory approaches to memory problems appear to be the treatment of choice.

Pizzamiglio et al. (1998) conducted imaging studies of the effects of rehabilitation for three patients with unilateral neglect from subcortical lesions, and recovery was reportedly associated with cerebral activation in right hemisphere cortical regions that subserve visuoperceptual functioning in normal individuals. Schiff et al. (2002) proposed the use of electrical stimulation of thalamic regions using deep brain stimulation (DBS). Subcortical brain structures were chronically stimulated at high frequencies to suppress neuronal activity and to amplify remaining cortical integrative functions. Widely distributed cortical and subcortical regions are activated according to magnetic resonance imaging (MRI) and positron emission tomography (PET) studies (Ceballos-Baumann, 2000; Rezai et al., 1999). DBS is used for cognitive impairment to selectively support impaired but partially functional brain networks primarily affecting selective attention and working memory. Further research in this area is suggested to support the utilization of this technique to assist with cognitive rehabilitation techniques.

Laatsch et al. (1999) compared single photon emission computed tomography (SPECT) imaging during cognitive rehabilitation programs of five patients. All patients revealed significant improvement following cognitive rehabilitation, which was maintained during a nontreatment period. SPECT data revealed the most significant increase in cerebral blood flow redistribution during the treatment period compared with the notreatment period even with individuals more than 2 years post–brain damage. Most changes in regional cerebral blood flow were related to improvements on neuropsychological tests.

Gordon and Hibbard (1991) suggested that treatment of cognitive processes focused on specific skill training is the most efficacious approach to training following traumatic brain injury. Treatment should include training of cognitive processes in conjunction with the learning of actual functional skills during simulated and community-based activities, as the cognitive processes provide a basic foundation that crosses over many skills and behaviors, and they are necessary if generalization is to occur. It is impossible to train every skill that a person will encounter following traumatic brain injury. Theories of learning suggest that learning occurs in a hierarchical fashion. Training of cognitive skills along with relevant functional skills should proceed in a step-by-step manner with a gradual increasing of the cognitive complexity of the tasks.

Techniques used to treat diffuse brain damage disturbances in attention, information processing, and cognition that most typically occur following closed head injury are described in this chapter (adapted from Adamovich et al., 1985). Behavioral observations to determine the functional consequences of cognitive deficits should be made on the rehabilitation unit, in the home, in the community, and at the work site. Generalization of treatment strategies is best accomplished when the clinical setting and treatment materials are as similar as possible to each person's real-life situation. Simulation of this real-life environment generally occurs first. The patient's ability to generalize should be tested by observing the use of compensatory techniques in settings in the home and the community.

Continuum of Care

The ideal way to provide care for patients who have suffered traumatic brain injury is through a continuum that includes acute inpatient rehabilitation and outpatient services. Subacute rehabilitation services are also appropriate prior to admission to a medical rehabilitation program for those patients who are at a level that is too low to allow them to fully participate in an active medical rehabilitation program. A subacute program also may be appropriate following medical rehabilitation when the patient needs continued, less intensive rehabilitation services prior to returning home. Outpatient programs include day treatment, which allows a patient to receive comprehensive, interdisciplinary outpatient services for a full or half day; comprehensive outpatient services; residential or transitional living services; supervised living facilities; comprehensive home health services; educational programs; vocational programs; and supported employment. Family members must be involved early in the rehabilitation process. The patient and family members must be given adequate knowledge, skill training, and resources that facilitate independence.

Treatment Techniques

Cognitive retraining can be provided in individual and group therapy sessions. Based on the results of a diagnostic assessment, treatment of cognitive skills begins when the patient first begins to experience difficulty and proceeds through a hierarchy of cognitive skills. Treatment ranges from a low-level stimulation programs to high-level treatment, which focuses on reasoning and problem solving. Specific cognitive activities are presented according to the hierarchy of skills suggested by Adamovich and Henderson (1992).

Attention

Head-injured patients have difficulty initiating, sustaining, shifting, and inhibiting the inappropriate shifting of attention. Attentional deficits include perseveration, distractibility, impulsivity, and disinhibition. Sohlberg and Mateer (2001) suggested that the majority of published articles about brain-injured adults have reported positive findings with attention process training, with significant improvement on unpracticed psychometric measures of attention. These investigators found improvement following training on attention, memory, learning, and on levels of independent living and return to work. Cicerone (2002) reported significant improvements of measures of attention, as well as reduction of self-reported attentional difficulties in daily functioning. Specific treatment techniques include varying concepts, rates, and sequences; varying length and intensity of work periods; utilizing techniques to focus attention and facilitate rehearsal; avoiding the presentation of repeating cues; and utilizing instructions to increase self-monitoring. Techniques that focus attention include addressing the person by name before initiating a task, waiting for eye contact, touching the patient, and using start-up phrases such as "Are you ready?" Therapy should begin utilizing pertinent, meaningful stimuli and gradually move to less familiar stimuli. If a person is capable of attending for 5 minutes, changing tasks at the end of a 5-minute period might help increase attentional duration and allow for a longer treatment session.

Perception

Visual and auditory perceptual tasks include tracking and scanning; perception of sounds, words, and objects; tracing or copying; following simple commands; and naming objects.

Discrimination

With discrimination tasks, the number and degree of similarity of stimuli that compete with the most pertinent or most salient stimulus or stimuli should be gradually increased. Activities begin with the visual discrimination of colors, shapes, and sizes followed by the discrimination of pictures, words, sentences, and situations. The level of cognitive functioning must be considered for all functional tasks. For example, if a patient is able to discriminate between only two items

at a time, only two foods should be placed on a food tray at a time, or only two articles of clothing should be given during a dressing activity.

Organization

Organizational activities include categorization, closure, and sequencing tasks. Categorization is the grouping of items by physical attributes, meaningful units, function, likenesses, and differences. Closure activities include the identification of missing elements of pictures, letters, words, sentences, stories, conversations, and situations. Sequencing activities include the sequencing of visual information from smallest to largest or lightest to darkest, with progression to the sequencing of letters, words, sentences, and steps, to functional activities, such as taking a shower, making coffee, and shopping.

Organizational skills are essential for all functional activities. An individual can be capable of completing the individual steps of an activity but be unable to sequence the entire activity. For example, a person might sit all day, intending to take a shower, get dressed, or make a sandwich but not know what to do first, second, and so on. What might appear, at first glance, to be an initiation problem is actually an inability to deal with the sequencing of a task that is too complex for that person.

Treatment must focus on the gradual progression from the sequencing of two steps such as taking the lid off the toothpaste and putting toothpaste on a toothbrush to three steps and so on. Patients will experience success and greater levels of independence if their level of cognitive functioning is considered during all activities.

Memory

Memory deficits occur due to ineffective encoding of information, inadequate storage of information, difficulty retrieving information, and the inability to cope with interferences. The two general approaches to the treatment of memory disturbances after traumatic brain injury are the development of internal retrieval strategies and the provision of external memory aids. Individuals who have experienced traumatic brain injury usually have long-lasting memory deficits that require both types of memory treatments. Recall strategies include verbal description, in which an adequate explanation of items and concepts to be recalled is provided by the client or clinician; visual imagery, in which objects, scenes of a story or situation, and maps or layouts in space are mentally pictured; chunking, in which information is visually or aurally organized into segments that coincide with the patient's memory span; categorization of information to improve recall of that information, for example, when required to remember items to be purchased at a grocery store, the patient should group the items into categories such as dairy products, frozen foods, meats, etc.; rehearsal, in which information to be recalled is drilled; temporal or special ordering, in which events in episodic and semantic memory are recalled by remembering certain landmark events associated with the event to be recalled or those that occurred at a similar point in time; and mnemonic devices, in which specific memory tricks are used to increase associative learning through paired association. For example, during encoding, new words or bits of information are chained or paired to a preestablished set of key words and phrases or a familiar sequence of known locations using several mnemonic systems. A peg system links or pegs new items to existing items, for example, rhyming peg: one = bun; or loci peg: items linked to familiar locations. The substitution word system is based on linking a visual image with a word; for example, to remember the name Cameron, visualize a camera on his balding head (outstanding facial feature). The link system links lists of items together in generally a funny way to facilitate retrieval, for example, to remember bologna and milk, picture a cow eating bologna as the farmer milks her.

Since medial temporal lobe injury is a frequent contributor to memory dysfunction in CHI, an acetylcholine deficit most likely contributes to memory dysfunction (Taverni et al., 1998). Donepezil, an acetylcholine-esterase inhibitor, was found to improve memory within 3 weeks for two patients. Although larger trials should be conducted, donepezil may prove to be a valuable tool for the treatment of memory dysfunction with CHI patients.

Memory aids are similar to the type of memory aids that non-brain-injured individuals utilize such as a calendar, appointment book, note pads, daily logs and diaries, memo books, lists, structured routines, alarms to remind a person to complete a task, tape recorders, and microcomputers. Patients with traumatic brain injury can often be extremely effective in dealing with a faulty memory if they are willing to utilize memory aids faithfully. Probably the least conspicuous and most effective memory aid is the use of a watch alarm to remind a person to look at his or her appointment book. This strategy works quite well if the patient remembers to write all necessary appointments and information in the appointment book.

Reasoning

Reasoning activities generally begin with practice in the clinic but must be extended to practice in real-life situations. Several types of reasoning should be addressed beginning with the most concrete and extending to the most abstract forms of reasoning. Patients with CHI have trouble identifying important relationships essential when effectively solving problems. They also have difficulty following the sequential, step-by-step reasoning process, generating alternatives, solution implementation, and verification. Convergent thinking involves the identification of main points or central themes. Deductive reasoning requires step-by-step problem solving. Inductive reasoning, more abstract, is a part of such diverse activities as cause-and-effect analysis, analogous thinking, and the formulation of antonyms and synonyms. Divergent thinking consists of unique abstract concepts, such as homo-graphs, absurdities, idioms, and proverbs.

Executive Functioning/ Metacognitive Skills

Executive functioning according to Lezak (1982) is the ability to formulate goals, develop a plan, and effectively execute a plan. Treatment of higher-level patients following traumatic brain injury should include the assessment and treatment of executive functioning. Impaired executive functioning can result in difficulty reintegrating into the home, community, school, or workplace. Ylvisaker and Szekeres (1989) suggested that seven concepts were specific to executive system problems or metacognitive dysfunctions: self-awareness and goal setting, planning, self-directing/initiating, self-inhibiting, self-monitoring, self-evaluating, and flexible problem solving.

Executive functioning deficits are thought to be a consequence of frontal lobe damage (Alexander et al., 1989). Levin and Kraus (1994) also discuss pathophysiologic and neuroimaging evidence that suggests that the frontal lobes are involved in closed head injury. They suggest that even though injury to the brain is often diffused in closed head injury, specific cognitive behavioral and mood disorders can be attributed to frontal lobe damage directly or indirectly. They suggest that treatment and rehabilitation require a multidisciplinary approach, which includes education of the patient and family and modification of the patient's home and work environments. Executive functioning deficits probably become most evident when the patient leaves the rehabilitation center and attempts to function in his or her home and community. These deficits should be a focus of all outpatient community reentry programs, and probably can best be treated with individual and group therapy, along with specific activities in the community, home, and work designed to provide for the practice of target behaviors. Individual and group therapy sessions should focus on the identification of individual strengths and weaknesses, insight, self-evaluation, self-monitoring, and utilization of feedback. According to Cicerone and Giacino (1992), the treatment of executive function deficits must, at some level, attempt to reestablish psychological processes that links social and environmental demands and the deliberate response of the individual (Dawson et al., 1999; Winocur et al., 2000). The goal, in other words, is a remediation of behavior that is initially under external control. The behavior is gradually internalized and brought under the patient's own control to be applied spontaneously in varied situations.

Use of Computers

Computers can be helpful in the treatment of attention, concentration/persistence, visual localization, visual scanning, visual tracking, reaction time, memory, hand-eye coordination, and specific cognitive tasks. Using computers, stimuli can be presented in a highly controlled manner, and the client is required to compete only with himself or herself, providing for a sense of control over therapy and progress that leads to increased motivation and feelings of self-worth. Accurate, objective, and immediate feedback is received, and people tend to enjoy using computers.

According to Wilson and Moffat (1984), clinicians should consider the following when selecting computer programs: consistent, controlled levels of difficulty within a task; lesson or file generating capability; concise, easy-to-follow instructions; consistent response format; accurate and age-appropriate content; degree of supervision required; friendly, unambiguous, and informative feedback; control of variables or parameters (i.e., length of time and stimulus is displayed, length of response delay time, task speed, number of trials per set, level of difficulty, type of prompts, size of stimuli, timing, and type of reinforcements); and method of keeping and reporting data.

Virtual environment (VE) computer-generated interactive three-dimensional (3D) scenarios have been suggested to be of value in the treatment of patients with psychological and cognitive impairments (Grealy et at., 1999). VE allows patients to be assessed and rehabilitated in life-like situations where there is total control over all content. Patient movements and interactions can be recorded in a database for analysis and comparisons. A virtual reality kitchen was found to benefit a patient with CHI (Gourlay et al., 2000).

Drawbacks in VE are cybersickness including motion sickness, visual disturbance, and problems with coordination and balance. All computer training should be selected and monitored by professional clinicians as part of a comprehensive treatment program for each individual.

Group Therapy

Group treatment allows for peer support, peer review, and the sharing of feelings and needs in a communication environment, which is more natural than the individual therapy setting. Group therapy provides individuals with opportunities to increase social interaction and self-monitoring skills in a more natural communication environment, increase self-esteem and self-motivation, increase the ability to develop short- and long-term goals that are meaningful, share feelings and needs, and provide and receive peer-review of behaviors.

Group therapy is appropriate at all levels along the treatment continuum. Tasks used at lower and middle cognitive levels are generally similar to tasks used in individual sessions. Group therapy activities that benefit head-injured persons with high-level thought processing and problem-solving deficits are described in the following section.

Interpersonal Interaction Group

The responsibility for presenting an assigned or selected topic is rotated among group members. A video recording should be made of each presentation. Utilizing the video recording, all group members should evaluate the session using an objective form. Each person should evaluate himself or herself regarding the roles placed as speakers and listeners during the group session. Specific areas to be evaluated include presentation of organized, sequential information; conveyance of main point; ability to use abstract information; ability to use feedback; too little or excessive information; irrelevant information; redundant information; observation of rules; appropriate topic switching; obscurity or ambiguity; and style of communication.

Pragmatic behaviors can also be evaluated, including behavior appropriate to situation, eye contact, turn taking, initiation of conversation, use of gestures, appropriate affect, speed of response, appropriate posture, appropriate rate, appropriate intonation, appropriate social distance, group support, an ability to profit from cuing, and willingness and ability to modify behaviors.

Listeners also can be evaluated for their use of appropriate questioning strategies, the ability to interpret information abstractly, requesting of repetitions when needed, the ability to identify missing information, the ability to give feedback, and the ability to identify the main point.

Social Skills Group

The ability of each group member to cooperate and accept group decisions should be evaluated following participation in an assigned social activity, such as planning special menus, birthday parties, outings, and family open houses. The ability of each group member to adjust behavior appropriately with regard to verbal output, dress, and gestures can be evaluated following assigned role-playing activities. Specific activities include a party with friends versus a job interview, or a family dinner versus dinner with a new date.

Empathic Abilities Group

On a rotating basis, the conflict-resolution skills of each group member should be evaluated following the role playing of a dispute between two friends according to a script prepared by the clinician or a subcommittee of group members. Specific abilities to be evaluated include the ability to determine reasons for the dispute (deductive reasoning), the ability to determine premises or assumptions of each person, the ability to establish compromise, the ability to test solutions, and the ability to negotiate a compromise (complementary reasoning).

PERSONAL AND SOCIAL ADJUSTMENT GROUP

In individual sessions, establish and rehearse various personal statements with each client. For example, a client might be required to make a statement regarding two personal strengths, for example, "I am a person who . . . " Video recordings should be made of the individual session and should be critiqued by the client and the clinician. After the client has mastered the individual session, a presentation should be made to the entire group. A self-evaluation and group evaluation should be made of the video recording of the group session using a system to score awareness, understanding, assimilation, and acceptance (adapted from Ben-Yishay and Diller, 1981).

LIFE SKILLS GROUP

The group members themselves may generate a list of activities to work on. Role playing in the group setting should be followed by actual community experiences. Activities include giving and following directions, shopping, using public transportation, emergency skills, meal preparation, household management, use of leisure and recreational time, time management, management of personal care attendants, and letter-writing skills.

Community Reentry

The most effective rehabilitation programs for patients with traumatic brain injury go beyond the walls of rehabilitation centers into their homes, communities, schools, and workplaces. After individual and group treatment, specific cognitive and executive skills must be assessed and treated in real-life situations. Practice in real-life situations

helps address difficulties with generalizations experienced by patients with traumatic brain injury and also brings difficulty into light that were anticipated in individual or group sessions (Adamovich and Henderson, 1992). Additional advantages of community-based treatment include the relevancy to the individual's life that is inherently motivating; the provision of opportunities to integrate various approaches to cognitive rehabilitation to achieve objectives and outcomes that are meaningful for the individual; opportunities to assess the individual's abilities to meet the unique demands of his or her environment; opportunities to observe, firsthand, the noninjury factors, for example, family dynamics, peer culture, etc., that affect the individual's ability to achieve his or her personal goals; increased generalization; higher level of success with meaningful activities; greater awareness of the individual consequences of actions; and the promotion of empowerment and inclusion (Kneipp, 1995). An evaluation of multidisciplinary community-based outreach rehabilitation after severe traumatic brain injury revealed that benefits were seen in the areas of personal care, mobility, and cognitive function years after injury, which outlasted the active treatment period with 48 patients (Powell et al., 2002).

Vocational and Return to School and/or Work

Premorbid levels of functioning must be considered when establishing educational and vocational goals. Premorbid considerations include level of educational history, previous occupation, employment history, hobbies and interests, history of substance abuse, and personality variables. It is unlikely that the person who is not a superstar educationally or vocationally premorbidly will be a superstar post-traumatic brain injury. MacMillan et al. (2002) studied 45 adults with moderate or severe CHI at least 2 years earlier. They found that preinjury psychiatric and substance abuse histories predicted employment status and that preinjury substance abuse predicted independent living status. Return to work is also affected by length of posttraumatic amnesia, cognitive level, disability level, functional status, length of acute stay, and prior occupation (Fleming et al., 1999). Common educational and vocational limitations following traumatic brain injury include the inability to delay gratification, an inability to cope with distractions, rigidity or an inability to modify tasks or behavior, an inability to identify salient or key factors, and a short attention span. Other factors that must be considered when selecting educational and vocational goals are the individual's planning skills, memory and cognitive abilities, the presence of a paralysis, the presence of visual and/or auditory limitations, and communication deficits. Community colleges, colleges, and universities generally have programs for students with hearing or visual deficits, yet these special programs are not as available for individuals with traumatic brain injury, and rehabilitation clinicians may need to take the lead in assisting in the development of special programs. Special educational programs should include cognitive remediation sessions, socialization groups, assistance with integration into regular or special classrooms that include assistance with transportation, tutors, adaptive equipment as necessary, and assistance with note taking. Special counselors and job placement counselors would also be of value.

When patients are returning to work, employers tend to be most concerned with the employee's speed, safety, and efficiency on the job; his or her ability to get along with his or her coworkers; and the potential overuse of sick benefits. A vocational emphasis is an extremely necessary component of all community reentry programs. Generally, return-to-work assessments and work hardening programs can be modified for patients with traumatic brain injury. Vocational evaluators and counselors must be educated regarding the typical cognitive deficits and behaviors that follow traumatic brain injury. A program must be determined that takes into account each individual's limitations and needs. The individuals

should undergo individual and group treatment that assists with the identification and acceptance of limitations pertaining to vocational limitations. Supervised work trials are essential, including job simulation, use of sheltered workshops, and finally, community work sites. Even though a return-to-work hierarchy is followed beginning with simulated trials and practice in a fairly controlled environment such as the shelter workshop or a clinic setting, when placed in a community on an actual work site, the traumatic brain injury patient will benefit greatly if a job coach is provided. The employer must be educated as to the specific limitations of the head-injured worker. They also must have the opportunity to request the services of the rehabilitation team or job coach, should it be necessary to modify the duties performed by the brain-injured worker.

Ruff et al. (1993) found that the three most important predictors for returning to work or school were intactness of the patient's verbal and intellectual power, speed of information processing, and age. A key to the successful return-to-work programs is the establishment of tax incentives for individuals with disabilities who work. Currently, it is very difficult for individuals to return to work if they are capable of performing on jobs that pay less than what they are currently earning from disability insurance or worker's compensation plans. It is difficult to convince a young father to give up a source of income even though the quality of his life would be enhanced by meaningful employment.

Conclusion

The treatment of patients with traumatic head injuries must extend beyond the inpatient setting to outpatient programs, which focus on community reentry. Speech-language pathologists must be prepared to treat a wide variety of behaviors including speech, language, voice, swallowing, and cognition. Additional skills necessary include the ability to function on an interdisciplinary team; the ability to do functional assessments, goal setting, and outcome measurements; knowledge of metacognitive and executive functioning skills assessment and treatment; the treatment of pragmatic skills; the provision of individual and group treatment; the ability to provide assessment and treatment in real-life settings in the community; and the ability to empower patients and families to regain control of their lives and to begin making their own decisions.

References

Adamovich, B.B. & Henderson, J. (1992). *Scales of Cognitive Ability for Traumatic Brain Injury (SCATBI)*. Chicago: Riverside.

Adamovich, B.B., Henderson, J.A. & Auerback, S. (1985). *Cognitive Rehabilitation of Closed Head Injured Patients, A Dynamic Approach*. Boston: Little, Brown.

Alexander, M.P., Benson, D.F. & Stuss, D.T. (1989). Frontal Lobes and Language. *Brain and language, 37*, 656–691.

Baker, H. & Leland, B. (1935). *Detroit Test of Learning Ability*. Indianapolis and Chicago: Bobbs-Merrill.

Ben-Yishay, Y. & Diller, L. (1981). Rehabilitation of Cognitive and Perceptual Defects in People with Traumatic Brain Damage. *International Journal of Rehabilitation Research, 4*, 208–210.

Bigler, E.D. (1990). Neuropathology of Traumatic Brain Injury. In: E.D. Bigler (Ed.), *Traumatic Brain Injury, Mechanisms of Damage, Assessment, Intervention, and Outcome* (p. 13). Austin, TX: Pro-Ed.

Boake, C., Millis, S.R., High, W.M., Jr., Delmonica, R.L., Kreutzer, J.S., Rosenthal, M., Sherer, M. & Ivanhoe, C.B. (2001). Using Early Neuropsychologic Testing to Predict Long-Term Productivity Outcome from Traumatic Brain Injury. *Archives of Physical Medicine and Rehabilitation, 82*, 761–768.

Ceballos-Baumann, A.O. (2000). Thalamic Stimulation for Essential Tremor Activates Motor and Deactivates Vestibular Cortex. *Neurology, 56*, 1347–1354.

Cicerone, K.D. (2002). Remediation of Working Attention in Mild Traumatic Brain Injury. *Brain Injury, 16*, 185–195.

Cicerone, K.D. & Giacino, J.T. (1992). Remediation of Executive Function Deficits After Traumatic Brain Injury. *Neuropsychological Rehabilitation, 2*, 12–22.

Dawson, D., Winocur, G. & Moscovitch, M. (1999). The Psychosocial Environment and Cognitive Rehabilitation in the Elderly. In: D.T. Stuss, G. Winocur, & I.H. Robertson (Eds.), *Cognitive Rehabilitation* (pp. 94–108). Cambridge, UK: Cambridge University Press.

Fleming, J., Tooth, L., Hassell, M. & Chan, W. (1999). Prediction of Community Integration and Vocational Outcome 2–5 Years After Traumatic Brain Injury Rehabilitation in Australia. *Brain Injury, 13*, 417–431.

Gordon, W.A. & Hibbard, M.K. (1991). The Theory and Practice of Cognitive Remediation. In: J.S. Kreutzer & P.H. Wehman (Eds.), *Cognitive Rehabilitation for Persons with Traumatic Brain Injury. A Functional Approach* (pp. 13–22). Baltimore, MD: Paul H. Brooks.

Gourlay, D., Lun, K.C. & Liya, G. (2000). Telemedicinal Virtual Reality for Cognitive Rehabilitation. *Medical Infobahn for Europe, 77*, 1181–1186.

Granger, C.V., Hamilton, B.B. & Keith, R.A. (1986). Advances in Functional Assessment for Medical Rehabilitation. *Topics in Geriatric Medicine, 1*, 59–74.

Grealy, M.A., Johnson, D.A. & Rushton, S.K. (1999). Improving Cognitive Function After Brain Injury: The Use of Exercise and Virtual Reality. *Archives of Physical Medicine and Rehabilitation, 80*, 661–667.

Hall, K.M., Hamilton, B.B. & Keith, R.A. (1993). Characteristics and Comparisons of Functional Assessment Indices: Disability Rating Scale, Functional Independence Measure, and Functional Assessment Measure. *Journal of Head Trauma Rehabilitation, 8*, 60–74.

Hawley, C.A., Taylor, R., Hellawell, D.J. & Pentland, B. (1999). Use of the Functional Assessment Measure (FIM+FAM) in Head Injury Rehabilitation: A Psychometric Analysis. *Journal of Neurology, Neurosurgery, and Psychiatry, 67*, 749–754.

Jackson, R.D., Mysiw, W.J. & Corrigan, J.D. (1989). Orientation Group Monitoring System: An Indicator of Reversible Impairments in Cognition During Post-Traumatic Amnesia. *Archives of Physical Medicine and Rehabilitation, 70*, 33–36.

Kneipp, S. (1995). *Real-World Cognitive Rehabilitation: Community-Based Interventions*. Workshop presented at Applied Cognitive Rehabilitation: A training seminar sponsored by the Society of Cognitive Rehabilitation, Inc.

Laatsch, L., Pavel, D. Jobe, T., Qing, L. & Quintana, J.C. (1999). Incorporation of SPECT Imaging in a Longitudinal Cognitive Rehabilitation Therapy Programme. *Brain Injury, 13*, 555–570.

Levin, H.S. (1987). The Neurobehavioral Rating Scale: Assessment of the Behavioural Sequelae of Head Injury by the Clinician. *Journal of Neurology and Neurosurgical Psychiatry, 50*, 183.

Levin, M.S. & Kraus, M.F. (1994). The Frontal Lobes and Traumatic Brain Injury. Special Issue: The Frontal Lobes and Neuropsychiatric Illness. *Journal of Neuropsychiatry and Clinical Neurosciences, 6*, 443–454.

Lezak, M.D. (1982). The Problem of Assessing Executive Function. *International Journal of Psychology, 17*, 231–297.

MacMillan, P.J., Hart, R.P., Martelli, M.F. & Zasler, N.D. (2002). Pre-Injury Statue and Adaptation Following Traumatic Brain Injury. *Brain Injury, 16*, 41–49.

Malec, J.D., Smigielski, J.S., DePompolo, R. & Thompson, J.M. (1993). Outcome Evaluation and Prediction in a Comprehensive-Integrated Post-Acute Outpatient Brain Injury Rehabilitation Programme. *Brain Injury, 7*, 15–29.

Pizzamiglio, L., Perani, D., Cappa, S.F., Vallar, G., Paolucci, S., Grassi, F., et al. (1998). Recovery of Neglect After Right Hemispheric Damage: H2150 Positron Emission Tomographic Activation Study. *Archives of Neurology, 55*, 561–568.

Powell, J., Heslin, J. & Greenwood, R. (2002). Community Based Rehabilitation After Severe Traumatic Brain Injury: A Randomized Controlled Trial. *Journal of Neurology, Neurosurgery and Psychiatry, 72*, 193–202.

Rezai, A. (1999). Thalamic Stimulation and Functional MRI: Localization of Cortical and Subcortical Activation with Implanted Electrodes. *Journal of Neurosurgery, 90,* 583–590.

Robertson, I.H. (1999). Setting Goals for Cognitive Rehabilitation. *Current Opinion in Neurology, 12,* 703–708.

Ross, J.D. & Ross, C.M. (1976). *Ross Test of Higher Cognitive Processes.* San Rafael, CA: Academic Therapy Publications.

Ruff, R.M., Marshall, L.F., Crouch, J. & Klauber, M.R. (1993). Predictors of Outcome Following Severe Head Trauma: Follow-up data from the Traumatic Coma Data Bank. *Brain Injury, 7,* 101–111.

Schiff, N.D., Plum, F. & Rezai, A.R. (2002). Developing Prosthetics to Treat Cognitive Disabilities Resulting from Acquired Brain Injuries. *Neurological Research, 24,* 116–124.

Sherer, M., Sander, A.M., Nick, T.G., High, W.M. Jr., Males, J.F. & Rosenthal, M. (2002). Early Cognitive Status and Productivity Outcome After Traumatic Brain Injury: Findings from the TBI Model Systems. *Archives of Physical Medicine and Rehabilitation, 83,* 183–192.

Sohlberg, M.M. & Mateer, C.A. (2001). Improving Attention and Managing Attentional Problems. *Annals of the New York Academy of Sciences, 931,* 359–375.

Taverni, J.P., Selinger, G. & Lichtman, S.W. (1998) Donepezil Mediated Memory Improvement in Traumatic Brain Injury During Post Acute Rehabilitation. *Brain Injury, 12,* 77–80.

Wechsler, D. (1981). *Wechsler Adult Intelligence Scale-Revised* (Manual). New York: Psychological Corporation.

Whiteneck, G., Charlifue, S., Gerhart, K., Overholser, J. & Richardson, G. (1992). Quantifying Handicap: A New Measure of Long-Term Rehabilitation Outcomes. *Archives of Physical Medical Rehabilitation, 73,* 519–526.

Wilson, B.A. & Moffat, N. (Eds.). (1984). *Clinical Management of Memory Problems.* Rockville, MD: Aspen Systems Corporation.

Winocur, G., Palmer, H., Stuss, D.T., Alexander, M.P., Craik, F.I.M., Levine, B. & Moscovitch, M. (2000). Cognitive Rehabilitation in Clinical Neuropsychology. *Brain and Cognition, 42,* 120–123.

Winslade, W.J. (1998). *Confronting Traumatic Brain Injury.* New Haven, CT: Yale University Press.

Ylvisaker, M. & Szekeres, S.F. (1989). Metacognitive and Executive Impairments in Head-Injured Children and Adults. *Topics in Language Disorders, 9,* 34–49.

16

Pragmatics

HEATHER HARRIS WRIGHT AND MARILYN NEWHOFF

The focus of this chapter differs somewhat from that of previous chapters, which focused on particular syndromes of brain damage and the resulting functional changes in speech and language abilities. In this chapter, the emphasis shifts from an etiologic focus based on the location of the disruption in the nervous system to a focus on one specific area of the language system, pragmatics, which can permeate syndromes of aphasia regardless of the location of the damage. This chapter discusses the overriding issue of communication.

Nature and Differentiating Features

Definition of Pragmatics

To better understand the pragmatic impairments evidenced by individuals with brain damage, the types of skills involved in pragmatics must be understood. *Pragmatics* refers to the set of rules that govern the *use* of language in context (Bates, 1976). This area of communication includes the ability to use language for a variety of functions, such as to comment, warn, request, protest, and acknowledge. Other pragmatic uses of language revolve around rules of discourse and include the ability to use linguistic and nonlinguistic devices to initiate and maintain topics, to request and respond to clarification, to take conversational turns, to adjust meaning and form for one's listener, and to use appropriate eye gaze and facial expressions. In short, the pragmatic dimension of language determines why a speaker says something, when the speaker says it, to whom the speaker says it, and how it is used.

Since the surge of interest in the pragmatic aspect of language in the 1970s, several authors have presented taxonomies that depict a wide range of pragmatic skills (Davis, 1989; Prutting & Kirchner, 1987). Although considerable agreement exists on the types of skills in question, authors often differ on how they organize or categorize these skills. In a very general sense, pragmatic skills can be divided into two major categories: *linguistic* and *nonlinguistic*. For example, pragmatic adaptations to a listener (i.e., changing the content or topic of a message depending on the listener) are often accomplished via specific syntactic forms (e.g., definite and indefinite articles, anaphoric pronouns) and specific lexical choices (e.g., listener-friendly vocabulary), representing a *linguistic* orientation. Conversely, changes in the suprasegmental aspects of speech or eye gaze can provide information to the listener regarding the intent of the speaker to maintain or relinquish his or her conversational turn, and these are clearly *nonlinguistic* behaviors (see Table 16–1 for a list of commonly identified pragmatic skills).

Linguistic Conversational Skills of Individuals with Aphasia

Traditionally, researchers have viewed pragmatic skills of adults with aphasia as better than their language skills (i.e., syntax and

Table 16–1. Pragmatic Skills

1. Linguistic conversational skills
   A. Speech act use (e.g., comment, request, warn, assert, promise, direct, acknowledge)
   B. Topic skills (e.g., initiation, maintenance, shift, shading)
   C. Turn-taking skills (e.g., initiation, response, interruption/overlap, pause time)
   D. Conversational repair skills (e.g., contingent responses, lexical selection, quantity and conciseness of information, requests for and responses to clarification)
   E. Presuppositional skills (e.g., appropriate use of pronouns, ellipsis, change in register)
   F. Speech act comprehension (e.g., indirect speech acts, emotional content)

2. Nonlinguistic conversational skills
   A. Paralinguistic aspects of communication (e.g., pitch and intensity, syllabic and juncture stress, intelligibility)
   B. Extralinguistic aspects of communication (e.g., eye gaze, proximity to conversational partner)

semantics), and have found that these individuals can present with appropriate pragmatic performance while having a significant language impairment (Avent et al., 1998; Wulfeck et al., 1989). Recent findings, however, have shown that adults with aphasia do not present with normal pragmatic performance for all linguistic skills; indeed, they often perform no better than adults with right hemisphere communication disorders, a group traditionally viewed as having pragmatic impairments (see Chapter 14 for review). This has led many researchers to conclude that both hemispheres are involved in "linguistic" pragmatics, not just the right hemisphere (Kasher et al., 1999; Zaidel et al., 2000).

It is also the case that pragmatic behaviors are evidenced during both production and comprehension tasks. In the case of productive pragmatic performance, variations may be due to aphasia type. Not surprisingly, during discourse, adults with severe Broca's aphasia initiate and shift topics less frequently, and produce fewer queries, than adults without brain damage (Dronkers et al., 1998). And, although adults with fluent aphasia produce a similar amount of language during conversation as do non-brain-damaged adults, less information is conveyed (Chapman et al., 1998). Deficit behaviors that seem free of aphasia-type influences include less specificity and accuracy of the message, inappropriate pause times during turn-taking, less quantity of information in the message, and less variety in the types of speech acts used (Borod et al., 2000; Kasher et al., 1999; Prutting & Kirchner, 1987; Zaidel et al., 2000). Though these are clearly weaknesses in the pragmatic skills of individuals with aphasia, *some* pragmatic skills seem less affected by the presence of aphasia: use of conversational repairs appropriately following breakdowns in conversation (Ulatowska et al., 1992) and adding new information during turn taking, as well as maintaining the conversation with turns (Ulatowska et al., 1992; Wulfeck et al., 1989). It may well be that aphasic individuals' deficits in productive pragmatic performance may be the result of their linguistic deficits. For example, word-retrieval deficits will likely impact their ability to add new information (resulting in increased burden on their conversation partner). However, these individuals do retain the knowledge of pragmatic constraints and demonstrate this, when they are able, such as during conversational turn-taking and maintenance.

Comprehension of indirect speech acts and emotional content is also a linguistic pragmatic skill that has been investigated in brain-damaged individuals. Indirect speech acts occur when a speaker makes a statement that is not intended for direct interpretation. For example, the phrase "Can you pass the salt?" has a direct interpretation of a question requiring a yes or no response; however, the indirect and intended interpretation for this phrase is a request requiring a physical act of passing the salt. Adults with aphasia, specifically Broca's aphasics who have difficulty comprehending the "Can you ___" syntactic form, are able to understand indirect speech acts rather well (Hirst et al., 1984).

Conveying emotion is typically considered a nonlinguistic, pragmatic skill, one that typically requires shifts in suprasegmentals for that conveyance. However, when communicating emotion with the use of words and sentences (e.g., "I feel like crying"), it can be considered a linguistic, pragmatic skill. Recently, researchers have devoted some attention to this linguistic communication of emotion and found that, in aphasia, inclusion of emotional content in a message actually facilitates comprehension abilities (Cicero et al., 1999; Reuterskiold, 1991). For example, in their study of oral word and sentence comprehension in aphasia, where tasks varied by the inclusion of emotional content, Cicero et al. (1999) determined that emotional content enhanced comprehension. Further, in a study of emotional content in reading passages, it was found that its inclusion in written language also improved reading comprehension by individuals with aphasia (Landis et al., 1982).

Nonlinguistic Conversational Skills of Individuals with Aphasia

Nonlinguistic conversational skills include *paralinguistic* contexts, such as prosodic changes, and *extralinguistic* contexts, such as formality of the setting, content knowledge of the speaker-listener, and emotional state of the speaker-listener (Davis, 1989). Prosodic changes can include variations in pitch, loudness, and syllabic and juncture stress and can provide for communication of emotional state as well as certain types of semantic and syntactic information. Relative to semantic/syntactic meaning, consider the word "convict," a noun when stress is placed on the first syllable, but a verb if stress is on the second syllable. Extralinguistic aspects of communication include external and internal contexts. Communication setting and knowledge of the topic, as well as the speaker's emotional state, are factors that will also influence conversational style and lexical choice.

In general, individuals with aphasia tend to comprehend and produce nonlinguistic

aspects of communication rather well, though much of the literature that has addressed this aspect of communication has focused only on comprehension of paralinguistic skills (Barrett et al., 1999; Geigenberger & Ziegler, 2001; Lorch et al., 1998). For one aspect, however, contradictory findings exist. Comprehension of emotional prosody by aphasic adults has been found to be much like that of non-brain-damaged adults on the experimental tasks of some researchers (Barrett et al., 1999; Geigenberger & Ziegler, 2001; Pell & Baum, 1997a). Still others have found that individuals with aphasia are impaired in processing emotional prosody (Pell, 1998; Pell & Baum, 1997b). Site of lesion may account for the contradictory findings. Now we have research results from Karow et al. (2001), as well as Cancelliere and Kertesz (1990), that suggest that adults with subcortical damage, in either hemisphere, have more difficulty with affective processing than adults with cortical damage. And, in their critical review of the literature regarding the neural bases of prosodic comprehension, Baum and Pell (1999) concluded that there is certainly evidence to indicate that the left hemisphere is involved in the production and comprehension of prosodic aspects of language. Regarding the use of some nonverbal skills, however, such as eye gaze and head nods, specific subgroups of left hemisphere brain-damaged individuals have shown themselves to be quite adequate in their performance (Prutting & Kirchner, 1987).

Summary

In general, individuals with aphasia present with a strength in pragmatics as compared with other language behaviors (i.e., comprehension and production). However, deficits may exist in specific pragmatic behaviors. These deficits may be due to underlying language impairments present in aphasia; for example, a word-retrieval deficit may reduce an aphasic individual's ability to initiate conversations or add new information to conversations. Or, as Karow et al. (2001) discovered, pragmatic deficits, such as impaired affective processing, may be a result of locale of damage.

Evaluation

As mentioned at the outset, pragmatics involves the use of language in context (Bates, 1976). That being the case, pragmatic skills must be evaluated within conversational contexts. The wealth of available linguistic and nonlinguistic information found in conversational settings can have a marked impact on comprehension and production capabilities of individuals with brain damage. One of the most valid measures of a person's pragmatic skills can be obtained by sampling language abilities in a naturalistic communicative setting. Additional information of a person's pragmatic skills can be obtained from questionnaires, communicative efficiency measures, and standardized tests. In the following section, pragmatic assessments are reviewed (see Table 16–2 for a list of pragmatic assessment tools).

Table 16–2. Pragmatic Assessment Tools

1. Observation and conversation profiles
   Pragmatic Protocol (Prutting & Kirchner, 1987)
   Profile of Communicative Appropriateness (Penn, 1988)
   Communication Profile (Gurland et al., 1982)
   Assessment Protocol of Pragmatic Linguistic Skills (Gerber & Gurland, 1989)
   Discourse Abilities Profile (Terrell & Ripich, 1989)

2. Communicative efficiency protocols
   Revised Edinburgh Functional Communication Profile (Wirz et al., 1990)
   Functional Communication Profile (Sarno, 1965)
   Communication/Competence Evaluation Instrument (Houghton et al., 1982)
   Communicative Efficiency Index (Lomas et al., 1989)

3. Standardized measures
   Communicative Abilities in Daily Living–2 (Holland et al., 1988)
   Amsterdam-Nijmegen Everyday Language Test (Blomert, 1990; Blomert et al., 1987, 1994)
   ASHA-FACS (Frattali et al., 1995)

Several of the assessment tools reviewed require a language sample. When collecting a language sample, clinicians engage clients in conversation to determine their pragmatic use of language. Although there is no agreed upon sample "size," the goal of the procedure should be to obtain a large enough sample so that a representative amount of communicative interaction is available for analysis. A sample of ~400 words in length is generally suggested as sufficient to yield reliable information (Doyle et al., 2000).

Observational and Conversational Profiles

After a representative sample of language is collected, the clinician can begin to judge the appropriateness of pragmatic skills. Several observational and conversational profiles are available and suitable for identifying pragmatic abilities of adults with neurologic impairments. These measures include the Pragmatic Protocol (Prutting & Kirchner, 1987), the Profile of Communicative Appropriateness (PCA) (Penn, 1988), the Communication Profile (Gurland et al., 1982), the Assessment Protocol of Pragmatic Linguistic Skills (APPLS) (Gerber & Gurland, 1989), and the Discourse Abilities Profile (DAP) (Terrell & Ripich, 1989). Both the Pragmatic Protocol and Communication Profile are designed to examine pragmatic behaviors exhibited in conversations. In the Pragmatic Protocol, 30 pragmatic skills, divided into three general measurement areas, are examined. *Verbal* aspects involve such skills as topic selection, initiation, maintenance, turn-taking, specificity of the message, and use of cohesive devices. *Paralinguistic* aspects include speech intelligibility, prosody, and vocal quality and intensity. Finally, *nonverbal* aspects include eye gaze, facial expressions, and physical proximity of the speaker and listener. If the client demonstrates one instance of a behavior that interferes with communication, that behavior is considered to be a possible impairment. The purpose of the Communication Profile is to examine linguistic behaviors such as initiation, maintenance, and termination of conversations as well as production of speech acts and presuppositions. It is a comprehensive measure of the aphasic client's conversational abilities (Manochipinig et al., 1992); however, it does not examine nonlinguistic behaviors.

Pragmatic behaviors exhibited during a client/clinician interaction, including conversation, narration, and procedural discourse components, are examined in both the PCA and DAP. Similar to the Pragmatic Protocol, the PCA is structured to examine pragmatic behaviors in several general areas: *response to interlocutor, control of semantic content, cohesion, fluency, sociolinguistic sensitivity,* and *nonverbal communication.* Appropriateness of the behaviors is judged by the clinician on a six-point rating scale. In the DAP, the examiner scores the presence or absence of various components of discourse. For example, taking turns is observed during conversation, whereas paralinguistic and extralinguistic behaviors are observed and rated during all forms of discourse.

The outcomes of linguistic and pragmatic behavioral, conversational breakdowns are examined in the APPLS. There are four parts to the analysis. In the first, breakdowns in the conversation are assessed and, in the second, breakdown-repair sequences are analyzed. The third part focuses on the linguistic structures and pragmatic functions that lead the client to successful portions of interactions, and the fourth is concerned with quantitative and qualitative summaries of the interactions. Breakdowns may include linguistic (e.g., word retrieval) or pragmatic (e.g., topic maintenance) problems. Breakdown-repair sequences may include client strategies or revisions (e.g., paraphrases) or partner strategies (e.g., requesting more specific information).

In summary, the Pragmatic Profile, PCA, and DAP are designed to examine linguistic and nonlinguistic pragmatic behaviors in discourse. Specifically, success of communication is the measure of both linguistic (i.e., word retrieval) and linguistic, pragmatic behaviors (i.e., turn-taking) in the APPLS. Whereas with the Pragmatic Profile and PCA appropriateness of the behaviors exhibited

is coded, with the DAP, presence or absence of the behaviors is coded. Each of these measures can be useful for treatment planning. For example, the APPLS can be used to measure both the client's strengths and weaknesses, lending itself quite well to planning remediation. Terrell and Ripich (1989) provide specific guidelines for planning treatment based on aphasic individual's performance on the DAP.

Communication Efficiency Protocols

This section discusses the protocols that measure the client's overall degree of communication efficiency. Individual pragmatic behaviors are not measured; rather, the combined effectiveness of the individual's pragmatic behaviors for communicative efficiency is measured. These measures could be considered functional communication measures, but are still included in this chapter because functional communication is a product of the effective use of several pragmatic behaviors (i.e., linguistic and nonlinguistic) (Penn, 1999). Protocols available for measuring communication efficiency include the Revised Edinburgh Functional Communication Profile (EFCP) (Wirz et al., 1990), the Functional Communication Profile (FCP) (Sarno, 1965), the Communication Competence Evaluation Instrument (CCEI) (Houghton et al., 1982), and the Communication Efficiency Index (CETI) (Lomas et al., 1989).

The EFCP and CETI are useful for determining an individual's functional communication strengths and weaknesses. With the EFCP, the clinician codes the client's use of speech, gesture, and writing in response to real-life situations (e.g., greeting). Because different modes of communication are observed, this measure is better with clients with severe communication impairments (Manochipinig et al., 1992). For the CETI, a significant other codes the aphasic individual's performance on 16 daily living situations. Performance is rated on a visual analog scale with "not at all able" at one end and "as able as before the illness" at the other. Example situations include getting someone's attention, communicating his or her emotions, and participating in conversations with strangers.

The FCP also measures aphasic individuals' functional communication, but in more natural communication settings. Performance of 45 behaviors, in five areas (movement, speaking, understanding, reading, and other), are rated on a nine-point scale. Though pragmatic skills are required for several of the behaviors measured, the FCP is designed to assess overall functional communication behaviors more than pragmatic ones (Gerber & Gurland, 1989). The CCEI is designed to assess functional communication and pragmatic behaviors in aphasic individuals. This measure was developed specifically for use with severely impaired aphasic individuals.

In summary, these measures are useful for assessing an aphasic individual's ability to communicate functionally, outside the treatment room. Though they are not intended to identify pragmatic deficit behaviors, they *do* provide information about the client's communicative effectiveness. And, to be communicatively effective, of course, requires the appropriate use of several pragmatic skills.

Standardized Measures

Although a language sample can provide information regarding pragmatic skills, there are standardized measures specifically designed to assess real-life communicative abilities. These include the Communicative Abilities in Daily Living–2 (CADL-2) (Holland et al., 1988), the American Speech-Language-Hearing Association (ASHA) Functional Assessment of Communication Skills for Adults (FACS) (Frattali et al., 1995), and the Amsterdam-Nijmegen Everyday Language Test (ANELT) (Blomert, 1990; Blomert et al., 1987, 1994). Holland et al.'s (1988) CADL-2 is designed to help clinicians better identify their clients' functional communicative abilities. The focus of this assessment tool is on communicative adequacy, not linguistic accuracy. The CADL-2 was constructed to incorporate daily living language contexts and

natural communicative skills of the client. The test is intended to examine a wide variety of behaviors including speech acts, humor and metaphor, numeric estimates and calculations, integration of verbal and nonverbal contexts to understand and relate information, and the use of social language. The CADL-2, then, allows for examination of several linguistic and nonlinguistic pragmatic behaviors not normally assessed in traditional diagnostic batteries.

The ASHA-FACS was designed to examine functional communication abilities in aphasic adults. Aphasic individuals are scored on their ability to complete several everyday communication activities across four different areas: social communication (e.g., "refers to familiar people by name"), communication of basic needs (e.g., "requests help when necessary"), reading, writing, and number sequences (e.g., "understands simple signs"), and daily planning (e.g., "knows what time it is"). The ANELT is also a measure of functional communication. Two rating scales (semantic comprehensibility and speech intelligibility) are used on the ANELT for measuring an individual's communicative efficiency with verbal expression. Ten situations (e.g., requesting that broken glass be fixed) are presented to the client, who then role-plays a conversation with the clinician for solving the situations. Neither the ANELT nor the ASHA-FACS is meant to examine specific linguistic or nonlinguistic pragmatic behaviors; however, the behaviors are indirectly examined as they are needed for functional communication. For example, if the situation of "fixing a broken glass" was presented from the ANELT, linguistic pragmatic skills such as turn-taking, topic maintenance, and topic initiation skills are required, and nonlinguistic skills such as eye gaze and prosody are required.

Summary

The context of assessment should be expanded to include interactions that comprise a wide variety of speech acts within a conversational setting. The assessment setting also should allow for observation of clients' abilities to regulate conversations linguistically (e.g., turn-taking, initiating topics) and nonlinguistically (e.g., use of appropriate eye contact). By establishing a conversational context, the clinician will be able to identify the pragmatic strengths and weaknesses of clients with aphasia and can establish appropriate treatment goals and activities based on these measures.

Treatment

Intervention for pragmatic impairments can be potentially successful when the clinical activities include all of the conversational functions and rules that normally underlie communicative interactions. Generally, the most efficient strategy for targeting pragmatic impairments in intervention involves two simple steps. First, the clinician should determine situations or contexts in which the impaired skills are normally used in a client's daily conversations. Second, similar settings should be constructed and/or made available in intervention to approximate the same context(s). For example, if a person has shown an impairment in the ability to request information during a conversational breakdown, then the first step in intervention might be to determine contexts in which most speakers provide requests for clarification. Examples of contexts in which this skill is used could include asking for directions to a new restaurant in town or participating in telephone conversations with grandchildren. Once several contexts are determined, the clinician can begin to incorporate and/or simulate these same contexts for intervention purposes. The intervention is pragmatic not only in the sense of incorporating the linguistic and nonlinguistic aspects of communication, but also in that the activities are of functional use. This last notion is not to be overlooked because it becomes easy to use preplanned activities from treatment manuals readily available on the market. This "cookbook" method of intervention is not considered respectful of client differences and specificities; thus, it rarely addresses the

needs and contexts of communication that individual clients have.

The following section presents brief descriptions of several approaches to pragmatic intervention with individuals with aphasia. The techniques we've selected have been used successfully in creating naturalistic communicative settings for targeting pragmatic deficits. Although pragmatic deficits are targeted, it should be noted that most goals for improving communication best occur in naturalistic contexts such as these.

Specific Treatment Tasks

PROMOTING APHASICS' COMMUNICATIVE EFFECTIVENESS

The notion of a naturalistic intervention setting served as the theoretical basis for the intervention protocol devised by Davis and Wilcox (1985), Promoting Aphasics' Communicative Effectiveness (PACE). PACE was developed from the recognition that traditional intervention techniques do not duplicate the structure of natural conversation. With PACE the client and clinician are focused on ideas to be conveyed rather than on the struggle for linguistic accuracy; divergent linguistic behavior is inherent in the interaction; and active listening (i.e., listening for the intent of the speaker) is required by both conversational partners. The four principles of PACE are as follows:

1. The clinician and client participate equally as senders and receivers of messages.
2. There is an exchange of new information between the clinician and client.
3. The speaker has free choice as to which modality is used to convey a message.
4. Feedback to the listener focuses on the *adequacy* of the message, that is, the degree to which it was communicated successfully.

PACE intervention frequently centers on the process of the clinician and client taking turns describing unknown pictures to each other. Typically, the clinician and client sit across from each other. A large stack of picture cards is placed face down on a table between them. The clinician and client then take turns choosing a card and describing the contents. For example, clients with problems in providing informative messages may describe pictures of simple objects or actions. If a client has difficulty in providing information in a logically ordered sequence of actions or events, the cards may contain a series of pictures that represent a simple story line or common event or procedure. The goal of the activity is to convey adequate information to the listener. The client's message is judged on how well the clinician is able to understand what's on the card being described. As a speaker, the clinician models the type of appropriate pragmatic behaviors that are being targeted for change in the activity. The important feature of this intervention protocol is that the use of conversational functions and rules is required of the client and modeled by the clinician.

Role Playing

A second useful intervention technique that can be used for pragmatic intervention is role playing, which provides opportunities to practice communication in situations that arise in everyday experiences, and enables the clinician to discuss and implement possible strategies useful outside the clinic environment. Role playing also allows for free exchange of information between the participants, thus emphasizing the use of language in context.

A role-playing activity typically involves three phases (Webster, 1977). During the first phase, the clinician and the client discuss the goal of the role-play activity as well as possible responses and behaviors that can be used during the activity. For example, if the goal is to initiate and maintain a topic across several conversational turns, one possible role-play situation might be the meeting of an old friend for the first time in several years. The clinician and the client first discuss possible "opening lines" that the client might use as

well as possible statements or questions that can serve to continue the topic.

After the clinician and the client have discussed the situation, role playing commences. The emphasis during this phase of role playing changes from practice and discussion of target pragmatic behaviors to using these skills in a "spontaneous" conversational setting. It is essential that the clinician retain his or her role throughout the role play so as to best represent a situation in which the client must use the target skills. If the clinician steps out of his or her role during this phase, he or she risks the chance of turning a functional, communicative setting into a nonfunctional, instructional setting.

The third intervention phase follows completion of the role play. After the role playing is completed, the clinician and the client discuss and evaluate the adequacy of the information exchanged. This last phase is particularly important because it enables the clinician and client to reflect on specific communicative behaviors. Additionally, it allows the clinician to reinforce those behaviors that contributed to the adequacy of the message conveyed, while providing possible alternative strategies for remediating inappropriate pragmatic skills. Although it is not a requirement, videotape playback enhances the evaluation of those communicative behaviors that have been targeted.

A role-playing treatment approach specifically designed for use with adults with neurogenic communication disorders is conversational coaching (Holland, 1991). It is an interactive approach consisting of practicing strategies in conversational simulations that were learned in treatment. The clinician prepares a script that is meaningful and relevant to the client, and that the client and clinician can follow. The script is just beyond the client's productive ability, thus encouraging use of strategies he or she has previously practiced. First, the clinician and client practice the script and the client is encouraged to use previously practiced strategies to convey the information. Then, the client communicates the script to others (i.e., family members or close friends) with the clinician coaching the client. Optimally, the coaching sessions are videotaped for later review. To promote generalization, the script is attempted with an unfamiliar communication partner.

Situations for role playing are many and varied and should be guided by the specific pragmatic goal of remediation, as well as by the usefulness of the content of the role play to the client's everyday living. Role playing may be useful in developing several pragmatic skills including making ambiguous messages understood, producing different speech acts, and practicing appropriate eye gaze and proximity. The main point is that role playing is a viable activity, not only for encouraging spontaneous communication, but also for providing a means of discussing and building pragmatic skills for effective communication.

BARRIER ACTIVITIES

The principles underlying PACE also can easily be incorporated into other types of intervention activities. Originally devised by researchers to examine children's ability to convey new versus old information (Glucksberg & Krauss, 1967), barrier games are communication settings that share with the PACE protocol the same underlying principle of creating a functional communicative setting. These activities, as the name implies, involve placing an opaque barrier between the clinician and the client so as to create a need for each individual to communicate. For most barrier activities, each participant has the same materials on his or her side of the barrier. The task usually requires each conversational partner to take a turn describing a move or change in the materials, requesting additional information about the materials, and/or commanding the other partner to move the materials. After a message is conveyed, the barrier is removed so that the two participants may judge the effectiveness of the speaker's message. As does PACE, these activities stress the importance of conveying new information adequately to a conversational partner, a principle that

often continues to be ignored in clinical intervention.

Barrier activities are general enough to use in remediation for a variety of pragmatic impairments (Busch et al., 1988). These activities provide numerous avenues for comprehending and producing various speech acts as well as conversational rules that serve to maintain the communication interaction. For example, in the manipulation of common objects on each side of the barrier, a client practices making and understanding requests for information, indirect requests for action, comments on actions, requests for clarification, and revisions of prior utterances. Other pragmatic goals can be targeted and accomplished through changes in the materials. For example, one commonly used barrier activity involves giving directions from one destination to another along a simple map. Clinicians can use this activity to work on clients' skills in providing adequate information to their listeners. To increase the quality and quantity of a client's conversational turn, a barrier activity might involve a description of the arrangement of similarly shaped objects that vary in size and color. This type of activity increases the need to provide more descriptive information to a listener. Whatever the activity, the use of a barrier between the speaker and the listener forces a conversational dialogue. These activities also remove emphasis on his or her role as an equal partner in the communicative event. This minimizes some of the problems inherent in a traditional didactic format.

Although most barrier activities require actual barriers to create a need for communicating, not all such activities require a physical barrier. Because the basic premise of the activity is to provide a reason to communicate, other physical settings can also be used. When available, a third person can act as the recipient of information that is known to the client and the clinician. For example, a client and clinician could view a photo album and then relate information about the photos to a third person who is not in visual range of the album. In this situation, then, distance alone is the barrier. Such an approach can be particularly useful because the clinician is free to cue the client as he or she provides information about a topic to a "naive" listener.

Speech-Language Groups

A third intervention technique for addressing pragmatic behaviors is group treatment. Groups are appropriate for adults with aphasia and are an excellent avenue for addressing pragmatic behaviors in naturalistic communicative situations. Further, groups may be used for clients to "practice" strategies learned in individual treatment in a more natural environment and with different communication partners. Several researchers have found that group intervention is an effective approach for treating speech and language deficits in adults with aphasia (Avent, 1997; Elman & Bernstein-Ellis, 1999a,b; Garrett & Ellis, 1999; Holland & Beeson, 1999). Indirect language treatment groups and sociolinguistic treatment groups are two types of groups in which pragmatic behaviors can be targeted.

Indirect treatment groups are less structured than direct group treatments (Davis, 1983). Activities in this type of group may include general conversations with topics ranging from current events, to vacations or trips recently taken or planned, to family stories. The groups may be primarily social groups; an opportunity for clients to meet one another and use learned strategies in a natural environment, but with less communication pressure. Or, the groups may consist of role playing. The approach is similar to what was explained in the previous section but with the clients partnering for role-playing situations and the clinician monitoring the exchanges as opposed to the client and clinician role-playing the situations.

Sociolinguistic treatment groups involve interactions between group participants, with the focus on client interaction and not clinician directives (Davis, 1983). Incorporating PACE (Davis & Wilcox, 1985) principles in group treatment is one way of doing this. PACE treatment addresses many pragmatic behaviors including turn-taking and initiating and maintaining conversation topics. Thus,

taking this approach to group intervention is one way of indirectly targeting linguistic, pragmatic behaviors. Additionally, this is also an opportunity for clients to use strategies learned in structured, individual treatment with individuals other than the clinician. Bollinger et al. (1993) investigated effects of group treatment on 10 chronically aphasic individuals' language abilities, using the Porch Index of Communicative Ability (PICA) (Porch, 1967) and CADL (Holland, 1980) as measures of language ability. Comparing pre- and postgroup treatment performance, Bollinger et al. found significant improvement on both measures, indicating that aphasic individuals' language behaviors can improve as a result of participating in sociolinguistic group treatment.

Bollinger et al. (1993) specifically discussed two group treatment approaches; however, there are many other types of groups that can be designed to address pragmatic and functional communication behaviors (cf. Kearns & Elman, 2001). Regardless of the type of group treatment employed, it is important for clinicians to consider several issues when planning treatment groups: (1) the goal of the treatment group; (2) the clients who will participate and how they will benefit from the groups; (3) how individual client goals will be addressed and measured; (4) how data will be taken and change in behavior measured; (5) when, in the course of recovery, clients will enroll in the groups (e.g., once individual treatment ceases or in addition to individual treatment); and (6) what activities/treatment programs will be part of the treatment groups. When clinicians design treatment for pragmatic impairments in aphasic adults, treatment groups can be optional or additional to individual activities.

Conclusion

Individuals with neurologic impairments demonstrate intact and impaired pragmatic skills. To most completely understand their communication deficits, all assessment plans should include a measure of their language use. Intervention goals can be established based on the results. Assessment and intervention for pragmatic impairments must take place in as naturalistic a setting as possible. The most opportune settings for examining and remediating pragmatic skills are within the person's real-life environments (e.g., social clubs, home). Realistically, however, to evaluate and/or treat pragmatic skills external to the clinical facility is an impractical approach for all but home-health clinicians. Typically, neither time nor resources support such an effort. The alternative advocated, then, is simulation of a natural conversational setting within the clinic itself. Either way, the use of functional, communicative procedures, often previously overlooked in traditional management paradigms, allow real communication to be experienced in the clinical setting. If a setting is created that fosters genuine communication, clients have a greater opportunity to improve their communicative effectiveness through conversational reinforcement of their pragmatic strengths, and through opportunities to develop skills and strategies that compensate for their weaknesses.

References

Avent, J.R. (1997). Group Treatment in Aphasia Using Cooperative Learning Methods. *Journal of Medical Speech Language Pathology, 5*, 9–26.

Avent, J.R., Wertz, R.T. & Auther, L.L. (1998). Relationship Between Language Impairment and Pragmatic Behavior in Aphasic Adults. *Journal of Neurolinguistics, 11*, 207–221.

Barrett, A.M., Crucian, G.P., Raymer, A.M. & Heilman, K.M. (1999). Spared Comprehension of Emotional Prosody in a Patient with Global Aphasia. *Neuropsychiatry, Neuropsychology and Behavioral Neurology, 12*, 117–120.

Bates, E. (1976). *Language Disorders and Language Development*. New York: Macmillan.

Baum, S.R. & Pell, M.D. (1999). The Neural Bases of Prosody: Insights from Lesion Studies and Neuroimaging. *Aphasiology, 13*, 581–608.

Blomert, L. (1990). What Functional Assessment Can Contribute to Setting Goals for Aphasia Therapy. *Aphasiology, 4*, 307–320.

Blomert, L., Kean, M.L., Koster, C. & Schokker, J. (1994). Amsterdam-Nijmegen Everyday Language Test: Construction, Reliability and Validity. *Aphasiology, 8*, 381–407.

Blomert, L., Koster, C., Mier, H.V. & Kean, M. (1987). Verbal Communication Abilities of Aphasic Patients: The Everyday Language Test. *Aphasiology, 6*, 463–474.

Bollinger, R., Musson, N. & Holland, A.L. (1993). A Study of Group Communication Intervention with Chronically Aphasic Persons. *Aphasiology, 7*, 301–313.

Borod, J.C., Rorie, K.D., Pick, L.H., Bloom, R.L., Andelman, F., Campbell, A.L., Obler, L.K., Tweedy, J.R., Welkowitz, J. & Sliwinski, M. (2000). Verbal Pragmatics Following Unilateral Stroke: Emotional Content and Valence. *Neuropsychology, 14*, 112–124.

Busch, C.R., Brookshire, R.H. & Nicholas, L.E. (1988). Referential Communication Abilities of Aphasic Speakers. *Journal of Speech and Hearing Disorders, 53*, 475–482.

Cancelliere, A.E.B. & Kertesz, A. (1990). Lesion Localization in Acquired Deficits of Emotional Expression and Comprehension. *Brain and Cognition, 13*, 133–147.

Chapman, S.B., Highley, A.P. & Thompson, J.L. (1998). Discourse in Fluent Aphasia and Alzheimer's Disease: Linguistic and Pragmatic Considerations. *Journal of Neurolinguistics, 11*, 55–78.

Cicero, B., Borod, J.C., Santschi, C., Erhan, H.M., Obler, L.K., Agosti, R.M., Welkowitz, J. & Grunwald, I. (1999). Emotional Versus Nonemotional Lexical Perception in Patients with Right and Left Brain Damage. *Neuropsychiatry, Neuropsychology and Behavioral Neurology, 12*, 255–264.

Davis, G.A. (1983). *A Survey of Adult Aphasia and Related Language Disorders*. Boston: Allyn & Bacon.

Davis, G.A. (1989). Pragmatics and Cognition in Treatment of Language Disorders. In: X. Seron & G. Deloche (Eds.), *Cognitive Approaches in Neuropsychological Rehabilitation: Neuropsychology and Neurolinguistics* (pp. 317–353). Hillsdale, NJ: Lawrence Erlbaum.

Davis, G.A. & Wilcox, M.J. (1985). *Adult Aphasia Rehabilitation: Applied Pragmatics*. San Diego: Singular.

Doyle, P.J., McNeil, M.R., Park, G., Goda, A., Rubenstein, E., Spencer, K., Carroll, B., Lustig, A. & Szwarc, L. (2000). Linguistic Validation of Four Parallel Forms of a Story Retelling Procedure. *Aphasiology, 15*, 537–549.

Dronkers, N.F., Ludy, C.A. & Redfern, B.B. (1998). Pragmatics in the Absence of Verbal Language: Descriptions of a Severe Aphasic and a Language Deprived Adult. *Journal of Neurolinguistics, 11*, 179–190.

Elman, R. & Bernstein-Ellis, E. (1999a). The Efficacy of Group Communication Treatment in Adults with Chronic Aphasia. *Journal of Speech, Language, and Hearing Research, 42*, 411–419.

Elman, R. & Bernstein-Ellis, E. (1999b). Psychosocial Aspects of Group Communication Treatment: Preliminary Findings. *Seminars in Speech and Language, 20*, 65–72.

Frattali, C., Thompson, C.M., Holland, A.L., Wohl, C.B. & Ferketic, M.M. (1995). *American Speech-Language-Hearing Association Functional Assessment of Communication Skills for Adults*. Rockville, MD: ASHA.

Garrett, K. & Ellis, G. (1999). Group Communication Therapy for People with Long-Term Aphasia: Scaffolding Thematic Discourse Activities. In: R. Elman (Ed.), *Group Treatment for Neurogenic Communication Disorders: The Expert Clinician's Approach* (pp. 85–96). Woburn, MA: Butterworth-Heinemann.

Geigenberger, A. & Ziegler, W. (2001). Receptive Prosodic Processing in Aphasia. *Aphasiology, 15*, 1169–1187.

Gerber, S. & Gurland, G.B. (1989). Applied Pragmatics in the Assessment of Aphasia. *Seminars in Speech and Language, 10,* 263–281.

Glucksberg, S. & Krauss, R. (1967). What Do People Say After They Have Learned to Talk? Studies to Development of Referential Communication. *Merrill-Palmer Quarterly, 13,* 309–316.

Gurland, G.B., Chwat, S.E. & Wollner, S.G. (1982). Establishing a Communication Profile in Adult Aphasia: Analysis of Communicative Acts and Conversations Sequences. In: R.H. Brookshire (Ed.), *Clinical Aphasiology: Conference Proceedings* (pp. 18–27). Minneapolis: BRK.

Hirst, W., LeDoux, J. & Stein, S. (1984). Constraints on the Processing of Indirect Speech Acts: Evidence from Aphasiology. *Brain and Language, 23,* 26–33.

Holland, A.L. (1980). *Communicative Abilities in Daily Living.* Baltimore: University Park Press.

Holland, A.L. (1991). Pragmatic Aspects of Intervention in Aphasia. *Journal of Neurolinguistics, 6,* 197–211.

Holland, A.L. & Beeson, P. (1999). Aphasia Groups: The Arizona Experience. In: R. Elman (Ed.), *Group Treatment for Neurogenic Communication Disorders: The Expert Clinician's Approach* (pp. 77–84). Woburn, MA: Butterworth-Heinemann.

Holland, A.L., Fratelli, C. & Fromm, D. (1988). *Communication Activities of Daily Living-2 (CADL-2).* Austin, TX: Pro-Ed.

Houghton, P.M., Pettit, J.M. & Towey, M.P. (1982). Measuring Communication Competence in Global Aphasia. In: R.H. Brookshire (Ed.), *Clinical Aphasiology: Conference Proceedings* (pp. 28–39). Minneapolis: BRK.

Karow, C.M., Marquardt, T.P. & Marshall, R.C. (2001). Affective Processing in Left and Right Hemisphere Brain-Damaged Subjects with and without Subject Involvement. *Aphasiology, 15,* 715–729.

Kasher, A., Batori, G., Soroker, N., Graves, D. & Zaidel, E. (1999). Effects of Right- and Left-Hemisphere Damage on Understanding Conversational Implicatures. *Brain and Language, 68,* 566–590.

Kearns, K.P. & Elman, R.J. (2001). Group Therapy for Aphasia: Theoretical and Practical Considerations. In: R. Chapey (Ed.), *Language Intervention Strategies in Aphasia and Related Neurogenic Communication Disorders* (4th ed., pp. 316–340). New York: Lippincott Williams & Wilkins.

Landis, T., Graves, R. & Goodglass, H. (1982). Aphasic Reading and Writing by the Lexical-Semantic Route. *Cortex, 18,* 105–112.

Lomas, J., Laura, P., Bester, S., Elbard, H., Finlayson, A. & Zoghaib, C. (1989). The Communicative Effectiveness Index: Development and Psychometric Evaluation of a Functional Communication Measure for Adult Aphasia. *Journal of Speech and Hearing Disorders, 54,* 113–124.

Lorch, M.P., Borod, J.C. & Koff, E. (1998). The Role of Emotion in the Linguistic and Pragmatic Aspects of Aphasic Performance. *Journal of Neurolinguistics, 11,* 103–118.

Manochipinig, S., Sheard, C. & Reed, V.A. (1992). Pragmatic Assessment in Adult Aphasia: A Clinical Review. *Aphasiology, 6,* 519–533.

Pell, M.D. (1998). Recognition of Prosody Following Unilateral Brain Lesion: Influence of Functional and Structural Attributes of Prosodic Contours. *Neuropsychologia, 36,* 710–715.

Pell, M.D. & Baum, S.R. (1997a). The Ability to Perceive and Comprehend Intonation in Linguistic and Affective Contexts by Brain Damaged Adults. *Brain and Language, 57,* 80–99.

Pell, M.D. & Baum, S.R. (1997b). Unilateral Brain Damage, Prosodic Comprehension, and the Acoustic Cues to Prosody. *Brain and Language, 57,* 195–214.

Penn, C. (1988). The Profiling of Syntax and Pragmatics in Aphasia. *Clinical Linguistics and Phonetics, 2,* 179–207.

Penn, C. (1999). Pragmatic Assessment and Therapy for Persons with Brain Damage: What Have Clinicians Gleaned in Two Decades? *Brain and Language, 68,* 535–552.

Porch, B.E. (1967). *The Porch Index of Communication Ability.* Palo Alto, CA: Consulting Psychologists Press.

Prutting, C.A. & Kirchner, D.M. (1987). A Clinical Appraisal of the Pragmatic Aspects of Language. *Journal of Speech and Hearing Disorders, 52,* 105–119.

Reuterskiold, C. (1991). The Effects of Emotionality on Auditory Comprehension in Aphasia. *Cortex, 27,* 595–604.

Sarno, M.T. (1965). *The Functional Communication Profile.* New York: NYU Medical Center, Institute of Rehabilitation Medicine.

Terrell, B.Y. & Ripich, D.N. (1989). Discourse Competence as a Variable in Intervention. *Seminars in Speech and Language, 10,* 282–297.

Ulatowska, H.K., Allard, L., Reyes, B.A., Ford, J. & Chapman, S. B. (1992). Conversational Discourse in Aphasia. *Aphasiology, 6,* 325–331.

Webster, E. (1977). *Counseling with Parents of Handicapped Children.* New York: Grune and Stratton.

Wirz, S., Skinner, C. & Dean, E. (1990). *Revised Edinburgh Functional Communication Profile.* Tucson, AZ: Communication Skills Builders.

Wulfeck, B.E.B., Juarez, L. & Opie, M. (1989). Pragmatics in Aphasia: Crosslinguistic Evidence. *Language and Speech, 32,* 315–336.

Zaidel, E., Kasher, A., Soroker, N., Batori, G., Giora, R. & Graves, D. (2000). Hemispheric Contributions to Pragmatics. *Brain and Cognition, 43,* 438–443.

17

Family, Caregiver, and Clinician Resources

ADRIENNE BLANCHARD

Health-care professionals serving persons with neurologic impairments realize that in order to fully serve a client, they must also serve the client's family. As LaPointe explained in Chapter 1, neurological events do not simply affect a physical or cognitive aspect of an individual. A quite insidious aspect of this life-changing experience is its impact on a family.

Family members and caregivers are a significant component of rehabilitation treatment. Providing a client with premium medical and physical care is not always enough; the family and caregivers are in need of services as well. Blaylock (2000) remarks that the scientific successes of modern medicine and technology highlight the need for effective communication and respectful collaboration with patients and families. Although the physical and emotional stress placed on families and caregivers is unique to each situation, professionals can help families through an often-difficult coping process.

Determining the specific type of service desired by the family is a crucial step in providing quality caregiver support. In a survey conducted by Wackerbarth and Johnson (2002), caregivers rated diagnosis and treatment information and legal and financial information as more important than general information such as how to provide care or current research and statistics. Caregivers also rated needs relating to supporting the care receiver as significantly more important than those addressing support for caregivers (Wackerbarth & Johnson, 2002). Health-care professionals using a family-centered intervention approach educate the family about the patient's diagnosis and treatment as well as available resources for support. Educational and other intervention programs should address the caregiver's confidence in problem solving and provide definition of difficult situations and sources of social support. These coping strategies significantly reduced reported caregiver burden in a study by Pratt et al. (1985).

Below is a list of organizations and references selected to direct the clinician, family, or caregiver of a person with neurologic impairment to sources of information and guidance. Unique and useful features of various resources are annotated. This by no means should be interpreted as an exhaustive list of available services. Most of the organizations listed offer support in forms of local support group directories, regular newsletters, and educational materials. The organizations are arranged by disease or condition; followed by general information available from Internet and video sources; organizations and literature specifically for family members and caregivers; literature with intervention implications for clinicians; and finally selected articles depicting life with a neurologic impairment from the perspectives of survivors and caregivers.

Organizations

American Speech-Language-Hearing
   Association
10801 Rockville Pike
Rockville, MD 20852
Toll-free, voice or TTY:
Professionals/Students: 800–498–2071
Public: 800–638–8255
www.asha.org

ASHA is the governing professional organization for audiologists and speech-language pathologists. It provides extensive resources related to human communication for professionals, students, and the public.

Alzheimer's Association
225 North Michigan Avenue, Floor 17
Chicago, IL 60611–1676
800–272–3900
www.alz.org

Call or write for an information packet including action series brochures (managing problem behaviors, structuring the day at home, understanding legal and financial issues, etc.) and topical series brochures (understanding Alzheimer's disease, long-distance caregiving, children and teens understanding Alzheimer's disease). "A Guide for Choosing a New Home" and a "Respite Care Guide" are also available.

ALS Association National Office
27001 Agoura Road, Suite 150
Calabasas Hills, CA 91301–5104
Information and Referral Service:
   800–782–4747
818–880–9007
www.alsa.org

ALSA provides statewide listings of support group and clinic locations, a guide to products and services for daily living, and an e-mail listserve for ALS updates.

National Aphasia Association
29 John St., Suite 1103
New York, NY 10038
800–922–4622
www.aphasia.org

The National Aphasia Association holds an annual "Speaking Out" conference for persons with aphasia, their families, and health-care professionals. Call or write for an information packet including pocket communication cards, aphasia fact sheets, dos and don'ts of communicating with a person with aphasia, regional community group listings, and helpful resources.

Aphasia Hope Foundation
2436 West 137th St.
Leawood, KS 66224
Phone: 913–402–8306
Fax: 913–402–8315
Toll free: 866–449–5804
www.aphasiahope.org

The Aphasia Hope Foundation provides resources including tips on communicating and living with aphasia, educational books and videos, and treatment software.

Brain Injury Association of America
8201 Greensboro Drive, Suite 611
McLean, VA 22102
703–761–0750
Family Helpline: 800–444–6443
www.biausa.org

The Brain Injury Association of America offers discussion of treatment and rehabilitation available in PDF format on-line. Call or write for "The Road to Rehabilitation" booklet series.

The Perspectives Network
P.O. Box 121012
W. Melbourne, FL 32912–1012
E-mail: *TPN@tbi.org*
www.tbi.org

The Perspectives Network has archives of articles related to brain injury, survivor tools, and reference material. A frequently asked questions (FAQ) section is also available in Chinese, French, German, Italian, Spanish, and other languages.

Huntington's Disease Society of America
158 West 29th Street, 7th Floor
New York, NY 10001–5300

Phone: 800–345–HDSA
Fax: 212–239–3430
www.hdsa.org

The Huntington's Disease Society of America offers national and chapter event listings, a family guide series, and a mailing list.

Caring for People with Huntington's Disease
www.kumc.edu/hospital/huntingtons/ index.html

This organization addresses specific care issues such as communication, swallowing, safety, and genetics, and has links to several informative sources.

Multiple Sclerosis Foundation
Ft. Lauderdale, FL
Program Services Department: 888-MS-FOCUS or e-mail: *support@msfocus.org*
www.msfocus.org

The Multiple Sclerosis Foundation Web site includes a multimedia page with video segments addressing MS treatment, research, cognitive issues, and personal stories.

Myasthenia Gravis Foundation of America
5841 Cedar Lake Road, Suite 204
Minneapolis, MN 55416
952–545–9438 or 800–541–5454
Fax: 952–545–6073
E-mail: *myasthenia@myasthenia.org*
www.myasthenia.org

The Myasthenia Gravis Foundation of America offers patient services, manuals for diagnosis and treatment, on-line videos, local chapter listings, and useful related links.

Myasthenia Gravis Association of Queensland, Australia
www.mg-qld.gil.com.au

This Web site offers Australian support groups, a monthly newsletter, and research fundraising.

Myasthenia Gravis
pages.prodigy.net/stanley.way/myasthenia

This Web site has listings of related links, including international organizations, medical information, personal support, and chat rooms.

National Parkinson Foundation
Bob Hope Parkinson Research Center
1501 N.W. 9th Avenue
Miami, FL 33136–1491
800–327–4545
www.parkinson.org

The National Parkinson Foundation, which has additional offices in California and New York, offers a guide to leading support groups, free publications available in English and Spanish, allows you to submit questions regarding medical issues, diet, care and coping, and speech therapy, to qualified professionals.

American Parkinson's Disease Association
1250 Hylan Blvd. Suite 4B
Staten Island, NY 10305–1946
718–981–8001
800–223–2732
www.apdaparkinson.com

The American Parkinson's Disease Association has videos available for loan. Topics include nutrition, exercise, caregiving, speech, treatment, and coping.

Parkinson's Web
pdweb.mgh.harvard.edu

This Web site offers links to national Parkinson's disease organizations and informative resources.

National Stroke Association
9707 E. Easter Lane
Englewood, Co. 80112
800–STROKES
303–649–9299
www.stroke.org

Call or write to request an information packet containing caregiver tips and educational brochures about stroke prevention and recovery.

American Stroke Association
National Center
7272 Greenville Avenue
Dallas TX 75231
ASA: 888–4–STROKE
or 888–478–7653

American Stroke Association offers educational information about strokes, treatment, recovery, and caregiver needs.

Different Strokes
9 Canon Harnett Court
Wolverton Mill
Milton Keynes
MK12 5NF
United Kingdom
info@differentstrokes.co.uk
www.differentstrokes.co.uk

Different Strokes offers support and information for young stroke survivors.

www.stroke-info.com

This Web site offers a stroke information directory that includes diagnostic and treatment research, facility locations, and on-line support.

www.stroke-survivors.co.uk

This stroke survivor's personal Web page focuses on cerebellar strokes and includes a glossary of stroke terminology and related Internet links.

General Information

www.communicationdisorders.com

This Web site offers an internet guide by Judith Maginnis Custer. Comprehensive is an understatement for this site, as it contains endless links addressing every area of speech-language pathology. Discussion forums, electronic newsletters, therapy and efficacy information, products, and businesses are listed.

www.speech-languagepathologist.org

The Web site offers live Internet chat room and posted discussion archive, message board,

resource list for various disorders, and free e-mail.

www.mayoclinic.com

The Mayo Clinic Web site lists health conditions A-Z, including the neurologic conditions discussed in this book. Diagnosis, treatment, and caregiving information are available for specific neurogenic disorders.

www.iog.wayne.edu/GeroWebd/Gero Web.html

Wayne State University's Institute of Gerontology provides numerous links and resources for researchers, educators, and practitioners involved with aging and older individuals. You may browse by category or search for a specific topic.

Health Professions Press

Books and resources on aging issues, Alzheimer's disease, activities, staff training, mental health, policy and ethics, and health administration are available. Browse at *www.healthpress.com* and order by phone, mail, or fax.

The Job Accommodation Network (JAN)

This network offers information about job accommodation and the employability of people with functional limitations. Online at *janweb.icdi.wvu.edu* or call 800–526–7234.

Videos and Materials

Home Care Companions has compiled two series of videos to address caregiver needs:
1. Communication Series:
How to Communicate Effectively with Someone Who Has Hearing Loss
How to Communicate Effectively with Someone Who Has Aphasia
How to Communicate Effectively with Someone Who Has Alzheimer's Disease
2. Caregiving Series:
How to Care for Someone on Bed Rest

How to Help Someone Who Uses A
  Wheelchair Without Hurting Yourself
Creating Healthy Home Care Conditions:
  Infection Control
How to Manage Medications
Fall Prevention
Fire Safety

The above are available at *www. homecarecompanion.com/videos.html* or by writing Healing Arts Communications, 33 North Central, Suite 211, Medford, OR 97501.

Norvartis Pharmaceuticals Corporation (East Hanover, NJ, 07936) produced an educational video about Alzheimer's disease, including warning signs, treatment, and tips for family members, entitled *Alzheimer's Disease: What Everyone Should Know.*

Alzheimer's: A Practical Guide for Sitters, Volumes 1 and 2 (Alabama Department of Mental Health and Mental Retardation, 1995) helps caregivers to understand dementia and the resulting impact on the family.

Recognizing and Responding to Emotions in Persons with Dementia, an instructional video to teach caregivers how to understand and decipher facial expressions, vocal signs, and body language, is available from:

Terra Nova Films, Inc.
9848 S. Winchester Avenue
Chicago, IL 60643
773–881–8491
tnf@terranova.org

Conversing with Memory Impaired Individuals Using Memory Aids, a workbook by Michelle S. Bourgeois, provides instructions for making and using memory aids with family members, children, or in day care and nursing home settings. This workbook is published by:

Northern Speech Services, Inc.
P.O. Box 1247
Gaylord, MI 49735
ISBN 0–941653–12–9

Judith Oetting's *Developing a Personal Memory Notebook: Techniques for Facilitating Memory and Orientation in Individuals with Dementia and Other Cognitive-Linguistic Im-*

pairments, offers reproducible pages for education, history, journal, calendar, health, and visitor divisions of a memory notebook. Published by Pro-Ed, this workbook may be ordered on-line at *http://www.proedinc.com* or

8700 Shoal Creek Boulevard
Austin, TX 78757–6897
800–897–3202

See *www.films.com* for detailed descriptions of the following videos, available from

Films for the Humanities and Sciences
P.O. Box 2053
Princeton, NJ 08543–2053
Phone: 800–257–5126
Fax: 609–275–3767
E-mail: *custserv@films.com*
Alzheimer's Disease
Alzheimer's Disease: The Long
  Nightmare
Alzheimer's Disease: Effects on Patients
  and Their Families
Caring for the Elderly
Nursing Home Care
Studies in Aging
Ageless America
Parenting Our Parents
The Aging Process
Factors in Healthy Aging
Strokes: New Treatments

Lunchbreak with Tony is a respite care video specifically oriented toward men. "Tony" visits with viewers as he talks about his workdays, old games, first cars, etc. Viewers reminisce with songs, movement, and conversation. For information about this and other respite care videos, contact:

Innovative Caregiving Resources, Inc.
P.O. Box 17332
Salt Lake City, UT 84117

What is Aphasia? (30 min.) and *Pathways: Moving Beyond Stroke and Aphasia* (30 min.), produced by Susan Adair Ewing and Beth Pfalzgraf (1991), are available from:

Wayne State University Press
5959 Woodward Avenue

Detroit, MI 48202
(313) 577–6120

The following two videos were developed particularly for persons and families who experienced a stroke recently.

Stroke: The Story of Treatment and Recovery, produced by the National Stroke Association (see address above).

The Healing Influence: Guidelines for Stroke Survivors and Family, with Patricia Neal, produced by the American Heart Association. Available from:

Danamar Productions
106 Monte Vista Place
Santa Fe, NM 87501
Phone: 800–578–6508
Fax: 505–989–4619
E-mail: *dana@cybermesa.com*

"Library Media Project: Video and Electronic Resources" offers a curated video collection on *Issues of the Aging*, including health concerns, policy issues, and social topics. Distributor's contact information is provided so that you can contact the distributor directly if your local library does not have the videos you want.

www.librarymedia.org/aging/Age_main.html

Resources Especially for Families and Caregivers

National Family Caregivers Association (NFCA)
10400 Connecticut Avenue, #500
Kensington, MD 20895–3944
800–896–3650
www.NFCAcares.org

This web site includes national organizations and programs for respite care and assisted living/nursing facilities, caregiver Web sites, and support programs.

Well Spouse Foundation
63 West Main Street, Suite H
Freehold, NJ 07728
800–838–0879

Membership benefits include monthly support meetings, newsletter, and conferences.

United States Department of Health and Human Services
Administration on Aging (AoA)
330 Independence Avenue, SW
Washington, DC 20201
(800) 677–1116 (Eldercare Locator: to find services for an older person in his or her locality)
(202) 619–7501 (AoA's National Aging Information Center: for technical information and public inquiries)
http://www.aoa.gov/default.htm

This Web site includes resources for all aspects of life (health care, housing, finances, exercise) during the later years of life.

"Resource Directory for Older People" containing names, addresses, phone numbers, and fax numbers of organizations that provide information and other resources on matters relating to the needs of older persons.

"Because We Care: A Guide for People Who Care" addresses common concerns of caregivers:

Available on-line in HTML or PDF format: *http://www.aoa.gov/eldfam/How_To_Find/ResourceDirectory/resource_directory.asp*

AARP
601 E St., NW
Washington, DC 20049
800–424–3410
www.aarp.org

Some AARP services require membership and a minimal annual fee.

National Adult Day Services Association, Inc.
722 Grant Street, Suite L
Herndon, VA 20170
Phone: 800–558–5301 or 703–435–8630
info@nadsa.org
www.nadsa.org

This Web site describes adult day services and provides a guide to selecting an adult day-care center. A database of adult day-care centers will be added to the Web site soon.

Alzwell Caregiver Support Web Site
www.alzwell.com

This Web site is devoted to caregivers. It offers eldercare information, live chatrooms, and discussion forums.

www.elderweb.com

You may want to begin at the site map page of the "ElderWeb" to navigate through information on finance and law, housing and care, medicine and wellness.

www.caregiver.com

This Web site offers topic-specific newsletters, on-line discussion and chats, and more, developed by caregivers for caregivers. The national magazine, *Today's Caregiver*, is also available on this Web site.

www.familycareamerica.com

Search here for local care facilities, eldercare resources, rehabilitation services, transportation, and more by entering a zip code.

www.caregiving.com

This Web site offers caregiver camaraderie in the form of support, seasoned advice, and counseling.

MU Extension, a division of the University of Missouri, aims to publicize the research and knowledge developed at the University of Missouri. Visit the EXPLOR page of the Web site (*muextension.missouri.edu/xplor*) to search by topic or keyword. Examples of useful publications include:

Clark, J.A. & Weber, K.A. (1997). Family Relationships: Elderly Caregiving. *Human Environmental Sciences*, GH 6657.
Isbell, L. & Halpert, B. (1985). Adult Day Care. *Human Environmental Sciences*, GH 6748.
Weagley, R.O. (1993). Staying Financially Able When Physically Disabled. *Human Environmental Sciences*, GH 3427.
Yost, A.C. & Martin, J. (1998). Bathroom Safety for Older People. *Human Environmental Sciences*, GH 7060.

Books for Caregivers

Acorn, S. & Offer, P. (1998). *Living with Brain Injury: A Guide for Families and Caregivers*. Toronto, ON: University of Toronto Press.

This book addresses issues resulting from brain injury, including physical abilities, relationships, psychological changes, family roles, school, employment, recreation, and leisure.

Baird, B. (1997). *Nana's Stroke*. Stow, OH: Interactive Therapeutics, Inc.

This illustrated children's book about strokes is available on-line: *www.interactivetherapy.com*, #W210.

Capossela, C. & Warnock, S. (1995). *Share the Care: How to Organize a Group to Care for Someone Who Is Seriously Ill*. New York: Fireside Books.

This book is a guide to sharing responsibility for caregiving as a means to alleviate caregiver stress

Davis, R.D. (2000). *The Nursing Home Handbook*. Holbrook, MA: Adams Media Corporation.

This book is a useful guide for selecting and enrolling in a nursing home facility. It addresses the impact of enrolling in a nursing home on individuals and family.

Lyon, J.G. (1998). *Coping with Aphasia*. San Diego: Singular. ISBN# 1879105756.
Mace, N.L. & Rabins, P.V. (2001). *The 36-Hour Day: A Family Guide to Caring for Persons with Alzheimer's Disease, Related Dementing Illnesses and Memory Loss Later in Life*. New York: Warner Books.

This book is a guide through the challenges related to dementia and memory loss.

Meyer, M.M., with Derr, P. (1998). *The Comfort of Home: An Illustrated Step-by-Step Guide for Caregivers*. Portland, OR: Care Trust Publications.

This book is particularly useful for home care patients with Alzheimer's disease or Parkinson's disease.

Rao, P.R., Ozer, M.N. & Toerge, M. (2001). *Managing Stroke: A Guide to Living Well After Stroke*. Washington, DC: NRH Press.

Strauss, C.J. (2001). *Talking to Alzheimer's.* Oakland, CA: New Harbinger.

This book addresses what to expect and how to interact with a person with dementia. Available on-line *www.interactivetherapy.com*, product number W200. ISBN: 1572242701

Tanner, D.C. (1999). *The Family Guide to Surviving Stroke and Communication Disorders.* Needham Heights, MA: Allyn & Bacon.
Visiting Nurse Associations of America. (1998). *Caregiver's Handbook: A Complete Guide to Home Health Care.* New York: DK Publishing.

This book offers tips on patient nutrition, transfer and hygiene, adapting the home, communication, legal and financial matters, and emotional needs of both patient and caregiver compiled by Visiting Nurse Associations of America.

Literature for Clinicians

Bakas, T. & Burgener, S.C. (2002). Predictors of Emotional Distress, General Health, and Caregiving Outcomes in Family Caregivers of Stroke Survivors. *Topics in Stroke Rehabilitation, 9,* 34–45.
Beisecker, A.E., Cobb, A.K. & Ziegler, D.K. (1998). Patient's Perspectives of the Role of Care Providers in Amyotrophic Lateral Sclerosis. *Archives of Neurology, 45,* 553–556.
Bourgeois, M.S. (1997). Families Caring for Elders at Home: Caregiver Training. In: B.B. Shadden & M.A. Toner (Eds.), *Aging and Communication for Clinicians by Clinicians* (pp. 227–249). Austin, TX: Pro-Ed.
Bourgeois, M.S. & Schulz, R. (1996). Interventions for Caregivers of Patients with Alzheimer's Disease: A Review and Analysis of Content, Process, and Outcomes. *International Journal of Aging and Human Development, 43,* 35–92.
Degeneffe, C.E. (2001). Family Caregiving and Traumatic Brain Injury. *Health and Social Work, 26,* 257–268.

This article reviews the nature of care needs, stress and burden experienced, and how families cope with caregiving demands. It concludes with a discussion of how the demands of family caregiving can be reduced.

Ellman, R. (Ed.). (1999). *Group Treatment of Neurogenic Communication Disorders: The Expert Clinician's Approach.* Woburn, MA: Butterworth-Heinemann.

This book offers approaches to group treatment in rehabilitation, subacute, outpatient, and community settings. Purchase on-line at *www.us.elsevierhealth.com*, ISBN 0750690844

Hinckley, J.J. (2000). Effective Tools for Family Education. *ADVANCE for Speech-Language Pathologists & Audiologists,* November.

This article explains how to educate family members about the nature and rehabilitative process involved in acquired neurologic communication disorders.

Hinckley, J.J. (2000). *What Is It Like to Have Trouble Communicating? A Series of Simulation Activities to Educate Family, Friends, and Caregivers.* Stow, OH: Interactive Therapeutics Inc.

This book is available on-line: *www.interactivetherapy.com*, product number W265.

Holland, A.L., Fromm, D.S., DeRuyter, F. & Stein, M. (1996). Treatment Efficacy: Aphasia. *Journal of Speech and Hearing Research, 39,* S27–36.
Kindig, M.N. & Carnes, M. (1993). *Coping with Alzhiemer's Disease and Other Dementing Illnesses.* San Diego: Singular. ISBN# 1565930975
Kriegsman, D.M.W., Pennix, B.W.J.H. & Van Eijk, J.T.M. (1994). Chronic Disease in the Elderly and Its Impact on the Family: A Review of the Literature. *Family Systems Medicine, 12,* 249–267.
Peterson, E.F. & Villegas, B.C. (1998). *Functional Learning for the Home and Community.* Gaylord, MI: Northern Speech Services.

This book offers functional therapy activities and goals addressing basic skills, memory, reading, writing, awareness, and executive skills as well as community reintegration and family education and training.

Rau, M.T. (1993). *Coping with Communication Challenges in Alzheimer's Disease.* San Diego: Singular. ISBN# 1879105764
Toner, M.A. & Shadden, B.B. (2002). Counseling Challenges: Working with Older Clients and Caregivers. *Contemporary Issues in Communication Science and Disorders, 29,* 68–78.
Vickers, C. (1998). *Communication Recovery: Group Conversation Activities for Adults.* Antonio, TX: Communication Skill Builders.

This book includes therapy exercises and discussion topics for "less fluent" and "more fluent" speakers.

Yorkston, K.M., Miller, R.M. & Strand, E.A. (1995). *Management of Speech and Swallowing in Degenerative Diseases.* Tucson, AZ: Psychological Corporation.

This book addresses the symptoms, speech characteristics, and swallowing disorders of amyotrophic lateral sclerosis, Parkinson's disease, Huntington's disease, and multiple sclerosis. It includes reproducible handouts for patients and families.

Important Perspectives

Hellgeth, A. (2002). Coping with Stroke: A Family's Perspective. *Topics in Stroke Rehabilitation, 9*, 80–84.

This article describes one family's challenges and strategies developed after the 50-year-old father's stroke.

Montgomery-West, P. (1995). A Spouse's Perspective on Life with Aphasia. *Topics in Stroke Rehabilitation, 2*, 1–4.

This article discusses another family's experience and coping strategies.

Quann, E.S. (2002). *By His Side: Life and Love After Stroke.* Highland, MD: Fastrak Press.

The author writes about her marriage after her husband suffered a stroke resulting in aphasia. This uplifting story provides encouragement and practical advice.

Young, J.M. & McNicoll, P. (1998). Against All Odds: Positive Life Experiences of People with Advanced Amyotrophic Lateral Sclerosis. *Health and Social Work, 23*, 35–43.

References

Blaylock, B.L. (2000). Patients and Families as Teachers: Inspiring an Empathetic Connection. *Families, Systems & Health, 18*, 161–175.

Pratt, C.C., Schmall, V.L., Wright, S. & Cleland, M. (1985). Burden and Coping Strategies of Caregivers to Alzheimer's Patients. *Family Relations, 34*, 27–33.

Wackerbarth, S.B. & Johnson, M.M.S. (2002). Essential Information and Support Needs of Family Caregivers. *Patient Education and Counseling, 47*, 95–100.

Index

Page numbers by "t" indicate that the entry on that page is in a table.

AAC
  treatment techniques of, 45–46
AARP, 254
ABCD, 204, 205
Abulic syndrome, 52
Acceleration-deceleration injuries, 225
Acoustic phonologic conversion system, 171
Acquired alexia, 87
Acquired brain damage
  in aphasia, 70
Acquired communication disorder, 2
Acquired disorders of writing, 97
Acquired dysgraphia
  assessing reasons for, 104
Acquired dyslexia
  brain functions of, 90
  classifications of, 87t
  compensatory strategies for, 94
  disorders of, 87t
  error type categories of, 88
  evaluation of, 86–90
  features of, 86
  reading disorders associated with, 83–95
  treatment for, 90–92
Acquired neurogenic agraphias
  anterior *vs.* posterior, 99
  clinical symptomatology of, 101
  cortical *vs.* subcortical, 100
  evaluation of, 104
  features of, 101–104
  functional architecture, 104
  left *vs.* right hemisphere, 99
  neurologic disorders of, 99
  pathophysiology of, 98
  treatment of, 106–111
  writing problems of, 97–112
Acquired reading disorders
  treatment for, 90
Activities
  in illness experience, 9
Activity-focused techniques, 208
Activity limitation, 40
ACTS, 131, 205

AD
  and dementia, 201–202
Adaptation, 13
Adaptation theory of agrammatism, 121
ADAS, 204
Addenbrooke's cognitive examination, 61t
Adjustments, 12
Administration on Aging (AoA)
  United States Department of Health and
    Human Services, 254
ADP, 128
ADRQL, 206
Adult literacy training
  functional activities of, 92
  reading skills of, 92
Advocacy and raising awareness
  of aphasia, 46–47
Afferent agraphia, 103
Age, 234
  aphasia, 31–32
  ICF framework, 39
  influencing recovery, 30
  traumatic brain injury, 234
Age of acquisition, 73
Agrammatic speech, 121
Agrammatism, 121, 134
  adaptation theory of, 121
Agraphic alexia, 86
  characteristics and physiology of, 87t
Agraphic performance, 98
Akinetic mutism, 56
Alexia with agraphia, 86
Alexia without agraphia, 86, 90
  characteristics and physiology of, 87t
Allographic impairment, 103
ALS Association National Office, 250
Alternative communication system (C-VIC), 186,
    196
Alzheimer Disease-Related Quality of Life
    (ADRQL), 206
Alzheimer's Association, 250
Alzheimer's disease
  and acquired neurogenic agraphias, 101

Alzheimer's disease (AD)
  and dementia, 201–202
Alzheimer's Disease Assessment Scale (ADAS), 204
Alzwell Caregiver Support Web Site, 255
American Heart Association, 254
American Parkinson's Disease Association, 251
American Speech Language Hearing Association (ASHA), 242, 250
  Committee on Communication Problems of Aging, 207
  FACS, 142, 205
    for adults, 130, 189
    for Wernicke's aphasia, 147
  Task Force on Treatment Outcome and Cost Effectiveness, 205
American Stroke Association National Center, 252
AMI, 204
Amsterdam-Nijmegan Everyday Language Test (ANELT), 242
  for Wernicke's aphasia, 147
Anatomic brain locations, 169
ANELT, 242
  for Wernicke's aphasia, 147
AoA
  United States Department of Health and Human Services, 254
Aphasia, 2, 118
  acquired brain damage, 70
  advocacy and raising awareness, 46–47
  applications for studying, 19–36
  applying functional neuroimaging to, 21
  behavioral patterns of, 144t
  causes of, 3–4
  chronicity of, 46
  considerations, 31–32
  design of experiment, 33–35
  education, 31–32
  etiologies of, 3–5
  foundations of, 2
  future directions, 36
  and gender, 31–32
  individuals
    caregivers for, 150–151
  interpretation of results, 35–36
  intervention
    approaches to, 39–47
    insider's perspective of, 42
  issues, 31–32
    steps for, 132
  of language impairments, 55
  language impairments of, 55
  neural mechanisms examining
    recovery of language, 24–26
  neuroimaging studies of, 32–33
  plan for, 133
  reading disorders associated with, 83–95
  recovery patterns, 30
  rehabilitation, 151

  social approach to, 42
  reorganizational processes, 27
  social factors of, 41
  subject selection, 31–32
  task performance, 33
  task selection, 32–33
  treatment
    in group, 78
    social approach, 43
  variables, 30t
  vascular compromises, 33–34
Aphasia Diagnostic Profiles (ADP), 128
Aphasia Hope Foundation, 250
Aphasia syndromes
  in naming impairments
    cognitive mechanism of, 69t
    neural correlates of, 69t
Aphasic alexia, 86
  characteristics and physiology of, 87t
Aphasic deficits, 158
Aphasic patients
  neuroimaging studies of, 31
Aphasic syndromes
  classification of, 125t
Aphasiology, 118
Aphemia, 118
Apraxia of speech, 127
  characteristics of, 127–128
  conduction aphasia
    comparison of characteristics, 156t
Apraxic agraphic, 100
Aprosodias, 218
Arcuate fasciculus, 155
Aricept, 207
Aristos, 15–17
  concept of, 15–16
Arizona Battery for Communication Disorders of Dementia (ABCD), 204, 205
Arthur Kopit, 8
Articulatory cues
  vs. linguistic cues, 158
ASHA. See American Speech Language Hearing Association (ASHA)
Assessment of Language Related Functional Abilities
  for Wernicke's aphasia, 147
Assessment of pragmatic aspects of language, 63t
AST
  for Wernicke's aphasia, 147
Asymmetric biposterior dysfunction, 172
Attaining mastery
  in illness experience, 10
Attentional control
  model, 59, 60
Attentional disorder
  neglect, 218–219
Attention disorder, 218
Attitudinal environment
  ICF framework, 40
Auditivo-verbal center, 171

Auditory comprehension, 117, 124
    conduction aphasia, 159, 160
Auditory Comprehension Test for Sentences
        (ACTS), 131, 205
Augmentative and alternative communication
        (AAC) techniques, 45–46
Authentic language, 42
Autobiographical Memory Interview (AMI), 204
Automatic processing
    in reading, 84

BADS, 61t
Barrier games, 245
Battery of Adult Reading Function, 88
BDAE. *See* Boston Diagnostic Aphasia
        Examination (BDAE)
BDS, 204
BEHAVE-AD, 205
Behavioral assessment of dysexecutive syndrome
        (BADS), 61t
Behavioral changes, 180
Behavioral Pathology in Alzheimer's Disease
        Rating Scale (BEHAVE-AD), 205
Behavioral patterns
    of aphasia, 144t
Belief in just world, 14
Benefit finding, 14
Benefit reminding, 14
Benton Revised Visual Retention Test (BVRT-R),
        204
BEST-2
    for Wernicke's aphasia, 147
Bimodal distribution model
    conduction aphasia, 156
Bitemporal lobe abnormality
    predilection for
        inferior middle, 172
        superior gyri, 172
        temporal pole, 172
Blessed Dementia Scale (BDS), 204
Block design, 33–34
    control conditions, 33–34
    definition of, 33–34
    strengths and weakness of, 34
Blood oxygen level-dependent (BOLD) signal, 20
Body Structure and Function Activity and
        Participation Framework
    for Wernicke's aphasia, 147
BOLD signal, 20
Boston Diagnostic Aphasia Examination (BDAE),
        105, 128, 129, 130, 160, 161, 177, 187, 204
    for Wernicke's aphasia, 147
Boston Naming Test, 72, 205
Boxcar design, 33–34
    definition of, 33–34
    strengths and weakness of, 34
Brain
    damage, 2
        foundations of, 2
        physiologic reorganization, 27

functions of, 4
    lobes of, 3f
Brain attack
    definition of, 3–5
Brain imaging studies
    conduction aphasia, 156
Brain injury, 70
    patients, 91
Brain Injury Association of America, 250
Broca, Pierre Paul, 117
Broca's aphasia, 27, 70, 117–137
    adaptation agrammatism in, 136
    agrammatism
        stress-salience hypothesis, 122
    anterior, 100
    aphasia batteries and patient classification,
        128–130
    apraxia of speech, 127
        comparison of characteristics, 156t
    associated signs and symptoms of, 126–128
    auditory comprehension impairments in, 131
    auditory stimulation treatment procedures, 134
    conduction aphasia
        comparison of characteristics, 156t
    differentiating features of, 124–126
    evaluation of, 128
    features of, 117, 120
    generic treatment strategies, 133–134
    language impairments in, 119
    linguistic hypotheses, 122–123, 123–124
    mapping therapy, 134
    nature of, 120–121
    nonlinguistic and linguistic hypotheses, 123–124
    nonlinguistic hypotheses, 121–122
    observations of, 118
    pathophysiology of, 118–120
    profile of, 126
    sentence production, 135
    specific treatment tasks, 134–137
    study of, 117
    supplemental evaluation procedures of, 130–132
    treatment, 132
        philosophy of, 132–133
    verbal impairments in, 130
    word-finding, 129
Broca's area, 4, 31, 118, 119
    for syntactic processing, 23
Broca's patients, 119
    central syntactic deficit hypothesis, 122
    dysarthric involvement of, 127
    improving communication abilities, 137
    self-generated cueing strategy
        deblocking, 133
Brodmann's areas
    neuropsychological behaviors of, 53t
Bromocriptine, 179
Burns Brief Inventory of Communication and
        Cognition, 187
Burns-Roe Informal Reading Inventory, 89
BVRT-R, 204

CADL, 130, 187, 189, 205
CADL-2, 63t, 242
Cambridge Cognitive Examination (CAMCOG),
    204
CAMCOG, 204
CAPPA, 161
Caregiver resources, 249–257
Caregivers, 14–15
    books for, 255–256
    and dementia, 206
Caring for People with Huntington's Disease, 251
CCEI, 241
CDR, 204
CEC, 189
Central syntactic deficit hypothesis
    Broca's patients, 122
CERAD, 204
Cerebral cortex, 2
Cerebral functions
    localization of, 117
Cerebral lobes
    illustration of, 2
Cerebral thromboses, 3f
Cerebrovascular accident (CVA), 173
    definition of, 3–5
    dissected brain, 4f
CETI, 241
    for Wernicke's aphasia, 147
CHI, 226
Cholinergic drugs
    effects of, 79
    in recovery of aphasia, 79
Chronic aphasia, 196
Chronic cognitive impairments, 199
Chronic illness, 12
    adaptation to, 11–12
Chronicity, 12–13
    fears of, 12
    stages of, 12–13
CIBI, 204
Client/clinician interaction, 241
Clinical decisions
    in aphasia, 72
Clinical Dementia Rating Scale (CDR), 204
Clinician Interview-Based Impression (CIBI), 204
Clinician resources, 249–257
Clinicians
    literature for, 256–257
Closed head injury (CHI), 226
Clots, 3f
CLOX (executive clock drawing task), 61t–62t
CNS, 97
Cognex, 206–207
Cognition, 226
Cognitive and reasoning skills
    in reading, 94
Cognitive-linguistic processes, 93
Cognitive processes, 228
Cognitive rehabilitation, 221
Cognitive skills training, 208

Cognitive system, 171
    components of, 32
    of word retrieval
        stages of, 68
Cohen-Mansfield Agitation Inventory, 205
Cohesion, 241
Colored Progressive Matrices, 186
COMFI, 205
Communication, 213
    guidelines for, 192
Communication boards
    attributes of
        familiarity, 196
        saliency, 196
Communication book
    global aphasia, 195–196
Communication Competence Evaluation
        Instrument (CCEI), 241
Communication disorders
    caused by, 2
    web site address of, 252
Communication exchange, 217
Communication Outcome Measure of Functional
        Independence (COMFI), 205
Communication Profile, 240
Communicative Abilities in Daily Living
        (CADL), 130, 187, 189, 205
Communicative Abilities in Daily Living 2
        (CADL-2), 63t, 242
Communicative boards
    global aphasia, 195–196
Communicative Competence Evaluation
        Instrument, 189
Communicative Effectiveness Index (CETI), 241
    for Wernicke's aphasia, 147
Communicative partners and volunteers, 44
Compensatory strategies, 134
Complex neuronal networks, 214
Comprehending speech acts, 245
Comprehension
    abilities, 71
    assessment
        in normal readers, 93
    loss vs. temporal lesion
        in Wernicke's area, 143
    of speech, 238
    targeting, 92
    training
        direction following, 93
Comprehension training
    direction following, 93
Computed tomography (CT), 119
    findings of, 119
    scans, 200
Computer generated interactive three-
        dimensional scenarios, 231
Computers
    for retraining reading, 94
Conduction aphasia, 155–166
    apraxia of speech

comparison of characteristics, 156t
associated problems, 159
auditory comprehension, 159, 160
bimodal distribution model, 156
brain imaging studies, 156
concept of, 155
criteria for, 157
disconnection model, 156
error recognition, 158
evaluation of, 159–160
facilitory channels, 164–165
features of, 157–159
functional communication, 165–166
gestural cues, 165
pathophysiology of, 155–156
phonetic errors of, 158
phonologic errors of, 158
prognosis of, 159
reading, 159, 164
repetition, 158–159, 160
rhythm and song, 165
salient characteristics of
    fluency, 157
    paraphasias, 157
    word finding, 157
sentence production, 164
spontaneous speech, 161
treatment of, 161–162
    specific targets, 162–164
two conduction aphasias, 156–159
verbal cues, 164–165
verbal repetition, 162–163
visual cues, 165
word finding, 160–161
    confrontation naming, 160
word retrieval, 163–164
writing, 164
Conduction aphasia characteristic
    fluency, 157
Confrontation, 124
Confusional states, 101
Connected speech, 161
Connected text
    reading of, 92
Consortium to Establish a Registry for
    Alzheimer's Disease (CERAD), 204
Constrained gesture, 195
Contention scheduler (CS), 60
Control conditions
    block designs, 33–34
Controlled processing
    in reading, 84–85
Control subjects, 213
Conventional speech therapy, 178
Conversation, 191
    focus on, 42
Conversational breakdowns, 241
Conversational coaching, 45
Conveying emotion, 239
Coping, 13–14

definition of, 13
    suggestions for, 16t
Cortical center for writing
    localization of, 98–99
Cortical stimulation mapping techniques, 21
Couples/family training, 44–45
Craig Handicap Assessment and Reporting Tool,
    226
C rule, 91
CS, 60
CT, 119
    findings of, 119
    scans, 200
Cue(s)
    types of, 75
Cueing hierarchy
    in aphasia, 74–75
    examples of, 75t
Cueing Verb Treatments (CVT) program, 135
CVA, 173
    definition of, 3–5
    dissected brain, 4f
C-VIC, 186, 196
CV pattern, 91
CVT program, 135

Danamar Productions, 254
DAP, 241
DBS, 227
DCT, 64t, 131, 148
Deblock, 133
Deep agraphia, 102
Deep brain stimulation (DBS), 227
Deep dyslexia
    characteristics and physiology of, 87t
Degenerative dementia
    in naming difficulties, 69
Degrees of Reading Power-Revised, 89
Delis-Kaplan executive function system (D-K
    EFS), 61t
Dementia, 199–209
    in Alzheimer's disease (AD), 201–202
    definition of, 199
    disorders of, 199
    environmental strategies, 208–209
    evaluation of, 203–206
    examination for
        physical and neurologic, 200
    features of, 201–203
    human immunodeficiency virus (HIV), 203
    impact on caregivers, 206
    language of, 1
    medication review, 200
    memory
        loss, 202
        training procedures, 208
        treatment strategies, 207–208
    Parkinson's disease, 203
    pathophysiology of, 200–201
    patient's medical condition, 200

Dementia *(continued)*
symptoms of
behavioral, 202, 207
chronic, 199
cognitive and noncognitive, 199
history, 200
treatment of, 206–207
specific tasks, 209t
Dementia with Lewy bodies (DLB), 203
Denial, 12–13
Detroit Test of Learning Aptitude, 226
Different Strokes, 252
Diffuse brain damage disturbances, 228
Direct impact forces, 225
Direction following
for comprehension training, 93
Disability, 5–6
World Health Organization (WHO)
classification schema of, 5
Discharge issues
criteria of, 46
planning of, 46
Discourse Comprehension Test (DCT), 64t, 131,
148
Discourse impairments, 56
Disease processes, 213
Disengaged, 14
Disinhibition syndrome, 52
Dispositional optimism, 14
Disruption stage
in illness experience, 7t, 8
Divergent word retrieval, 163
D-K EFS, 61t
DLB, 203
Documentation, 188
Donepezil (Aricept), 207
Dorsolateral frontal-subcortical circuit, 54
Dorsolateral syndrome. *See* Dorsolateral frontal-
subcortical circuit
Dynamic aphasia, 55–56
features of, 55
Dysarthria, 127
Dysexecutive syndrome. *See* Dorsolateral frontal-
subcortical circuit
Dysgraphia
published and experimental tests for, 104–106
treatment
literature for, 107
strengths and weaknesses of, 111
Dysgraphia Battery, 149
Dysgraphia subtype, 102
Dysgraphia treatment studies
outcomes of, 108t–110t

Early intervention, 191
Early visual analysis (EVA), 83
Edinburgh Functional Communication Profile
(EFCP)
revised, 241

Education
and aphasia, 31–32
global aphasia
patient, family, and staff, 191–192
influencing recovery, 30
EEG, 19, 200
EFCP
revised, 241
ElderWeb, 255
Electroencephalography (EEG), 19, 200
Emotional intelligence
concept of, 13
Enmeshed, 14
Environmental factors
ICF framework, 39–40
ERPs, 19
Error analyses, 73–74
EVA, 83
Event-related designs, 34
Event-related potentials (ERPs), 19
Executive clock drawing task, 61t–62t
Exelon, 207
Experimental conditions
block design for, 33–34
Experimental Neurogenic Dysgraphia Battery,
149
Experimental sequences
task arrangement of, 33–34
EXPLOR, 255
External environment
organism-external variables, 30t
Extralinguistic contexts, 239
Extralinguistic deficits, 221–222

FAB, 62t
Facilitory channels
conduction aphasia, 164–165
FACS. *See* Functional Assessment of
Communication Skills (FACS)
FACT, 131, 148
FAM, 226
Familiarity, 73
Families
healthy and vulnerable
characteristics of, 15t
Families and caregivers resources, 254–255
videos and materials, 252–254
Family, caregiver, and clinician resources
organizations, 250–252
Family Care America, 255
Family resources, 249–257
Family systems, 14–15
Family training, 44–45
FAS Word Fluency Measure, 205
FCCA, 204
FCM, 205
for Wernicke's aphasia, 147
FCP, 189, 241
Films for Humanities and Sciences, 253

FIM, 226
Final Comprehension Consensus Assessment
      (FCCA), 204
Flash cards, 93
FLCI, 205
Florida Semantics Battery, 72
Fluency, 241
   conduction aphasia characteristic, 157
Fluent aphasia, 124, 125t, 157
Fluent aphasic patients, 125
   speech rate, 125
fMRI. *See* Functional magnetic resonance
      imaging (fMRI)
Focal cortical contusions, 225
Franklin Learning Resources, 94
French Anthropology Society, 117
Frontal abulia syndrome. *See* Dorsolateral
      frontal-subcortical circuit
Frontal alexia
   characteristics and physiology of, 87t
Frontal assessment battery (FAB), 62t
Frontal cerebral lobe dysfunction, 1
Frontal disinhibition. *See* Orbitofrontal-
      subcortical circuit
Frontal lobe damage, 231
Frontal lobe function
   clinical tests of, 60
      characteristics of, 61t–64t
   rehabilitation
      methods of, 65
   treatment for, 60, 65
   treatment strategies, 65
Frontal lobe syndrome, 52
Fronto-subcortical circuitry
   neuropsychological behaviors of, 53t
Frontotemporal dementias (FTD), 202–203
Fry Readability Scale, 92
FTD, 202–203
Fuld Object Memory Evaluation, 204
Functional assessment measure (FAM), 226
Functional Assessment of Communication Skills
      (FACS), 130, 242
   ASHA, 142, 205
      for adults, 130, 189
      for Wernicke's aphasia, 147
Functional Auditory Comprehension Test
      (FACT), 131, 148
Functional communication abilities, 242
Functional Communication Measures (FCM), 205
Functional Communication Profile (FCP), 189,
      241
Functional independence measure (FIM), 226
Functional Linguistic Communication Inventory
      (FLCI), 205
Functional magnetic resonance imaging (fMRI),
      19, 85, 120, 201
   activation
      nonfluent aphasic patent, 28f
   brain examinations of, 20

limitations of, 20
principles of, 19–21
problem for, 20
procedure for, 20
results
   primary progressive aphasia (PPA), 35f
strengths and weaknesses, 19–21
study
   semantic judgments of, 58–59
Functional neuroimaging, 19–36
   applying, 21
   effects of treatment, 26–27

Galantamine (Reminyl), 207
GDS
   for Age-Related Cognitive Decline and
      Alzheimer's Disease, 204
Gender
   and aphasia, 31–32
   ICF framework, 39
Gerstmann's syndrome, 100–101
Gestural cues
   conduction aphasia, 165
Gesture, 77
GIL, 84
Global aphasia, 186–198
   assessment, 187–189
   augmented communication program, 197
   communication environment
      establishing conditions for, 191–192
   communication partners, 197
   communicative boards, 195–196
   definition of, 186–187
   education
      patient, family, and staff, 191–192
   evaluation of, 187
   functional communication assessment of, 189
   gestural communication, 193–194
      strengthening response, 193–194
   intersystemic reorganization, 195
   patients
      ability determination, 188–189
      interaction with clinicians, 188
      speech, 195
   performance variables in, 187t
   programs, 196
   recovery
      prediction of, 189–190
   response, 193
   treatment, 192–193
      computer-assisted, 197
      decisions, 190–191
      ending cues, 197
      equivocal response, 193
      goals in, 192
      group, 196
      residential, 196–197
   visual action therapy, 194–195
   writing, 194

Global Deterioration Scale (GDS)
  for Age-Related Cognitive Decline and
    Alzheimer's Disease, 204
Government and binding theory of Chomsky
  Broca's aphasia linguistic hypotheses, 123
GPC, 84
Grammatical categories, 73
Grapheme to phoneme (GPC), 84
Graphemic buffer impairment, 102–103
Graphemic input lexicon (GIL), 84
Graphemic output lexicon, 102
Group members, 232
Group treatment, 43–44
  benefits of, 44
  pragmatics, 246
  strengths and weaknesses of, 44
  traumatic brain injury, 232
G rule, 91

Handicap, 5–6
  World Health Organization (WHO)
    classification schema of, 5
Handwriting assessment, 104
HD
  and dementia, 203
Head injury, 213
Health care
  models of, 39–41
Healthcare professionals
  and patient care, 11
Healthy families
  characteristics of, 15t
Helm Elicited Language Program for Syntax
    Stimulation (HELPSS), 135
HELPSS, 135
Hemisphere
  anterior *vs.* posterior, 99–100
  left *vs.* right, 99
Hemodynamic response function (HRF), 34f
HIV, 203
HRF, 34f
Human communication
  foundations of, 2
Human immunodeficiency virus (HIV)
  and dementia, 203
Huntington's disease (HD)
  and dementia, 203
Huntington's Disease Caregiver Directory, 251
Huntington's Disease Society of America, 250
Hyperresponsivity, 214
Hyporesponsivity, 214

ICF. *See* International Classification of
    Functioning, Disability, and Health (ICF)
ICIDH-2, 5
IFG
  left, 85
Illness constellation model, 7
Illness experience, 6–7
  stages of, 7–11, 7t

Imageability, 73
Imaging, 201
Imaging studies, 227
Impaired performance
  in naming tasks, 71
Impairment, 5–6, 40
  World Health Organization (WHO)
    classification schema of, 5
Inferential comprehension
  tasks of, 89
Inferior frontal gyrus (IFG)
  left, 85
Inferior parietotemporo-occipital area, 172
Information processing, 226
  speed of, 234
Initial phoneme cues, 163
Innovative Caregiving Resources, Inc., 253
Instructional level, 92
Insula, 155
Interactional strategies, 134
Internal locus of control, 14
International Classification of Functioning,
    Disability, and Health (ICF), 39
  framework, 39
    components of, 40
    and gender, 39
    social environment, 40
  interaction of components, 40f
International Classification of Impairments,
    Disabilities, and Handicaps revision
    (ICIDH-2), 5
Internet training
  in treatment approaches, 46
Intersystemic gestural reorganization, 77
Intrinsic environment
  organism-internal variables, 30t

Jackson, Hughlings, 55, 213
JAN
  web site address of, 252
Job Accommodation Network (JAN)
  web site address of, 252
John Fowles, 15
John Hopkins Dysgraphia Battery, 149

Key words, 230

Language
  assessment of pragmatic aspects of, 63t
  cognitive processes of, 32
Language Care Center (LCC), 186, 196
Language comprehension, 27
Language examination
  for Wernicke's aphasia, 146
Language impairments
  of aphasia, 55
  in PFC damage, 55
Language of dementia, 1
Language processing, 30
  neural correlates of, 21–23

Language recovery
   neurobiology of, 32
LCC, 186, 196
Left hemisphere-damaged patients, 99
Left hemisphere temporoparietal cortex, 69
Left inferior frontal gyrus, 85
Left temporal lobe, 85
Length, 73
Letter representation (LR), 83
Lexical agraphia, 99, 101–102
Lexical assessment tasks
   in input modality, 72t
   in output modality, 72t
Lexical Comprehension Test, 177
Lexical retrieval, 180
Lexical route, 84
Lexical routes, 102
Lexical-semantic route, 84
Lexical task
   comparisons of, 72–73
Life participation approach to aphasia (LPAA),
      41
Lifestyle
   ICF framework, 39
Limb movements
   in word-retrieval training, 78
Limited functional capacities, 227
Lingraphica, 186
   system, 196
Linguistic cues, 213
   vs. articulatory cues, 158
Linguistic hypotheses
   Broca's aphasia, 123–124
Linguistic skills, 237
Linguistic-specific treatment
   definition of, 27
Listeners, 232
Literacy history, 86
LPAA, 41
LR, 83

Magnetic resonance imaging (MRI), 200, 201
   in mental operations, 58
   structural, 200
Magnetoencephalography (MEG), 19
Mayo Clinic
   web site address of, 252
Mayo-Portland Adaptability Inventory, 226
McNeil and Tseng's Experimental Neurogenic
      Dysgraphia Battery, 149
Meaningful social intervention, 166
Medial frontal-subcortical circuit, 55
Medial temporal lobe injury, 230
Medical model, 39
MEG, 19
Melodic Intonation Therapy (MIT), 135
Memory
   aids, 230
   dementia
      loss of memory, 202

training procedures, 208
   treatment strategies, 207–208
   traumatic brain injury, 229–230
   working memory system, 103
Micrographia, 100
Microsoft Word
   readability statistics, 92
Mildly impaired readers, 93–94
Mini-Mental Status Exam (MMSE), 204
MIT, 135
MMSE, 204
Moderately impaired reader, 92–93
MOSES, 205
Motivation
   influencing recovery, 30
Motor planning
   in apraxia of speech, 103
Mourning, 13
MRI. *See* Magnetic resonance imaging (MRI)
Multidimensional Observation Scale for Elderly
      Subjects (MOSES), 205
Multiple Sclerosis Foundation, 251
Myasthenia Gravis, 251
Myasthenia Gravis Association of Queensland,
      Australia, 251
Myasthenia Gravis Foundation of America, 251

Name training
   in context, 78
Naming, 68
   assessment
      errors of, 73
      purpose of, 74
   assessment of, 72
   characteristics of, 73
   classification scheme of, 70
   cognitive mechanisms of, 68
   disorders of, 69f
   disruption
      in anomic aphasia, 70
   error
      examination of, 73
      sources of, 73
   impairments
      differentiating features of, 70–72
      nature of, 70–72
      neural substrates of, 68–70
      pathophysiology of, 68
   mechanisms of, 72
   pattern
      in conduction aphasia, 70
   treatment
      individualized approach to, 74
   and word retrieval
      problems of, 68–79
NART, 148
National Adult Day Services Association, Inc., 254
National Aphasia Association, 195, 250
National Family Caregivers Association, 254
National Parkinson Foundation, 251

National Stroke Association, 251
Natural communication, 161
Natural communication settings, 165
Naturalistic intervention setting, 243
Neglect agraphia
    attentional disorder, 218–219
    in language abilities, 219
    treatments for, 222
    in writing, 219
Neglect dyslexia
    in reading, 219
Nelson Reading Skills Test (NRST), 148
Neural network, 69
    in language recovery, 26–27
Neural patterns
    associated with recovery, 28–29
Neural recruitment
    effects of treatment, 26–30
Neural tissue
    variables related to, 30t
Neurobehavioral Rating Scale, 226
Neurobehavioral sequelae
    classes of, 225–226
Neurocognitive conditions, 97
Neurogenic communication disorders
    social context of, 5
Neurogenic dysgraphia
    heuristics for, 106
Neuroimaging studies
    of regional brain activity, 22–23
    task development for, 32
Neurological substrate
    of reading, 85–86
Neurologic impairment, 174
    organizations, 249–252
    reading material, 255–257
    resources, 249–257
    videos, 252–254
Neuroplastic processes
    factors related to, 30–31
Neuropsychological tests, 227
Neuropsychologic classification system
    assessment purposes of, 105t
Neuroradiographic techniques, 119
New Adult Reading Test (NART), 148
Noncanonic sentences, 27
Nonfluent aphasia, 124, 125t
Nonfluent aphasic patent
    fMRI activation, 28f
Nonfluent aphasic patients, 125
Nonlexical route, 102
Nonlinguistic skills, 237
Nonliteral language
    misinterpretation of, 215
Nonmeaningful limb movements, 78
Nonverbal aspects, 240
Nonverbal communication, 241
Northern Speech Services, Inc., 253
Northwestern University Sentence
    Comprehension Test, 130
NRST, 148

Nursing Home Behavior Problem Scale, 205

Object and Action Naming Battery, 72
Object and action naming battery, 63t
Object recognition system, 70
Observation, 188
Occipital lobe, 85
Oliver Sacks, 11
Openness to experience, 14
Optic aphasia
    cognitive scheme of, 71
Optimism, 191
Optimized conditions, 195
Oral naming impairments
    self-cueing process of, 77
Oral naming tasks, 71
Oral reading, 88
    improvements in, 77
Oral reading process
    model of, 84f
Orbitofrontal-subcortical circuit, 54–55
Orbitomedial syndrome, 54–55
Organism-external variables, 31
    external environment, 30t
Organism-internal variables, 30
    intrinsic environment, 30t
Organism-specific variables, 30–31
    intrinsic environment, 30t
Orientation Group Monitoring System, 226
Orthographic knowledge, 102
Orthographic system, 98

PACE. See Promoting Aphasic Communicative
    Effectiveness (PACE)
Paired associate learning, 91
PALPA. See Psycholinguistic Assessments of
    Language Processing in Aphasia
    (PALPA)
Pantomimes
    in naming failures, 77–78
Paragraph level, 93
Paralinguistic aspects, 240
Paralinguistic contexts, 239
Parallel distributed processing (PDP), 158
Paraphasias
    conduction aphasia characteristics, 157
Parietal/temporal/occipital (PTO) cortex, 4
Parkinson's disease
    and dementia, 203
Parkinson's Web, 251
Participation restriction, 40
Pathophysiology
    of PFC, 51–52
Patient, 11
Patient-initiated responses
    in RET, 136
PB, 84
PCA, 241
PDP, 158
Peabody Picture Vocabulary Test, 205
Peripheral agraphias, 103–104

Peripheral and central nervous system (PNS/CNS), 97
Peripheral commissural aphasia, 171
Personal factors
    ICF framework, 39
Perspectives Network, 250
PES-AD, 206
PET. *See* Positron emission tomography (PET)
PFC. *See* Prefrontal cortex (PFC)
PFCD. *See* Prefrontal cortex damage (PFCD)
Pharmacologic treatment, 78–79
Pharmacotherapy, 179
Philadelphia Geriatric Center Affect Rating Scale, 206
Phoneme-to-grapheme route, 102
Phonetic errors
    of conduction aphasia, 158
Phonic rules
    in teaching children, 91
Phonologic agraphia, 101, 102
Phonologic alexia
    characteristics and physiology of, 87t
Phonologic buffer (PB), 84
Phonologic cueing, 180
Phonologic dysgraphia, 102
Phonologic dyslexia
    characteristics and physiology of, 87t
Phonologic errors
    of conduction aphasia, 158
Phonologic-level processing deficits, 163
Phonologic output lexicon (POL), 70, 84
Phonologic representations
    of naming impairments, 71
Phonologic route, 84
Phonologic stage, 68
Phonologic treatments, 76
Physical environment
    ICF framework, 40
Physiological processes, 179
Physiologic principle
    definition of, 19
PICA. *See* Porch Index of Communicative Ability (PICA)
Picture card
    for name training, 78
Picture naming
    semantic errors in, 73
Pittsburgh Aphasia Treatment Research and Education Center, 196
Planning
    in illness experience, 9
Pleasant Events Schedule-AD (PES-AD), 206
PNS/CNS, 97
POL, 70, 84
Porch Index of Communicative Ability (PICA), 187, 188
    scores, 189
    for Wernicke's aphasia, 147
Positron emission tomography (PET), 19, 24, 119, 179
    activation

stroke patient, 25f
    brain examinations of, 20
    data analysis for, 20
    in mental operations, 58
    principles of, 19–21
    procedure for, 20
    strengths and weaknesses, 19–21
    study
        activation patterns from, 24f
        semantic analysis of, 58
Posttreatment activation patterns, 27–28
Posttreatment scans, 28–29
PPA
    fMRI results, 35f
Pragmatic behaviors, 232, 241
Pragmatic Profile, 241
Pragmatic Protocol, 241
Pragmatics, 237–247
    assessment tools, 240t
    barrier activities, 245–246
    behaviors, 238
    communication efficiency protocols, 241–242
    conversational profiles, 240–241
    conversational skills, 238t
    definition of, 237
    direct group treatments, 246
    evaluation of, 240
    features of, 237–240
    indirect treatment groups, 246
    individuals with aphasia
        linguistic conversational skills of, 237–239
        nonlinguistic conversational skills of, 239
    observational profiles, 240–241
    promoting aphasics' communicative effectiveness, 243–244
    role playing, 244–245
    social groups, 246
    sociolinguistic groups, 246
    specific treatment tasks, 243–246
    speech-language groups, 246
    standardized measures, 242
    treatment of, 243
Prefrontal aphasia. *See* Dynamic aphasia
Prefrontal cortex (PFC), 51
    classic behavioral sequelae of, 52–54
    components of
        heteromodal sector, 52
        motor-premotor sector, 52
        paralimbic sector, 52
    events of, 59
    functions
        models of, 59
        theories of, 59
    neural pathways of, 51
    neuroanatomical features of, 51
    pathophysiology of, 51–52
    semantic processing of, 58
Prefrontal cortex damage (PFCD)
    ambiguities
        processing of, 57
        results of, 57

Prefrontal cortex damage (PFCD) *(continued)*
  clinical evaluation of, 51
  clinical identification of, 51
  differentiating features of, 52
  in discourse comprehension, 56
  discourse deficits of, 55
  in discourse processing, 56
  in discourse production, 56
  in language deficits, 51–66
  language deficits of, 55
  in language impairments, 55
  language process studies, 58
  in story comprehension
    characteristics of, 57
    framework of, 57
    studies of, 57
  supporting research findings, 58–59
Prefrontal functions
  evaluation of, 59
Prefrontal lesions, 55
Prefrontal mediation
  testing of, 59
Prefrontal neuroanatomic areas
  neuropsychological behaviors of, 53t
Prefrontal regions
  dorsolateral view of, 54f
  medial/cingulate view of, 54f
  orbital view of, 54f
Preinjury psychiatric history, 233–234
Premotor systems
  lateral, 170
  medial, 170
Press of speech, 149
Primary progressive aphasia (PPA)
  fMRI results, 35f
Processing ambiguity in text, 57–58
Processing tasks
  breakdown of, 72
Producing speech acts, 245
Productive circumlocution, 163
Pro-Ed, 253
Profile of Speech Characteristics, 161
Promoting Aphasic Communicative
    Effectiveness (PACE), 152, 165, 197, 245
  naming protocol, 78
  principles of, 243
  therapy, 134
Pseudoword repetition, 24f
Psycholinguistic Assessments of Language
    Processing in Aphasia (PALPA), 72, 88,
    105, 130, 160
Psychological and cognitive impairments, 232
PTO cortex, 4
Pure agraphia, 101
Pure alexia
  characteristics and physiology of, 87t
Pyramids and Palm Trees, 72
Pyramids and Palm Trees Test, 204

Quality of life (QOL), 13–14, 205, 208
  indicators, 206

Quality of Life Assessment Schedule (QOLAS),
    206
Quick Assessment for Aphasia
  for Wernicke's aphasia, 147

Race
  ICF framework, 39
Radiologic assessment procedures
  limitations of, 201
RAP, 196
Rapid scanning, 93
Rating Scale Profile of Speech Characteristics, 129
Raven's Colored Progressive Matrices, 187
RBMT, 204
RCBA-2, 88, 148
rCBF
  in Wernicke's and Broca's areas, 143–144
Reading
  ability, 124
  areas of, 85
  and automatic processing, 84
  cognitive and reasoning skills, 94
  comprehension, 91
  conduction aphasia, 159, 164
  of connected text, 92
  in controlled processing, 84–85
  and neglect dyslexia, 219
  and neurological substrate, 85–86
  partner, 94
  process
    pathophysiology of, 83–84
  retraining of, 83
  skills
    and adult literacy training, 92
  and writing, 77
Reading Comprehension Battery for Aphasia,
    187
Reading Comprehension Battery for Aphasia-2
    (RCBA-2), 88, 148
Reading disorders
  acquired
    treatment for, 90
  associated with acquired dyslexia, 83–95
  associated with aphasia, 83–95
  traditional and psycholinguistic classifications
    of, 87t
Reagan, Ronald
  Alzheimer diagnosis, 199
Realistic activities, 165
Realization, 12
Reasoning skills
  in reading, 94
Recall strategies, 230
Recognition Span Test, 204
Recovery
  early stages of, 188
Recovery of function
  clinical evidence of, 24
Recovery of language
  underlying mechanisms in, 24
Regaining self stage

in illness experience, 7t, 8–10
Regaining wellness stage
  in illness experience, 7t, 10–11
Regional cerebral blood flow (rCBF)
  in Wernicke's and Broca's areas, 143–144
Rehabilitation, 179
  in aphasia, 151
    conversational therapy, 151
    Schuell's stimulation, 151
    social approach, 151
Relinquish control
  in illness experience, 10
Reminyl, 207
Renegotiate roles
  in illness experience, 9
Reorganization approach, 91
Reorganizing technique, 178
Repetition, 124
  cognitive-linguistic model of, 172f
Repetition conduction aphasia, 156
Repetition errors
  transcortical sensory aphasia, 171
Repetition tasks, 176
Reproduction conduction aphasia, 156
Residential Aphasia Program (RAP), 196
Response elaboration training (RET), 136
  clinician-patient interactions, 136
Response to interlocutor, 241
Restitutive naming treatments, 74–75
Restitutive treatments
  investigations of, 76–77
Restriction of gesture, 195
RET, 136
Retraining reading
  computers for, 94
Revised Edinburgh Functional Communication
    Profile, 241
Revised Token Test, 148
Revised Wechsler Memory Scale (WMS-R), 204
RHD. See Right hemisphere brain damage (RHD)
Rhyming task, 73
RIC evaluation of communication problems, 64t
Right hemisphere brain damage (RHD), 213
  communication deficits, 214
  deficits
    categories of, 215
  disorders of, 213
  patients, 99
  priming study, 219
Right hemisphere communicative and cognitive
    disorders, 220
Right hemisphere syndrome, 1, 213–222
  affect, 218
  anosognosia, 219–220
  attention, 218
  cognition, 220
  communication, 215–218
  comprehension problems, 216
  discourse organization (macrostructure), 216
  discourse production, 216
  evaluation of, 220–221

figurative, 215–216
  humor, 216–217
  inferencing, 216
  nature and differentiating features of, 214–215
  neglect, 218–219
  nonliteral language, 215–216
    misinterpretation of, 215
  pathophysiology of, 213–214
  perception, 218–220
  pragmatics, 217
  prosody, 217–218
  specific treatment tasks, 221–222
  treatment of, 221–222
    facilitation of visual scanning, 222
    process oriented, 221
    suppression deficit hypothesis, 221–222
    task oriented, 221
  visuoperception, 220
Rivastigmine (Exelon), 207
Rivermead Behavioral Memory Test (RBMT), 204
Role playing
  activity
    phases of, 244
  in naming treatment, 78
Ross Test of Higher Cognitive Processes, 226
R rule, 91

Salient subject, 195
SALT, 148
SAS, 60
Scales of Cognitive Ability for Traumatic Brain
    Injury (SCATBI), 226
SCATBI, 226
SCRT, 76
SEC
  framework, 65
  knowledge of, 60
  model, 59–60
Selecting computer programs, 231
Self-advocacy training, 45
Self-cueing, 133, 163
Self-monitoring, 150
Semantic categories, 73
Semantic category rhyme therapy (SCRT), 76
Semantic comprehension training, 75
Semantic content
  control of, 241
Semantic cueing, 180
Semantic distinctions treatment, 76
Semantic dysfunction
  in naming difficulties, 69
Semantic feature analysis (SFA) training, 76
Semantic level breakdown, 71
Semantic level deficit, 163
Semantic mediation, 71
Semantic representations (SR), 84
Semantic stage, 68
Semantic treatments, 75–76
Sensory aphasia, 143
Sentence level, 92
Sentence processing, 23

Sentence production
  conduction aphasia, 164
Sentences
  phonologic processing of, 85
  semantic processing of, 85
Severe Impairment Battery (SIB), 204
Severely impaired reader, 92
Severe-moderate brain injury, 227
SFA training, 76
Shock, 12
Short term auditory comprehension treatment
  on brain activation, 27
SIB, 204
Silent reading, 88
Single brain center
  opponents and proponents of, 98
Single photon emission computed tomography
  (SPECT), 24, 120, 170, 200, 201, 227
Single word reading
  analysis of, 90
  features of, 87
Slosson Oral Reading Test-Revised, 89
SMA, 170
Social approach
  in aphasia intervention, 41
  evaluation of, 42–43
  evolution of, 41
Social environment
  ICF framework, 40
Social model, 39
Sociolinguistic sensitivity, 241
Somatic marker theory, 59, 60
Spatial agraphia, 103
Spatial resolution, 19
Specific environments, 208
Specific treatment approaches, 74–75
SPECT. See Single photon emission computed
  tomography (SPECT)
Speech acts, 180
Speech-language-pathologist
  web site address of, 252
Speech production, 217
Speech rate
  fluent aphasic patients, 125
Speed reading
  training in, 93
SPM. See Statistical parametric mapping (SPM)
Spontaneous speech
  conduction aphasia, 161
SR, 84
Statistical parametric mapping (SPM)
  images, 28f
    areas of activation, 29f
Stimulus characteristics, 73
Stop technique, 149
Story comprehension, 56–57
Strategies for Obtaining Information from
  Aphasic Persons, 151
Stroke, 213
  definition of, 3–5

Stroke patient
  PET activation, 25f
Stroop color and word test, 62t
Structural MRI, 200
Structured event complex (SEC)
  framework, 65
  knowledge of, 60
  model, 59–60
Study skills, 94
Sublexical route, 102
Substance abuse history, 233–234
Summary Profile of Standardized subtests, 129
Supervisory attention system (SAS), 60
Supplementary motor area (SMA), 170
Support groups, 15, 191
Support language recovery, 30t
Supramarginal gyrus, 155
Surface agraphia, 101–102
Surface alexia
  characteristics and physiology of, 87t
Surface dyslexia
  characteristics and physiology of, 87t
Survival reading skill, 92
Synonymy Test, 177
Systematic Analysis of Language Transcripts
  (SALT), 148

Tachistoscopic program, 93
Tacrine (Cognex), 206–207
Tape players
  for retraining reading, 94
Target word
  function of, 133
TBI. See Traumatic brain injury (TBI)
TEA, 62t
Temporal lobe regions
  and word production, 22
Temporal resolution, 19
Terra Nova Films, Inc., 253
Testing
  direction of, 131
Test of everyday attention (TEA), 62t
Test of Reading Comprehension, 148
Test of Written Language-3, 149
Theoretical distinctions, 158
Third alexia
  characteristics and physiology of, 87t
Token Test, 131, 148, 205
Traditional language retraining, 178
Transactional strategies, 134
Transcortical aphasia, 169–182
  Alzheimer's type, 174
  evaluation of, 175–177
  mixed transcortical aphasia, 173, 175, 177,
    179–180, 181
  nature and differentiating features of, 173–175
  pathophysiology of, 169–173
  specific treatment tasks, 180
  transcortical motor aphasia, 169–180
  transcortical sensory aphasia, 171–181

treatment for, 177–180
Transcortical motor aphasia, 56, 70, 126, 169–180
Transcortical sensory aphasia, 169, 171–181
    repetition errors, 171
Transient transcortical sensory aphasias, 172
Traumatic brain injury (TBI), 1, 3, 90, 225–235
    age, 234
    assessment of, 226
    attention, 228–229
    community reentry, 233
    continuum of care, 228
    cost per year to society, 225
    discrimination, 229
    educational goals, 234
    empathic abilities group, 232–233
    executive functioning, 231–233
    features of, 225–226
    functional outcome measures, 226–227
    group therapy, 232
    interpersonal interaction group, 232
    life skills group, 233
    memory, 229–230
    metacognitive skills, 231–233
    organization, 229
    pathophysiology of, 225
    perception, 229
    personal adjustment group, 233
    reasoning, 230–231
    return to school or work, 233–234
    social adjustment group, 233
    social skills group, 232
    treatment, 227–228
        techniques, 228–234
    use of computers, 231–232
    vocational goals, 233–234
Tumors, 213

Uncertainty stage
    in illness experience, 7t, 8
Unilateral left lobe abnormality
    predilection for
        inferior middle, 172
        superior gyri, 172
        temporal pole, 172
United States Department of Health and Human
        Services Administration on Aging, 254
Use of language, 237

Vascular dementia (VaD), 202
VAT, 194
    purpose of, 194
VCE pattern, 91
VC pattern, 91
VE, 231
Verbal aspects, 240
Verbal cues
    conduction aphasia, 164–165
Verbal imitation, 162
Verbal output, 124
Verbal paraphasias, 176

Verbal production, 133
Verbal repetition
    conduction aphasia, 162–163
Verb generation, 24f
Verbo-motor center, 171
Verb Production Battery, 130
Vicariative naming treatments, 77
Virtual environment (VE), 231
Visual action therapy
    global aphasia, 194–195
Visual action therapy (VAT), 194
    purpose of, 194
Visual cues
    conduction aphasia, 165
Visuospatial neglect, 219
Vulnerable families
    characteristics of, 15t
VV pattern, 91

WAB. *See* Western Aphasia Battery (WAB)
Wada technique, 21
Wayne State University Press, 254
Wayne State University's Institute of Gerontology
    web site address of, 252
WCST, 63t
Wechsler Adult Intelligence Scale, 226
Wellness and quality of life
    emphasis on, 41–42
Well Spouse Foundation, 254
Wernicke, Carl, 142, 155
Wernicke area activation, 23
Wernicke's aphasia, 70, 125, 142–152
    comprehension deficit, 144
    conversational coaching, 151
    definition of, 143
    evaluation of, 146–147
    family inclusion, 150–151
    features of, 144–146
    history/pathophysiology of, 142–144
    paraphasic speech, 145
    patient's lack of concern, 146
    posterior, 100
    reading comprehension, 145
    recovery resistance, 143–144
    redistribution of function, 144
    specific treatment methodologies, 151–152
    supplemental tests of, 147
    supported conversation, 151–152
    treatment planning for, 150
    treatment principles, 149–150
    writing deficits, 145
Wernicke's area, 4
Western Aphasia Battery (WAB), 64t, 128, 161,
        177, 187, 204
    for Wernicke's aphasia, 147
WHO
    health classification system, 39
Wings, 8
Wisconsin card sorting test (WCST), 63t
WMS-R, 204

Woodcock Reading Mastery Tests, 88–89
Word(s)
  phonologic processing of, 85
  semantic processing of, 85
Word finding
  conduction aphasia, 160–161
  conduction aphasia characteristics, 157
Word production
  neural correlates of, 22
Word recognition, 87
Word repetition treatment, 76
Word retrieval, 68
  abilities
    treatments of, 75
  cognitive system
    stages of, 68
  conduction aphasia, 163–164
  factors of, 73
  psycholinguistic variables of, 73
Word retrieval difficulties

  in aphasia, 68
  treatment for, 74
    compensatory strategies, 74
    vicariative approaches to, 74
Word-stem completion, 25
Work environment
  targeting of, 45
Working memory system, 103
World Health Organization (WHO)
  health classification system, 39
Writing, 97
  conduction aphasia, 164
  global aphasia, 194
  and neglect agraphia, 219
  subskills of, 97
Writing ability, 124
Writing disturbances, 98
Writing problems
  with acquired neurogenic agraphias,
    97–112